YOUR ALL-IN-ONE GUIDE TO
FAST, EASY CALORIE COUNTING

The millions of readers of *The All-in-One Calorie Counter* can attest to the advantages of having such a valuable resource at your fingertips. Now, renowned nutrition expert Jean Carper has completely revised and updated this book with the latest information available from food manufacturers and from the U.S. Department of Agriculture.

This convenient and important book, often imitated but never matched, contains more than 10,000 entries on just about every kind of food imaginable—including fast foods, ethnic dishes, brand-name products, and more.

THE
ALL-IN-ONE
CALORIE
COUNTER

Jean Carper

3rd Revised Edition

BANTAM BOOKS

NEW YORK • TORONTO • LONDON • SYDNEY • AUCKLAND

THE ALL-IN-ONE CALORIE COUNTER

A Bantam Book / published by arrangement with
Workman Publishing Co., Inc.

PUBLISHING HISTORY

Bantam edition / January 1974
Revised Bantam edition / July 1980
2nd revised edition / March 1987
3rd revised edition / February 1994

ISBN 0-553-29843-7

Published simultaneously in the United States and Canada

Bantam Books are published by Bantam Books, a division of Bantam Doubleday Dell
Publishing Group, Inc. Its trademark, consisting of the words "Bantam Books" and the
portrayal of a rooster, is Registered in U.S. Patent and Trademark Office and in other
countries. Marca Registrada. Bantam Books, 1540 Broadway, New York, New York 10036.

PRINTED IN THE UNITED STATES OF AMERICA

OPM   10 9 8 7 6 5 4

Acknowledgments

Many thanks to Judy Carper, the research coordinator for this book, for her expert job of gathering information, putting it in the computer with such accuracy and making it come out totally organized.

Contents

CONTENTS

Introduction

"Counting calories is not just the best way to long-term weight maintenance—it's the only way," according to the late internationally noted nutritionist Dr. Jean Mayer. It is that unit of energy—the calorie—that determines how much weight you put on and take off, he says. And certainly there are hundreds of thousands of successful calorie-counting dieters who would agree. Take in fewer calories than you burn up each day, and you're bound to shed pounds.

But how to do it? Unfortunately, there aren't any mysterious secrets for making dieting actually fun. But in this book you'll find loads of information that I hope will take some of the monotony out of dieting, boost your chances of success, enable you to eat some foods on your diet you never dreamed possible and clear up some misconceptions you may have about which foods are high in calorie content and which aren't. For example, many calorie-conscious persons avoid potatoes and spaghetti like the plague (which by themselves are fairly low in calories) and load up on "protein" foods such as beef (which is comparatively much higher in calories). At the same time I have heard people say Japanese sushi (rice and vegetables or raw fish) is high in calories. It is not, as you will see in this book.

In the case of potatoes and pasta, it is not the basic food itself but the way it is prepared or the embellishments that make the caloric difference. A medium-sized boiled potato weighs in with only 104 calories, whereas only ten French fries have 137 calories. Of course, if you want to splurge occasionally and eat French fries or load up your baked potato with butter and sour cream or cheese sauce, you should consider the calorie difference.

And why shouldn't you eat a Mars bar occasionally if you want one? Or a slice of Sara Lee's rich cake? Or Jeno's pizza? Dieting—even if you are counting calories—doesn't have to be a monklike experience—ascetic and uninteresting. However, overindulging in sweet or high-fat foods at the expense of well-balanced nutrition is not in your best interest.

A stumbling block may be that you don't know how many calories are present in food products. For unlike pure, fresh foods, when the ingredients get into a company chef's kitchen, they are all mixed any which way according to the company's special recipe. Only the company can tell you how many calories are in their foods. And that's the kind of information you will find in this book: a comprehensive listing of not only all common "generic-type" foods, but also commercially prepared foods—from Apple Jacks to Ore-Ida's fried, frozen zucchini sticks.

You will see that the number of calories in similar grocery products can vary greatly, and you will find that simple knowledge can trim calories off a product quickly. For example, it is almost startling to realize that two ounces of Chicken of the Sea light tuna in oil contains 170 calories, but that two ounces of the same brand tuna canned in water has only 60—a saving of 110 calories!

If you've bought or are thinking of buying this book, you're probably already committed to losing or maintaining your weight, so there's no use wasting time telling you why you should be weight-conscious, or all about the terrible medical problems you may confront if you aren't. But there are some facts about calories that you may find valuable. A calorie is a unit of energy in foods. Technically, it is the amount of heat needed to raise the temperature of one liter (about a quart) of water by one degree centigrade. The body constantly takes in calories through food and expends them through activity.

Theoretically, if you took in precisely as many calories in a day as you used up in energy, you wouldn't gain or lose a smidgen of an ounce that day. But when you take in more calories than your body can use, you store them as fat. The rule of thumb is that a moderately active person needs about 15 calories per day per pound of body weight to "stay as is." That is, if you weigh 120 pounds and want to stay that way, you should consume about 1800 calories a day. If you're happy at 150 pounds, you should take in 2250 calories a day. (Of course, this assumes a constant level of exercise. If you increase your level of activity, as experts advise as part of a weight-loss program, you expend additional calories.) If you want to get rid of some of that stored fat by counting calories, the calorie intake should dip considerably. How much you want to lose and how fast are up to you.

According to the American Medical Association, there are about 3500 calories in each stored pound of fat. So if you want to take off a pound, you have to get rid of that 3500 somehow. One way to do it is to shave 500 calories a day for seven days off your caloric intake. Thus, if you're 120 pounds and want to take off a pound a week, you would cut your regular 1800-calorie daily count to 1300; and if you weigh 150, you would want to go down from 2250 calories daily to 1750. Theoretically, that's the formula that should work for most people. Your scales will track your own success. It's okay, too—in fact, many experts say preferable—to lose only a half pound a week. Losing weight slowly means you are more apt to keep it off longer.

As far as giving you the basic facts necessary to follow your diet, you'll find in this book the calorie counts on all kinds of foods—both fresh and processed (by brand name, of course)—from A to Z. Included also is a special section on calorie counts of restaurant foods. New surveys show that Americans now eat about 50 percent of their meals outside the home—in restaurants of all types, including fast-food chains. It is not easy to know the exact calorie counts in general restaurant foods, but we have obtained approximate figures from the U.S. Department of Agriculture, used in its national nutritional surveys and compilations. We consider these figures an exciting addition to this book, making it even more comprehensive and helpful.

A word about the figures in the book: This book was first published in 1974 and has been an enormous success. It was completely revised and updated in 1980, 1987, and 1994. Hundreds of people have written to say how much it helped them lose weight, and it is used in numerous organized weight-loss clinics. We are convinced it is the most comprehensive and easy-to-use guide available. It has sold about two million copies. Since the last revision, some of the calorie counts have changed because of new analyses or reformulation of products and new products have been introduced. We simply did the book over from start to finish. Of course, some of the calorie counts are the same or similar, since the calories in many basic foods, such as milk, cheese, bread, as well as alcoholic drinks, don't change much. A few companies we contacted did not have new information; thus we used their previous figures.

The figures bearing brand names in this book were provided by food companies and are the latest the company advised us were available. Only a few companies we contacted declined to send available information; a few companies reported they did not have such information and a few said they were in the process of doing new analyses that were not ready at the time of publication.

We used the calorie figures and serving sizes as provided by the companies. Many companies, notably those using nutritional labeling, provide calorie counts rounded off. For example, a food with 109 calories, according to a chemical analysis, may be rounded up to 110. On the other hand, many companies still report figures without rounding off, which accounts for more precise counts. Since similar foods may vary slightly—by a few calories—anyway, such rounding off is insignificant. Some companies have asked us to point out that their figures are the best average calculations or analyses they have on specific products, but because of normal variations beyond their control, there may be ever-so-slight variations from batch to batch for the same manufacturer. Even such factors as seasonal conditions or soil composition may influence final food nutritional values.

Although companies now put nutritional labels on their foods, it is still difficult to make comparisons among various brand name foods without running all around the supermarket. Thus, one benefit of this book: you can pick out the lower-calorie item *before* you go shopping.

Important: Most calorie counts remain exceedingly stable over the years. However, a food maker may change the composition of a product, changing the calorie count. In that case, the calorie count on the label will differ from that in this book. To avoid confusion, check the label, and if such contradictions exist, you should assume the *label is correct*.

The accuracy of a food company's labeling and dissemination of nutritional information is regulated by the federal Food and Drug Administration, and a company would be subject to severe penalties for putting out a food label that is grossly inaccurate. If you wish, you can contact the companies directly for more information.

All the calorie counts without any brand name or company attribution are from the U.S. Department of Agriculture.

To sum up, the new revised *All-in-One Calorie Counter* will provide you with the latest, most accurate, comprehensive data available about fresh foods, processed foods and restaurant foods.

Jean Carper

How to Use This Book

The most important organizational fact about *The All-in-One Calorie Counter*, as you will quickly see, is that it is alphabetized for easy use according to food categories. That is, you don't have to look in the front of the book under B for bean soup and then flip to the T's to find out if tomato soup is lower in calories. The supermarket portion of the book runs through the alphabet, starting with baby food and ending with yogurt. After that, you will find our special section on restaurant foods, including fast-food chains.

All the breads are listed together in the B section, all the fruits are grouped together under F, the vegetables under V and so on. Simply by looking at the Contents in the front of the book, you can quickly spot which category a food is in and turn directly to that section. You will then find the foods alphabetized within the sections. Some foods, to be sure, just don't fit easily into categories, and rather than force them into some artificial grouping, we have listed them alphabetically too, even though there may be only one or two of a kind; for example, thickeners have a listing of their own.

In other words, the book is akin to a dictionary—with headings at the top of each page, too, to help you out. If you get stuck and can't decide where a food might be, just consult the index.

We have tried to standardize the language and the serving sizes as much as possible to make them useful, but here again we haven't strained the point. We have tried to be practical. For example, under cereals you won't find all of them in either 1-cup or ½-cup portions. The reason: Cereals vary greatly in their density and weight. Thus, the typical 1-ounce serving size for cereals varies in cup measurements, depending on the type of cereal. An ounce of puffed rice will fill a 1-cup measuring cup, but an ounce of heavier All-Bran fills about ⅓ of a measuring cup. In all cases, we have followed the manufacturers' recommendations and provided single-serving sizes they believe appropriate.

For listings using the word "prepared," the calories are based on the assumption that the food has been prepared according to the manufacturer's directions. If you alter the preparation, for example, by adding meat drippings instead of water to a gravy mix or using milk when water is called for on the package or adding other embellishments of your own, you must figure in these extras. Whenever milk is called for in a preparation, we assume it is whole milk—not skim or nonfat or condensed milk. If you use other ingredients—either raising or lowering the calorie content in the finished product—you should make provision for them.

In most cases, companies prefer to tell you how many calories are in the finished prepared product—for example, a cup of pudding from a pudding mix—because it is rare that the powder would be used in any other way. But in some instances you will find the calorie count for the dry mix only—*before* preparation. That way, if you want to add another ingredient to your mix, you can do so and add up the extra calories. Also on this note: Whenever you merely add water to a mix, you are not adding calories—for example, when you prepare a Lipton's dry soup mix. If you use the dry soup mix in any other fashion, say as a dip mix, there are the same number of calories in the dry mix as in the cup of prepared soup.

In keeping with our determination to make this book easy to use, we have taken due note of the power of identity of brand names. Whenever possible, without interfering with the organization, we have used brand names for quick identification. Thus, when you look up a certain cookie, cracker or cereal, you don't have to peruse the whole list searching for a description of your cookie. We don't have Cheez-Its listed under "Crackers, cheese"; it is alphabetized simply under Cheez-Its. Similarly, we have Oreo cookies under O and not under "Chocolate creme sandwich." The same goes for Froot Loops (under F in the cereal section). At the same time, it was not always possible to do this without creating a chaotic organization, and in many cases the only identifying factor is a description of the product (chocolate chip cookies, for example) and the name of the manufacturer.

Within the listings, we repeat the measurements frequently. However, on items such as cookies, bread and frozen dinners, where the portion size is almost always one cookie, one slice, or complete dinner, we have simply noted the portion at the head of the section. This has also been done on fairly short listings. However, if you do not see a portion size for a certain food, look for it at the head of the section.

To avoid confusion, whenever possible, we have stated the measurement in the most easily used terms: cups, tablespoons and fluid ounces for liquids and items such as canned fruits and vegetables; and weight ounces for items such as cheese and frozen fish fillets. On some of the candy bars, we have noted the calories per ounce, so you can figure calories if the sizes of the candy bars change. Since many candy companies report calories for their current-size bars, we urge you to check the weight of the candy bar on the wrapper to be sure it corresponds with the weight noted in this book.

A few other words of advice: On certain basic products, even though the brand names differ, the calorie counts are essentially the same. For example, the caloric content of milk, cheese, butter and oils depends primarily on the fat content. That is why all standard margarines have the same calorie count: 100 per tablespoon. Cheeses of the same type, for example cheddar, have virtually the same fat content no matter who makes it. Thus, you can assume that the calorie counts for such basic natural cheeses are standard despite the brand name. On the other hand, when companies make their own cheese products or low-calorie cheeses and spreads, the calorie count depends upon their special recipes.

In this revision, we have retained our "health foods" section, even though such foods have become increasingly popular and widely purchased. The line between such "health and natural" foods and general foods is growing less clear, as Americans become more nutrition-conscious and many food companies respond by formulating and promoting so-called "health foods." Even so, some companies and some ingredients, such as carob, are still closely associated in the public's mind with "health and natural" foods and we think it is easier for readers who want to find those products to look them up in a special section. Some of the products are still sold only in specialty or "health food" stores. However, we have to admit that some such foods may have slipped over into other sections. So if you don't find them in one place, check elsewhere.

For our readers who have used the previous editions, here is what's new about this revision. It has many more items both by brand name and generic. We are listing more than 10,000 foods, compared with 8800 in our last edition.

Despite our best efforts, there is no way we can save you from doing some figuring on your own, simply because no one, including yourself, wants to eat the food company's designated serving size all the time. And obviously, when you use your own recipes, you can obtain the calorie counts for only the basic ingredients. You have to take it from there.

For doing your own conversions, here is an equivalency table that may help:

$$1 \text{ tablespoon} = 3 \text{ teaspoons}$$
$$2 \text{ tablespoons} = 1 \text{ fluid ounce}$$
$$4 \text{ tablespoons} = \frac{1}{4} \text{ cup}$$
$$5\frac{1}{3} \text{ tablespoons} = \frac{1}{3} \text{ cup}$$
$$16 \text{ tablespoons} = 1 \text{ cup}$$
$$1 \text{ cup} = 8 \text{ fluid ounces}$$
$$2 \text{ cups} = 1 \text{ pint}$$
$$2 \text{ pints} = 1 \text{ quart}$$
$$1 \text{ pound} = 16 \text{ ounces}$$

Happy calorie counting!

Abbreviations

art	artificial
diam	diameter
fl	fluid
in	inch
lb	pound
med	medium
na	not available
oz	ounce
pkg	package
swt	sweetened
tbsp	tablespoon
tsp	teaspoon
unswt	unsweetened
w	with
wo	without

THE
ALL-IN-ONE
CALORIE
COUNTER

Baby Food

BAKED GOODS

	CALORIES
Biscuit / 1 piece / **Gerber**	50
Cookie animal shaped / 2 pieces / **Gerber**	60
Cookie arrowroot / 2 pieces / **Gerber**	50
Cracker animal shaped / 4 pieces / **Gerber**	50
Pretzel / 2 pieces / **Gerber**	45
Zwieback toast / 2 pieces / **Gerber**	70

STRAINED BABY FOODS

Cereal, Dry: ½ ounce unless noted (½ ounce is about 6 tablespoons dry.)

Barley/ **Beech-Nut** Stage 1	60
Barley / **Gerber**	60
Barley / **Heinz**	60
Hi Protein / **Heinz**	60
High Protein / **Gerber**	50
High Protein w apple and orange / **Gerber**	60
Mixed / **Beech-Nut** Stage 2	60
Mixed / **Gerber**	60
Mixed / **Heinz**	60
Mixed w banana / **Gerber**	60
Oatmeal / **Beech-Nut** Stage 1	70
Oatmeal / **Gerber**	60
Oatmeal / **Heinz**	60
Oatmeal and bananas / **Beech-Nut** Stage 2	70
Oatmeal w banana / **Gerber**	60

CALORIES

Rice / **Beech-Nut** Stage 1	60
Rice / **Gerber**	60
Rice / **Heinz**	60
Rice and apples / **Beech-Nut** Stage 2	70
Rice and bananas / **Beech-Nut** Stage 2	70
Rice w banana / **Gerber**	60

Cereal: 1 jar

Mixed w apples and bananas / **Beech-Nut** Stage 2	90
Mixed w apples and bananas / **Heinz**	100
Mixed w applesauce and bananas / **Gerber** Second Foods	90
Oatmeal w apples and bananas / **Beech-Nut** Stage 2	90
Oatmeal w apples and bananas / **Heinz**	110
Oatmeal w applesauce and bananas / **Gerber** Second Foods	90
Rice w apples and bananas / **Beech-Nut** Stage 2	90
Rice w apples and bananas / **Heinz**	110
Rice w applesauce and bananas / **Gerber** Second Foods	90

Desserts: 1 jar

Apple and strawberry / **Beech-Nut** Stage 2	90
Apple, peach and strawberry / **Beech-Nut** Stage 2	100
Apple yogurt / **Beech-Nut** Stage 2	120
Apricot yogurt / **Heinz**	110
Banana apple / **Gerber** Second Foods	80
Banana pineapple / **Beech-Nut** Stage 2	110
Banana yogurt / **Beech-Nut** Stage 2	120
Banana yogurt / **Heinz**	120
Blueberry yogurt / **Heinz**	100
Cottage cheese w pineapple / **Beech-Nut** Stage 2	130
Dutch apple / **Beech-Nut** Stage 2	100
Dutch apple / **Gerber** Second Foods	80
Dutch apples / **Heinz**	110
Fruit / **Gerber** Second Foods	90
Fruit / **Heinz**	100
Guava tropical fruit / **Beech-Nut** Stage 2	100
Hawaiian delight / **Gerber** Second Foods	100
Island fruit / **Beech-Nut** Stage 2	90

CALORIES

Mango tropical fruit / **Beech-Nut** Stage 2	110
Mixed fruit / **Heinz**	110
Mixed fruit yogurt / **Beech-Nut** Stage 2	130
Papaya tropical fruit / **Beech-Nut** Stage 2	100
Peach cobbler / **Gerber** Second Foods	80
Peach cobbler / **Heinz**	100
Peach yogurt / **Beech-Nut** Stage 2	120
Peach yogurt / **Heinz**	110
Pear yogurt / **Beech-Nut** Stage 2	130
Pear yogurt / **Heinz**	110
Pineapple orange / **Heinz**	90
Pudding banana / **Beech-Nut** Stage 2	100
Pudding banana / **Heinz**	110
Pudding cherry vanilla / **Gerber** Second Foods	80
Pudding custard / **Heinz**	110
Pudding vanilla custard / **Beech-Nut** Stage 2	140
Pudding vanilla custard / **Gerber** Second Foods	100
Strawberry banana yogurt / **Heinz**	130
Strawberry yogurt / **Heinz**	120
Tutti Frutti / **Heinz**	100

Fruit: 1 jar

Apple blueberry / **Gerber** Second Foods	50
Apples and apricots / **Beech-Nut** Stage 2	80
Apples and apricots / **Heinz**	80
Apples and bananas / **Beech-Nut** Stage 2	80
Apples and cherries / **Beech-Nut** Stage 2	70
Apples and cranberries / **Heinz**	100
Apples and pears / **Beech-Nut** Stage 2	80
Apples and pears / **Heinz**	80
Apples, pears and bananas / **Beech-Nut** Stage 2	90
Applesauce / **Beech-Nut** Baby's First	50
Applesauce / **Beech-Nut** Stage 1	70
Applesauce / **Gerber** First Foods	35
Applesauce / **Gerber** Second Foods	50
Applesauce / **Heinz**	70
Applesauce / **Heinz** Beginner Foods	50
Applesauce apricot / **Gerber** Second Foods	50
Apricots, pears and apples / **Beech-Nut** Stage 2	90
Apricots w tapioca / **Gerber** Second Foods	70

CALORIES

Apricots w tapioca / **Heinz**	100
Bananas / **Beech-Nut** Baby's First	70
Bananas / **Beech-Nut** Stage 1	120
Bananas / **Gerber** First Foods	70
Bananas / **Heinz** Beginner Foods	90
Bananas and fruit juice w tapioca / **Gerber** Second Foods	80
Bananas and pineapple / **Heinz**	100
Bananas, pears and apples / **Beech-Nut** Stage 2	100
Bananas w pineapple and tapioca / **Gerber** Second Foods	60
Bananas w tapioca / **Gerber** Second Foods	80
Bananas w tapioca / **Heinz**	100
Fruit dessert / **Beech-Nut** Stage 2	80
Guava w tapioca / **Gerber** Second Foods	80
Mango w tapioca / **Gerber** Second Foods	80
Papaya w tapioca / **Gerber** Second Foods	70
Peaches / **Beech-Nut** Baby's First	45
Peaches / **Beech-Nut** Stage 1	70
Peaches / **Gerber** First Foods	40
Peaches / **Gerber** Second Foods	80
Peaches / **Heinz**	100
Peaches / **Heinz** Beginner Foods	70
Peaches mango w tapioca / **Gerber** Second Foods	80
Pears / **Beech-Nut** Baby's First	50
Pears / **Beech-Nut** Stage 1	80
Pears / **Gerber** First Foods	45
Pears / **Gerber** Second Foods	60
Pears / **Heinz**	80
Pears / **Heinz** Beginner Foods	70
Pears and pineapple / **Beech-Nut** Stage 2	90
Pears and pineapple / **Heinz**	90
Pears and pineapple / **Gerber** Second Foods	60
Plums, apples and rice / **Beech-Nut** Stage 2	70
Plums w tapioca / **Gerber** Second Foods	80
Plums w tapioca / **Heinz**	90
Prunes / **Gerber** First Foods	70
Prunes and rice / **Beech-Nut** Stage 2	110
Prunes w tapioca / **Gerber** Second Foods	80
Prunes w tapioca / **Heinz**	130
Tropical fruits w tapioca / **Gerber** Second Foods	70

CALORIES

Juices, Strained: 1 jar or can

Apple / **Beech-Nut** Stage 1	60
Apple / **Gerber**	60
Apple / **Heinz**	70
Apple-apricot / **Heinz**	70
Apple-banana / **Gerber**	60
Apple-banana / **Heinz**	70
Apple-cherry / **Beech-Nut** Stage 2	70
Apple-cherry / **Gerber**	60
Apple-cherry / **Heinz**	70
Apple-cranberry / **Beech-Nut** Stage 2	60
Apple-cranberry / **Heinz**	70
Apple-grape / **Beech-Nut** Stage 2	70
Apple-grape / **Gerber**	60
Apple-grape / **Heinz**	70
Apple-peach / **Gerber**	60
Apple-peach / **Heinz**	70
Apple-pineapple / **Heinz**	70
Apple-plum / **Gerber**	60
Apple-prune / **Gerber**	60
Apple-prune / **Heinz**	70
Grape white / **Beech-Nut** Stage 1	90
Grape white / **Gerber**	80
Juice plus / **Beech-Nut** Stage 2	90
Mango w grape and pear / **Beech-Nut** Stage 2	80
Mixed / **Heinz**	70
Mixed fruit / **Beech-Nut** Stage 2	70
Mixed fruit / **Gerber**	60
Orange / **Gerber**	60
Orange / **Heinz**	70
Orange-apple / **Heinz**	70
Orange-apple-banana / **Heinz**	70
Papaya w pear and grape / **Beech-Nut** Stage 2	70
Peach w pear and grape / **Beech-Nut** Stage 2	70
Pear / **Beech-Nut** Stage 1	70
Pear / **Gerber**	60
Pear / **Heinz**	70
Tropical blend / **Beech-Nut** Stage 2	90
Tropical blend nectar / **Beech-Nut** Stage 2	90

CALORIES

Main Dishes, Strained: 1 jar

Beef and egg noodle / **Beech-Nut** Stage 2	90
Beef and egg noodle / **Gerber** Second Foods	80
Beef and egg noodle / **Heinz**	na
Beef Dinner Supreme / **Beech-Nut** Stage 2	130
Beef w vegetables / **Gerber** Second Foods Lean Meat	80
Chicken and rice / **Beech-Nut** Stage 2	80
Chicken noodle / **Beech-Nut** Stage 2	90
Chicken noodle / **Gerber** Second Foods	70
Chicken noodle / **Heinz**	na
Chicken soup / **Beech-Nut** Stage 2	90
Chicken soup / **Heinz**	na
Chicken w vegetables / **Gerber** Second Foods Lean Meat	70
Ham w vegetables / **Gerber** Second Foods Lean Meat	100
Macaroni and beef / **Beech-Nut** Stage 2	100
Macaroni cheese / **Gerber** Second Foods	70
Macaroni tomato beef / **Gerber** Second Foods	70
Macaroni, tomato and beef / **Heinz**	na
Turkey Dinner Supreme / **Beech-Nut** Stage 2	110
Turkey rice / **Beech-Nut** Stage 2	70
Turkey rice / **Gerber** Second Foods	70
Turkey rice w vegetables / **Heinz**	na
Turkey w vegetables / **Gerber** Second Foods Lean Meat	80
Vegetable bacon / **Gerber** Second Foods	90
Vegetable beef / **Beech-Nut** Stage 2	80
Vegetable beef / **Gerber** Second Foods	70
Vegetable chicken / **Beech-Nut** Stage 2	90
Vegetable chicken / **Gerber** Second Foods	70
Vegetable ham / **Beech-Nut** Stage 2	90
Vegetable ham / **Gerber** Second Foods	70
Vegetable lamb / **Beech-Nut** Stage 2	100
Vegetable turkey / **Gerber** Second Foods	60
Vegetables and bacon / **Heinz**	na
Vegetables and beef / **Heinz**	na
Vegetables and ham / **Heinz**	na
Vegetables and lamb / **Heinz**	na
Vegetables dumplings and beef / **Heinz**	na

Vegetables egg noodles and chicken / **Heinz**	na
Vegetables egg noodles and turkey / **Heinz**	na

Meat and Eggs, Strained: 1 jar

Beef / **Gerber** Second Foods	80
Beef and beef broth / **Heinz**	na
Beef and broth / **Beech-Nut** Stage 1	80
Chicken / **Gerber** Second Foods	90
Chicken and broth / **Beech-Nut** Stage 1	70
Chicken and chicken broth / **Heinz**	na
Egg yolks / **Gerber** Second Foods	130
Ham / **Gerber** Second Foods	90
Lamb / **Gerber** Second Foods	80
Lamb and broth / **Beech-Nut** Stage 1	60
Lamb and lamb broth / **Heinz**	na
Liver and liver broth / **Heinz**	na
Turkey / **Gerber** Second Foods	80
Turkey and broth / **Beech-Nut** Stage 1	90
Turkey and turkey broth / **Heinz**	na
Veal / **Gerber** Second Foods	70
Veal and broth / **Beech-Nut** Stage 1	70

Vegetables, Strained: 1 jar

Beets / **Gerber** Second Foods	45
Beets / **Heinz**	70
Carrots / **Beech-Nut** Baby's First	25
Carrots / **Beech-Nut** Stage 1	45
Carrots / **Gerber** First Foods	30
Carrots / **Gerber** Second Foods	30
Carrots / **Heinz**	35
Carrots / **Heinz** Beginner Foods	30
Carrots and peas / **Beech-Nut** Stage 2	50
Corn, creamed / **Beech-Nut** Stage 2	100
Corn, creamed / **Gerber** Second Foods	80
Corn, creamed / **Heinz**	100
Garden / **Beech-Nut** Stage 2	60
Garden / **Gerber** Second Foods	50
Green beans / **Beech-Nut** Stage 1	40
Green beans / **Gerber** First Foods	25
Green beans / **Gerber** Second Foods	35

Green beans / **Heinz**	40
Green beans / **Heinz** Beginner Foods	30
Mixed / **Beech-Nut** Stage 2	60
Mixed / **Gerber** Second Foods	50
Mixed / **Heinz**	60
Peas / **Beech-Nut** Baby's First	40
Peas / **Beech-Nut** Stage 1	70
Peas / **Gerber** First Foods	30
Peas / **Gerber** Second Foods	60
Peas / **Heinz** Beginner Foods	50
Peas, creamed / **Heinz**	90
Spinach, creamed / **Gerber** Second Foods	50
Squash / **Beech-Nut** Baby's First	30
Squash / **Beech-Nut** Stage 1	60
Squash / **Gerber** First Foods	25
Squash / **Gerber** Second Foods	30
Squash / **Heinz**	60
Squash / **Heinz** Beginner Foods	30
Sweet potatoes / **Beech-Nut** Baby's First	50
Sweet potatoes / **Beech-Nut** Stage 1	90
Sweet potatoes / **Gerber** First Foods	50
Sweet potatoes / **Gerber** Second Foods	70
Sweet potatoes / **Heinz**	100
Sweet potatoes / **Heinz** Beginner Foods	60

JUNIOR BABY FOODS

Cereal: 1 jar

Mixed w applesauce and bananas / **Gerber** Third Foods	140
Oatmeal w applesauce and bananas / **Gerber** Third Foods	140
Rice w mixed fruit / **Gerber** Third Foods	130

Desserts: 1 jar

Cottage cheese w pineapple / **Beech-Nut** Stage 3	170
Dutch apple / **Gerber** Third Foods	130
Dutch apple / **Heinz**	150
Fruit / **Gerber** Third Foods	120
Fruit / **Heinz**	140

CALORIES

Hawaiian Delight / **Gerber** Third Foods	150
Mixed fruit yogurt / **Beech-Nut** Stage 3	160
Peach cobbler / **Gerber** Third Foods	120
Pineapple-orange / **Heinz**	140
Pudding, custard / **Heinz**	160
Pudding, vanilla custard / **Beech-Nut** Stage 3	180
Pudding, vanilla custard / **Gerber** Third Foods	150
Tutti-Frutti / **Heinz**	150

Fruit: 1 jar

Apple-blueberry / **Gerber** Third Foods	80
Apples and apricots / **Heinz**	110
Apples and bananas / **Beech-Nut** Stage 3	100
Apples and cherries / **Beech-Nut** Stage 3	100
Apples and cranberries / **Heinz**	150
Apples and pears / **Heinz**	120
Applesauce / **Beech-Nut** Stage 3	90
Applesauce / **Gerber** Third Foods	90
Applesauce / **Heinz**	110
Apricots, pears and apples / **Beech-Nut** Stage 3	120
Apricots w tapioca / **Gerber** Third Foods	110
Apricots w tapioca / **Heinz**	140
Bananas, pears and apples / **Beech-Nut** Stage 3	130
Bananas w pineapple / **Heinz**	140
Bananas w pineapple and tapioca / **Gerber** Third Foods	80
Bananas w tapioca / **Gerber** Third Foods	130
Bananas w tapioca / **Heinz**	150
Fruit dessert / **Beech-Nut** Stage 3	120
Peaches / **Beech-Nut** Stage 3	90
Peaches / **Gerber** Third Foods	110
Peaches / **Heinz**	140
Pear-pineapple / **Gerber** Third Foods	100
Pears / **Beech-Nut** Stage 3	100
Pears / **Gerber** Third Foods	100
Pears / **Heinz**	120
Plums w tapioca / **Gerber** Third Foods	120

Fruit Juices: 1 jar or can

Apple / **Gerber** Third Foods	60
Apple / **Gerber** Third Foods w Lofat Yogurt	100
Apple-cherry / **Gerber** Third Foods	60
Apple-grape / **Gerber** Third Foods	60
Banana / **Gerber** Third Foods w Lofat Yogurt	110
Grape / **Gerber** Third Foods	80
Mixed / **Gerber** Third Foods	60
Mixed / **Gerber** Third Foods w Lofat Yogurt	100
Orange / **Beech-Nut** Stage 3	70
Pear / **Gerber** Third Foods	60
Pear peach / **Gerber** Third Foods w Lofat Yogurt	90

Main Dishes: 1 jar

Beef and egg noodle / **Beech-Nut** Stage 3	120
Beef and egg noodle / **Gerber** Third Foods	110
Beef w vegetables / **Gerber** Third Foods Lean Meat	90
Chicken noodle / **Beech-Nut** Stage 3	100
Chicken noodle / **Gerber** Third Foods	100
Chicken noodle / **Heinz**	60
Chicken rice / **Heinz**	70
Chicken w vegetables / **Gerber** Third Foods Lean Meat	70
Ham w vegetables / **Gerber** Third Foods Lean Meat	100
Macaroni w beef and tomato sauce / **Gerber** Chunky	140
Macaroni and beef / **Beech-Nut** Stage 3	130
Macaroni, tomato and beef / **Gerber** Third Foods	110
Noodles and beef / **Gerber** Chunky	150
Noodles and chicken w carrots and peas / **Gerber** Chunky	110
Rice w beef and tomato sauce / **Gerber** Chunky	140
Rice w chicken / **Gerber** Chunky	120
Spaghetti and beef / **Beech-Nut** Stage 3	130
Spaghetti, tomato and beef / **Gerber** Third Foods	120
Spaghetti w tomato sauce and beef / **Gerber** Chunky	150
Turkey and rice / **Beech-Nut** Stage 3	100
Turkey and rice / **Gerber** Third Foods	100
Turkey w vegetables / **Gerber** Third Foods Lean Meat	90
Vegetable bacon / **Gerber** Third Foods	130

CALORIES

Vegetable beef / **Beech-Nut** Stage 3	120
Vegetable beef / **Gerber** Third Foods	120
Vegetable chicken / **Beech-Nut** Stage 3	110
Vegetable chicken / **Gerber** Third Foods	100
Vegetable ham / **Gerber** Third Foods	110
Vegetable turkey / **Gerber** Third Foods	100
Vegetables and beef / **Gerber** Chunky	130
Vegetables and beef / **Heinz**	60
Vegetables and chicken / **Gerber** Chunky	140
Vegetables and chicken / **Heinz**	60
Vegetables and ham / **Gerber** Chunky	130
Vegetables and ham / **Heinz**	70
Vegetables and turkey / **Gerber** Chunky	110
Vegetables and turkey / **Heinz**	60

Meats: 1 jar

Beef / **Gerber** Third Foods	80
Chicken / **Gerber** Third Foods	90
Chicken sticks / **Gerber**	120
Ham / **Gerber** Third Foods	90
Meat sticks / **Gerber**	110
Turkey / **Gerber** Third Foods	90
Turkey sticks / **Gerber**	120
Veal / **Gerber** Third Foods	80

Vegetables: 1 jar

Broccoli, carrots and cheese / **Gerber** Third Foods	80
Carrots / **Beech-Nut** Stage 3	60
Carrots / **Gerber** Third Foods	45
Carrots / **Heinz**	45
Corn, creamed / **Heinz**	140
Green beans / **Beech-Nut** Stage 3	45
Green beans, creamed / **Gerber** Third Foods	80
Green beans, creamed / **Heinz**	90
Mixed / **Gerber** Third Foods	70
Peas / **Gerber** Third Foods	90
Squash / **Gerber** Third Foods	60
Sweet potatoes / **Beech-Nut** Stage 3	110
Sweet potatoes / **Gerber** Third Foods	100
Sweet potatoes / **Heinz**	130

Beer, Malt Liquor, Nonalcoholic Beer

12 fluid ounces

CALORIES

BEER

Augsburger	168
Budweiser	142
Budweiser Dry Draft	130
Budweiser Light	110
Busch	143
Busch Light Draft	110
Carlsberg	150
Carlsberg Light	110
Coors	137
Coors 3.2%	119
Coors Dry	119
Coors Dry 3.2%	101
Coors Light	103
Coors Light 3.2%	98
Cutter	76
Extra Gold	151
Extra Gold 3.2%	120
Goebel	138
Hamms	139
Keystone	121
Keystone 3.2%	104
Keystone Dry	121
Keystone Light	100
Keystone Light 3.2%	99
Killian's	161
Killian's 3.2%	127

CALORIES

King Cobra	180
Löwenbräu Dark	158
Löwenbräu Light	98
Löwenbräu Special	158
Magnum	160
Meisterbrau	141
Meisterbrau Light	98
Michelob	152
Michelob Classic Dark	154
Michelob Dry	130
Michelob Golden Draft	152
Michelob Golden Draft Light	110
Michelob Light	134
Miller Genuine Draft	147
Miller Genuine Draft Light	98
Miller High Life	147
Miller Lite	96
Miller Reserve	133
Miller Reserve Light	106
Miller Sharp's	68
Milwaukee's Best	133
Milwaukee's Best Light	98
Natural Light	144
Natural Pilsner	110
O'Doul's	70
Old Milwaukee	145
Old Milwaukee Light	122
Pabst Blue Ribbon	144
Pabst Extra Light	69.2
Pabst Light	110
Piels	138
Schaefer	138
Schaefer Light	111
Schlitz	145
Schlitz Light	99
Signature	150
Strohs	142
Strohs Light	115

MALT LIQUOR

Elephant Malt	212
Olde English 800	165
Schlitz	177

NONALCOHOLIC BEER

Hamms	55
Pabst	55

Biscuits

BISCUITS, MIX

	CALORIES
Arrowhead Mills / 2 oz	100
Bisquick / ½ cup	240
Gold Medal Pouch Mixes / ⅛ mix prepared	90

BISCUITS, REFRIGERATED

1 biscuit

Pillsbury Butter Tastin	100
Pillsbury Butter Tastin Big Country	100
Pillsbury Butter Tastin Grands	190
Pillsbury Butter Tastin Hungry Jack	100
Pillsbury Country	50
Pillsbury Flaky Grands	190
Pillsbury Flaky Hungry Jack	80
Pillsbury Good 'n Buttery	90
Pillsbury Heat 'n Serve	280
Pillsbury Ovenready Extra Lights	50
Pillsbury Southern Style Big Country	100
Pillsbury Southern Style Hungry Jack	80

CALORIES

Baking powder / **Pillsbury**	100
Butter / **Pillsbury**	50
Buttermilk	
Pillsbury	50
Pillsbury 1869 Brand	100
Pillsbury Big Country	100
Pillsbury Extra Rich Hungry Jack	50
Pillsbury Flaky Hungry Jack	90
Pillsbury Fluffy Hungry Jack	90
Pillsbury Heat 'n Serve	170
Pillsbury Ovenready Extra Lights	50
Pillsbury Tender Layer	50
Cinnamon raisin **Pillsbury** Grands	190
Honey **Pillsbury** Flaky Hungry Jack	90

Bread

CALORIES

1 slice unless noted

Apple cinnamon / **Pritikin**	80
Autumn grain / **Merita**	70
Barbecue / **Millbrook**	100
Black / **Mrs. Wright's** Old World	60
Brown, plain, canned / ½-in slice / **B&M**	92
Brown, plain, canned / ½-in slice / **Friends**	92
Brown w raisins, canned / ½-in slice / **B&M**	94
Brown w raisins, canned / ½-in slice / **Friends**	94
Butter and egg / **Mrs. Wright's**	70
Buttermilk	
Butternut	80
Dutch Hearth	80
Eddy's	80
Holsum	80
Mrs. Wright's	70
Sweetheart	80
Weber's	80

CALORIES

Buttertop	
Butternut	70
Eddy's	70
Sweetheart	70
Cereal grain / **Mrs. Wright's Grainbelt**	140
Cinnamon / 2 slices / **Pepperidge Farm**	180
Dark 'n Grainy / **Less**	40
D'Italiano / **Merita**	70
French	
Dutch Hearth / 1-oz slice	70
Dutch Hearth / 1.5-oz slice	110
Eddy's / 1-oz slice	70
Eddy's / 1.5-oz slice	110
Holsum / 1-oz slice	70
Holsum / 1.5-oz slice	110
Holsum French Stix	140
Pepperidge Farm / 2-oz slice	150
Pepperidge Farm French Twin / 1-oz slice	80
Sweetheart / 1-oz slice	70
Sweetheart / 1.5-oz slice	110
Grain	
Country Farms Hunter's Grain	120
Mrs. Wright's Unsalted	70
Granola bran	
Mrs. Wright's	80
Honey and oat bran / **Roman Meal**	70
Honey bran	
Mrs. Wright's	90
Pepperidge Farm / 2 slices	180
Honey, molasses and graham / **Mrs. Wright's**	100
Honey oatberry / **Mrs. Wright's**	130
Honey wheatberry / **Mrs. Wright's**	70
Italian	
Butternut	60
Dutch Hearth	60
Less	40
Millbrook	60
Mrs. Wright's Old Fashioned	100
Roman Meal Light	40

CALORIES

Low Sodium	
Butternut	80
Eddy's	80
Multigrain	
Country Farms	80
Pritikin	70
Weight Watchers	40
Oat	
Country Farms	130
Pepperidge Farm Hearty Crunchy / 2 slices	190
Oat bran	
Betterway	80
Weight Watchers	40
Oat bran and honey / **Roman Meal** Light	40
Oatmeal	
Mrs. Wright's	80
Pepperidge Farm / 2 slices	140
Pepperidge Farm Light / 2 slices	90
Pepperidge Farm Very Thin Sliced / 2 slices	80
Onion dill / **Pritikin**	70
Pita / **Sahara** / 1 oz	80
Pita oat bran / **Sahara** / 1 oz	70
Pita whole wheat / **Sahara** / 1 oz	70
Potato / **Sweetheart**	70
Pumpernickel	
Pepperidge Farm Family / 2 slices	160
Pepperidge Farm Party / 4 slices	60
Raisin	
Butternut	80
Mrs. Wright's Lite	40
Mrs. Wright's Unsalted	80
Roman Meal	70
Sunmaid	80
Raisin nut / **Mrs. Wright's**	70
Raisin w cinnamon / **Pepperidge Farm** / 2 slices	180
Roman Meal / **Roman Meal**	70
Rye	
Pepperidge Farm Dijon / 2 slices	100
Pepperidge Farm Dijon Hearty / 2 slices	140
Pepperidge Farm Family / 2 slices	160

Pepperidge Farm Family Seedless / 2 slices	160
Pepperidge Farm Party / 4 slices	60
Pritikin	70
Weight Watchers	40
Rye, dill / **Mrs. Wright's**	100
Rye, Jewish w seeds / **Mrs. Wright's**	60
Rye, Swedish / **Mrs. Wright's**	80
Rye w seeds / **Mrs. Wright's**	60
Rye wo seeds / **Mrs. Wright's**	60
Sesame, butter and egg / **Mrs. Wright's**	70
Sesame, Vienna / **Mrs. Wright's**	70
Sesame wheat	
Mrs. Wright's	70
Pepperidge Farm / 2 slices	190
Seven grain	
Betterway	80
Mrs. Wright's	130
Mrs. Wright's Lite	40
Pepperidge Farm Hearty/ 2 slices	180
Roman Meal	70
Roman Meal Light	40
Sourdough / **Roman Meal**	40
Sourdough, French	
Eddy's / 1-oz slice	70
Eddy's / 1.5-oz slice	110
Eddy's / 2.4-oz slice	170
Holsum / 1-oz slice	70
Holsum / 1.5-oz slice	110
Holsum / 2.4-oz slice	170
Mrs. Wright's	80
Sweetheart / 1-oz slice	70
Sweetheart / 1.5-oz slice	110
Sweetheart / 2.4-oz slice	170
Sourdough white / **Mrs. Wright's**	80
Split top / **Merita**	60
Sun grain	
Roman Meal / 1-oz slice	70
Roman Meal / 1.3-oz slice	90
Texas toast	
Butternut	110
Holsum	110

CALORIES

Merita	90
Vienna	
Mrs. Wright's	70
Pepperidge Farm	70
Pepperidge Farm Light / 2 slices	90
Wheat	
Betterway 100% Wheat	80
Betterway Wheat Nugget	80
Butternut	70
Butternut Butter Split	80
Butternut Lite Loaf	40
Butternut Sweet	80
Country Farms 100% Whole Wheat	120
Dutch Hearth Very Thin / .6-oz slice	45
Dutch Hearth Very Thin / .8-oz slice	60
Holsum Lite	40
Holsum Premium	70
Less	40
Merita 100% Whole Wheat / .9-oz slice	70
Merita 100% Whole Wheat / 1-oz slice	70
Merita Lite	40
Millbrook Buttercrown	80
Millbrook Lite Loaf	40
Mrs. Karl's Butter Split	80
Mrs. Karl's Sweet	80
Mrs. Wright's	70
Pepperidge Farm / 2 slices	180
Pepperidge Farm Family / 2 slices	140
Pepperidge Farm Light / 2 slices	90
Pepperidge Farm Very Thin Sliced / 2 slices	70
Pritikin	70
Roman Meal 100% Whole Wheat / 1.3-oz slice	80
Roman Meal 100% Whole Wheat / 1-oz slice	70
Roman Meal Hearty Light	40
Roman Meal Light	40
Sweetheart Lite Loaf	40
Weber's Lite Loaf	40
Weight Watchers	40
Wheat, cracked / **Pepperidge Farm** / 2 slices	140
Wheat, honey berry / **Country Farms**	120

CALORIES

Wheat, sprouted / **Pepperidge Farm** / 2 slices	140
Wheat, stoneground / **Mrs. Wright's**	130
Wheat, stoneground 100% / **Mrs. Wright's**	70
White	
Butternut	70
Butternut Lite Loaf	40
Cookbook	70
Cotton/Holsum	70
Cotton/Holsum Lite	40
Country Farms Old Fashioned	120
Dutch Hearth Very Thin	70
Eddy's	70
Holsum	70
Holsum Heavenly	70
Holsum Thin Sliced	60
Less	40
Merita	70
Merita Lite	40
Merita Old Fashioned	70
Millbrook Lite Loaf	40
Millbrook Old Fashioned	70
Millbrook Thin Sliced	60
Mrs. Karl's	70
Mrs. Wright's Soft Twist	80
Mrs. Wright's Texas Toastin	130
Mrs. Wright's Unsalted	70
Pepperidge Farm Family / 2 slices	140
Pepperidge Farm Hearty Country / 2 slices	190
Pepperidge Farm Sandwich / 2 slices	130
Pepperidge Farm Thin Sliced / 2 slices	160
Pepperidge Farm Toasting White / 2 slices	180
Pepperidge Farm Very Thin Sliced / 2 slices	80
Sweetheart	70
Weber's	70
Weight Watchers	40

BREAD AND CRACKER CRUMBS

Corn flake crumbs / 1 oz / **Kellogg's**	100
Italian style / 2 tbsp / **Progresso**	60

CALORIES

Plain / 2 tbsp / **Progresso**	60
Seasoned / 1 rounded tbsp / **Contadina**	35

BREAD MIXES

Prepared unless noted

Apple cinnamon	
⅟₁₂ mix w egg substitute / **Pillsbury**	190
⅟₁₂ mix / **Pillsbury**	180
Banana	
⅟₁₂ mix w egg substitute / **Pillsbury**	170
⅟₁₂ mix / **Pillsbury**	170
Blueberry	
⅟₁₂ mix w egg substitute / **Pillsbury**	180
⅟₁₂ mix / **Pillsbury**	180
Corn	
Arrowhead Mills / 1 oz	100
Aunt Jemima Easy Mix / 1.7 oz	196
Gold Medal White / ⅙ mix	140
Gold Medal Yellow / ⅙ mix	150
⅟₁₆ mix / **Pillsbury** Ballard	150
Cranberry	
⅟₁₂ mix w egg substitute / **Pillsbury**	170
⅟₁₂ mix / **Pillsbury**	160
Date	
⅟₁₂ mix w egg substitute / **Pillsbury**	160
⅟₁₂ mix / **Pillsbury**	160
Nut	
⅟₁₂ mix w egg substitute / **Pillsbury**	170
⅟₁₂ mix / **Pillsbury**	170
Oatmeal raisin	
⅟₁₂ mix w egg substitute **Pillsbury**	190
⅟₁₂ mix / **Pillsbury**	190

BREAD, REFRIGERATED

Corn / ⅟₁₀ pkg / **Pillsbury** Twists	70
French / 1-in slice / **Pillsbury**	60
Italian / 1 oz / **Pepperidge Farm** Brown and Serve	80

CALORIES

Multigrain / ⅛ loaf / **Pillsbury**	80
Oatmeal / ¹⁄₁₀ pkg / **Pillsbury** Twists	80
Oatmeal raisin / ⅛ loaf / **Pillsbury**	90
Wheat / 1-in slice / **Pillsbury**	70
Wheat and honey / ¹⁄₁₀ pkg / **Pillsbury** Twists	80
White / 1-in slice / **Pillsbury**	70

BREAD STICKS

1 stick unless noted

Onion / **Stella D'Oro**	40
Pizza / **Stella D'Oro**	45
Regular	
Stella D'Oro	40
Stella D'Oro Dietetic	45
Sesame / **Stella D'Oro**	50
Sesame / **Stella D'Oro** Dietetic	50
Soft / ⅛ pkg / **Pillsbury**	100
Wheat / **Stella D'Oro**	40

CROUTONS

½ oz unless noted

Cheddar and Romano cheese / **Pepperidge Farm**	60
Cheese and garlic / **Pepperidge Farm**	70
Croutettes / **Kellogg's**	70
Italian style / **Progresso**	30
Onion and garlic / **Pepperidge Farm**	70
Seasoned	
Pepperidge Farm	70
Weight Watchers / 1 pouch	30
Sour cream and chive / **Pepperidge Farm**	70

STUFFING MIXES

½ cup prepared unless noted

Americana San Francisco / **Stove Top**	170
Apple and raisin / dry / 1 oz / **Pepperidge Farm**	
Distinctive Stuffings	110

CALORIES

Beef / **Stove Top**	180
Broccoli and cheese / **Stove Top** Microwave	170
Chicken	
Betty Crocker / ⅙ serv	180
Pepperidge Farm Distinctive Stuffings / 1 oz dry	110
Chicken-flavored	
Golden Grain / 1 oz dry	106
Stove Top	180
Stove Top Flexible Serving	170
Stove Top Microwave	160
Town House	180
Corn bread	
Golden Grain / 1 oz dry	105
Pepperidge Farm / 1 oz dry	110
Stove Top	170
Town House	170
Corn-bread flavored / **Stove Top** Flexible Serving	180
Corn bread, homestyle / **Stove Top** Microwave	160
Country style / dry / 1 oz / **Pepperidge Farm**	100
Cube / dry / 1 oz / **Pepperidge Farm**	110
Garden herb / dry / 1 oz / **Pepperidge Farm** Distinctive Stuffings	120
Herb / ⅙ serv / **Betty Crocker**	180
Herb and butter / dry / 1 oz / **Golden Grain**	104
Herb, homestyle / **Stove Top** Flexible Serving	170
Herb, savory / **Stove Top**	170
Herb, seasoned / dry / 1 oz / **Pepperidge Farm**	110
Long grain and wild rice / **Stove Top**	180
Mushroom and onion / **Stove Top**	180
Mushroom and onion flavored / **Stove Top** Microwave	170
Pork / **Stove Top**	170
Pork flavored / **Stove Top** Flexible Serving	170
Stuffing bread / dry / 1 oz / **Mrs. Wright's**	80
Turkey / **Stove Top**	170
Vegetable and almond / dry / 1 oz / **Pepperidge Farm** Distinctive Stuffings	110
w rice / **Stove Top**	180
w wild rice / dry / 1 oz / **Golden Grain**	108
Wild rice and mushroom / dry / 1 oz / **Pepperidge Farm** Distinctive Stuffings	130

Butter, Margarine and Oils

BUTTER

	CALORIES
½ cup (¼ lb stick)	810
1 tbsp	100
1 pat (1 in sq ⅓ in high)	35

MARGARINE

1 tablespoon unless noted

Imitation
Weight Watchers Cooking Spray / 1 second	2

Regular and Soft
Blue Bonnet Soft	100
Fleischmann's	100
Fleischmann's Diet	50
Fleischmann's Light Corn Oil	80
Fleischmann's Soft	100
Fleischmann's Soft Unsalted	100
Fleischmann's Unsalted	100
Hollywood Safflower Oil	100
Hollywood Safflower Sweet Unsalted	100
Imperial	100
Kraft Chiffon Soft	90
Kraft Chiffon Soft Stick	100
Kraft Chiffon Soft Unsalted	90
Kraft Parkay	100
Kraft Parkay Soft	100
Kraft Parkay Soft Diet	50
Land O Lakes	35
Mazola	100

CALORIES

Promise Extra Light   70
Shedd's   80
Weight Watchers Reduced Calorie Stick   60
Weight Watchers Reduced Calorie Tub   50
Weight Watchers Sweet Unsalted   50

Spread
Blue Bonnet Better Blend   90
Blue Bonnet Better Blend Soft   90
Blue Bonnet Better Blend Unsalted   90
Blue Bonnet Whipped   80
Fleischmann's Extra Light Corn Oil   50
Fleischmann's Light Corn Oil   80
Hollywood Soft   90
Kraft Parkay   60
Kraft Parkay Squeeze   90
Kraft Touch of Butter Bowl   50
Kraft Touch of Butter Stick   90
Promise   90
Promise Extra Light   32
Shedd's Corn Oil   60
Shedd's Vegetable Oil   60

Whipped
Blue Bonnet   70
Fleischmann's Lightly Salted   70
Fleischmann's Unsalted   70
Kraft Chiffon   70
Kraft Miracle Brand Cup   60
Kraft Miracle Brand Stick   70
Kraft Parkay   70
Kraft Parkay Stick   70

Cakes

FROZEN

	CALORIES
Apple spice bake / 4-¼ oz / **Pepperidge Farm**	170
Applesauce / 2.5 oz / **Aunt Fanny's**	234
Boston cream supreme / 2-⅞ oz / **Pepperidge Farm**	290
Carrot / 2-½ oz / **Pepperidge Farm**	260
Carrot / 3 oz / **Weight Watchers**	170
Carrot w cream cheese / 1-½ oz / **Pepperidge Farm**	150
Cheesecake / 3.90 oz / **Weight Watchers**	210
Cheesecake, brownie / 3.50 oz / **Weight Watchers**	200
Cheesecake, strawberry / 3.90 oz / **Weight Watchers**	180
Cheesecake, strawberry / 4-¼ oz / **Pepperidge Farm**	300
Cherries and cream / 3 oz / **Weight Watchers**	190
Cherries supreme / 3-¼ oz / **Pepperidge Farm**	170
Chocolate / 2.50 oz / **Weight Watchers**	180
Chocolate brownie / 1.25 oz / **Weight Watchers**	100
Chocolate fudge / 1-⅝ oz / **Pepperidge Farm**	180
Chocolate fudge stripe / 1-⅝ oz / **Pepperidge Farm**	170
Chocolate mousse / 2-½ oz / **Pepperidge Farm**	190
Chocolate mousse / 2.50 oz / **Weight Watchers**	170
Chocolate supreme / 2-⅞ oz / **Pepperidge Farm**	300
Coconut / 2-¼ oz / **Pepperidge Farm**	230
Coconut layer / 1-⅝ oz / **Pepperidge Farm**	180
Coffee w cinnamon streusel / 2.25 oz / **Weight Watchers**	190
Devil's food / 1-⅝ oz / **Pepperidge Farm**	180
Double chocolate / 2-¼ oz / **Pepperidge Farm**	250

CALORIES

Double fudge / 2.75 oz / **Weight Watchers**	200
Fudge / 2.5 oz / **Aunt Fanny's**	222
German chocolate / 2-¼ oz / **Pepperidge Farm**	250
German chocolate / 2.50 oz / **Weight Watchers**	200
German chocolate layer / 1-⅝ oz / **Pepperidge Farm**	180
Golden layer / 1-⅝ oz / **Pepperidge Farm**	180
Hot fudge brownie / 3-¼ oz / **Pepperidge Farm**	400
Lemon coconut / 3 oz / **Pepperidge Farm**	280
Lemon cream / 1-⅝ oz / **Pepperidge Farm**	170
Lemon supreme / 2-¾ oz / **Pepperidge Farm**	170
Peach parfait / 4-¼ oz / **Pepperidge Farm**	150
Pineapple cream / 2 oz / **Pepperidge Farm**	190
Pound / 2.5 oz / **Aunt Fanny's**	260
Pound / 1 oz / **Pepperidge Farm** Cholesterol Free	110
Praline pecan mousse / 2.71 oz / **Weight Watchers**	190
Raspberry vanilla swirl / 3-¼ oz / **Pepperidge Farm**	160
Strawberry cream / 2 oz / **Pepperidge Farm**	190
Strawberry shortcake / 3 oz / **Pepperidge Farm**	170
Strawberry stripe / 1-½ oz / **Pepperidge Farm**	160
Vanilla fudge swirl / 2-¼ oz / **Pepperidge Farm**	250
Vanilla layer / 1-⅝ oz / **Pepperidge Farm**	190

PREPARED

Angel food / 1-oz slice / **Dolly Madison**	90
Pound / 2-⅓-oz slice / **Dolly Madison**	220

MIXES

¹⁄₁₂ cake unless noted. Prepared according to package directions

Angel food
Betty Crocker Confetti	150
Betty Crocker Lemon Custard	150
Betty Crocker Traditional	130
Betty Crocker White	150
Duncan Hines	140
Mrs. Wright's	130
Pillsbury / ⅛ cake	90

Banana
    Duncan Hines 260
    Duncan Hines, no cholesterol 250
    Mix dry / **Fearn** / ⅙ cake 130
    Pillsbury Plus 250
    prepared w egg whites / **Pillsbury** Plus 190
Banana w frosting / **Pillsbury** Microwave Snack Cake 170
Bundt / ¹⁄₁₆ cake
    Black forest cherry / **Pillsbury** 270
    Black forest cherry / prepared w egg whites /
      Pillsbury 260
    Boston cream / **Pillsbury** 260
    Boston cream / prepared w egg whites / **Pillsbury** 250
    Chocolate caramel / **Pillsbury** 290
    Chocolate caramel / prepared w egg whites /
      Pillsbury 280
    Chocolate eclair / **Pillsbury** 260
    Chocolate eclair / prepared w egg whites / **Pillsbury** 250
    Chocolate macaroon / **Pillsbury** 280
    Chocolate macaroon / prepared w egg whites /
      Pillsbury 270
    Chocolate mousse / **Pillsbury** 260
    Chocolate mousse / prepared w egg whites /
      Pillsbury 250
    Fudge / **Pillsbury** 310
    Fudge / prepared w egg whites / **Pillsbury** 300
    Lemon / **Pillsbury** 270
    Lemon / prepared w egg whites / **Pillsbury** 260
    Pineapple cream / **Pillsbury** 280
    Pineapple cream / prepared w egg whites /
      Pillsbury 270
Butter chocolate / **Betty Crocker** SuperMoist 280
Butter pecan / **Betty Crocker** SuperMoist 250
Butter pecan / no cholesterol / **Betty Crocker**
  SuperMoist 220
Butter recipe / **Pillsbury** Plus 260
Butter recipe / prepared w egg whites / **Pillsbury** Plus 250
Butter recipe, chocolate / **Pillsbury** Plus 250
Butter recipe, chocolate / prepared w egg whites /
  Pillsbury Plus 240
Butter recipe, fudge / **Duncan Hines** 270

CALORIES

Butter recipe, golden / **Duncan Hines**	270
Butter yellow / **Betty Crocker** SuperMoist	260
Carob / mix dry / ⅙ cake / **Fearn**	120
Carrot	
Betty Crocker SuperMoist	250
Betty Crocker SuperMoist, no cholesterol	210
Fearn / mix dry / ⅙ cake	140
Pillsbury Plus	260
Pillsbury Plus, prepared w egg whites	190
Carrot w frosting / ⅑ cake / **Pillsbury** Microwave Snack Cake	170
Cheesecake / ⅛ cake / **Royal**	160
Cheesecake / ⅛ cake / **Royal** Lite	130
Cherry chip / **Betty Crocker** SuperMoist	190
Chocolate w frosting / ⅑ cake / **Pillsbury** Microwave Snack Cake	160
Chocolate chip	
Betty Crocker SuperMoist	290
Betty Crocker SuperMoist, no cholesterol	220
Pillsbury Plus	240
Pillsbury Plus, prepared w egg whites	190
Chocolate chocolate chip / **Betty Crocker** SuperMoist	260
Chocolate fudge / **Betty Crocker** SuperMoist	260
Chocolate pudding / ⅙ cake / **Betty Crocker**	230
Coffee cake	
Aunt Jemima Easy Mixes / 1 serv	156
Cinnamon streusel / ⅙ cake / **Pillsbury**	230
Pecan streusel / ⅙ cake / **Pillsbury**	230
Dark chocolate / **Pillsbury** Plus	250
Dark chocolate / prepared w egg whites / **Pillsbury** Plus	180
Dark dutch fudge	
Betty Crocker SuperMoist	260
Duncan Hines	280
Duncan Hines, no cholesterol	270
Devil's food	
Betty Crocker SuperMoist, no cholesterol	220
Betty Crocker SuperMoist Light	200
Betty Crocker SuperMoist Light, no cholesterol	180
Duncan Hines	280
Duncan Hines, no cholesterol	270
Mrs. Wright's	190

CALORIES

Pillsbury   170
Pillsbury, prepared w egg whites   160
Pillsbury Plus   270
Pillsbury Plus, prepared w egg whites   180
Devil's food w chocolate frosting / ⅙ cake
   Betty Crocker MicroRave   310
   Betty Crocker MicroRave, no cholesterol   240
   Betty Crocker MicroRave Singles / 1 serv   440
French vanilla / **Duncan Hines**   260
French vanilla / no cholesterol / **Duncan Hines**   250
Fudge marble / **Duncan Hines**   260
Fudge marble / no cholesterol / **Duncan Hines**   250
Fudge swirl / **Pillsbury** Plus   270
Fudge swirl / prepared w egg whites / **Pillsbury** Plus   200
Funfetti / **Pillsbury** Plus   230
Funfetti / prepared w egg whites / **Pillsbury** Plus   190
Funfetti / chocolate w frosting / 1 cake / **Pillsbury** Microwave Cupcake Mix   160
Funfetti / yellow w frosting / 1 cake / **Pillsbury** Microwave Cupcake Mix   180
German chocolate
   Betty Crocker SuperMoist   260
   Betty Crocker SuperMoist, no cholesterol   220
   Pillsbury Plus   250
   Pillsbury Plus, prepared w egg whites   180
German chocolate w coconut pecan frosting / ⅙ cake / **Betty Crocker** MicroRave   320
German chocolate w coconut pecan frosting / ⅙ cake / **Betty Crocker** MicroRave   320
Gingerbread / ⅑ cake
   Betty Crocker   220
   Betty Crocker, no cholesterol   210
   Pillsbury   180
Golden vanilla / **Betty Crocker** SuperMoist   280
Golden vanilla / no cholesterol / **Betty Crocker** SuperMoist   220
Lemon
   Betty Crocker SuperMoist   260
   Betty Crocker SuperMoist, no cholesterol   220
   Pillsbury Plus   240
   Pillsbury Plus, prepared w egg whites   180

Lemon chiffon / **Betty Crocker**	200
Lemon pudding / ⅙ cake / **Betty Crocker**	230
Lemon supreme / **Duncan Hines**	260
Lemon supreme / no cholesterol / **Duncan Hines**	250
Marble / **Betty Crocker** SuperMoist	260
Marble / no cholesterol / **Betty Crocker** SuperMoist	220
Milk chocolate / **Betty Crocker** SuperMoist	260
Milk chocolate / no cholesterol / **Betty Crocker** Super-Moist	210
Orange supreme / **Duncan Hines**	260
Orange supreme / no cholesterol / **Duncan Hines**	250
Pineapple supreme / **Duncan Hines**	260
Pineapple supreme / no cholesterol / **Duncan Hines**	250
Pineapple upside-down / ⅑ cake / **Betty Crocker**	250
Pineapple upside-down / no cholesterol / ⅑ cake / **Betty Crocker**	240
Pound / **Betty Crocker**	200
Pound / **Mrs. Wright's**	200
Rainbow chip / **Betty Crocker** SuperMoist	250
Sour cream chocolate / **Betty Crocker** SuperMoist	260
Sour cream chocolate / no cholesterol / **Betty Crocker** SuperMoist	220
Sour cream white / **Betty Crocker** SuperMoist	180
Spice	
Betty Crocker SuperMoist	260
Betty Crocker SuperMoist, no cholesterol	220
Duncan Hines	260
Duncan Hines, no cholesterol	250
Fearn / ⅙ cake / mix dry	140
Strawberry **Pillsbury** Plus	250
Strawberry / prepared w egg whites / **Pillsbury** Plus	190
Strawberry supreme / **Duncan Hines**	260
Strawberry supreme / no cholesterol / **Duncan Hines**	250
Streusel	
Apple / **Betty Crocker** MicroRave / ⅙ cake	240
Apple / **Betty Crocker** MicroRave / ⅙ cake, no cholesterol	210
Blueberry / **Pillsbury**	260
Blueberry / **Pillsbury**, prepared w egg whites	250
Cinnamon / **Pillsbury**	260
Cinnamon / **Pillsbury**, prepared w egg whites	250

CALORIES

Cinnamon pecan / **Betty Crocker** MicroRave / ⅙
  cake   280
Cinnamon pecan / **Betty Crocker** MicroRave / ⅙
  cake, no cholesterol   230
Lemon / **Pillsbury**   260
Lemon / **Pillsbury**, prepared w egg whites   250
Swiss chocolate / **Duncan Hines**   280
Swiss chocolate / no cholesterol / **Duncan Hines**   270
Vanilla / **Pillsbury** Plus   260
Vanilla / prepared w egg whites / **Pillsbury** Plus   190
White
  Betty Crocker SuperMoist   240
  Betty Crocker SuperMoist, no cholesterol   220
  Betty Crocker SuperMoist Light   180
  Duncan Hines   250
  Duncan Hines, no cholesterol   240
  Mrs. Wright's   180
  Pillsbury   180
  Pillsbury, prepared w egg whites   170
  Pillsbury Plus   220
  Pillsbury Plus, prepared w egg whites   190
Yellow
  Betty Crocker SuperMoist   260
  Betty Crocker SuperMoist, no cholesterol   220
  Betty Crocker SueprMoist Light   200
  Betty Crocker SuperMoist Light, no cholesterol   180
  Duncan Hines   260
  Duncan Hines, no cholesterol   250
  Mrs. Wright's   190
  Pillsbury   180
  Pillsbury, prepared w egg whites   170
  Pillsbury Plus   260
  Pillsbury Plus, prepared w egg whites   190
Yellow w chocolate frosting / ⅙ cake / **Betty Crocker**
  MicroRave   300
Yellow w chocolate frosting / no cholesterol / ⅙ cake /
  Betty Crocker MicroRave   230
Yellow w hot fudge frosting / 1 serv / **Betty Crocker**
  MicroRave Singles   440

SNACK CAKES

1 piece unless noted

Banana dream / **Dolly Madison**	340
Banana flips / **Aunt Fanny's**	300
Brownie / **Dolly Madison**	330
Brownie / **Tastykake**	340
Butter streusel / **Dolly Madison**	150
Carrot cake / **Dolly Madison**	400
Chip Tops snack bar / **Dolly Madison**	460
Cinnamon swirl / **Dolly Madison**	170
Creamie, banana / **Tastykake**	170
Creamie, chocolate / **Tastykake**	170
Creamie, vanilla / **Tastykake**	180
Creme boats / **Dolly Madison**	160
Cupcakes	
Buttercream, cream-filled / **Tastykake**	120
Chocolate / **Dolly Madison**	170
Chocolate / **Tastykake**	100
Chocolate, cream-filled / **Tastykake**	120
Chocolate, cream-filled / **Tastykake** Tastylite	100
Chocolate royale / **Tastykake**	170
Orange / **Aunt Fanny's**	334
Vanilla, cream-filled / **Tastykake** Tastylite	100
Dessert cups / **Dolly Madison**	100
Dessert roll / **Dolly Madison**	220
Dipsie, cream-filled / **Aunt Fanny's**	230
Dutch apple / **Dolly Madison**	170
Fingers	
Devil's food / **Aunt Fanny's**	288
Raspberry / **Aunt Fanny's**	303
Spice / **Aunt Fanny's**	290
Vanilla / **Aunt Fanny's**	301
Frosty angel / **Dolly Madison**	310
Fudge nut brownie / **Frito-Lay**	360
Honey 'n spice / **Dolly Madison**	360
Junior	
Chocolate / **Tastykake**	340
Coconut / **Tastykake**	300

CALORIES

Koffee Kake / **Tastykake**	260
Orange / **Tastykake**	340
Lemon / **Tastykake**	310
Kandy Kake	
Chocolate / **Tastykake**	80
Coconut / **Tastykake**	80
Peanut butter / **Tastykake**	90
Koffee Kake, cream-filled / **Tastykake**	110
Kreme Kup / **Tastykake**	90
Krimpet	
Butterscotch / **Tastykake**	100
Jelly / **Tastykake**	90
Strawberry / **Tastykake**	100
Vanilla, cream-filled / **Tastykake**	120
Peanut butter bar / **Frito-Lay**	270
Pound cake mini / **Dolly Madison**	300
Snack squares / **Dolly Madison**	200
Strudels, apple / **Aunt Fanny's**	315
Strudels, cherry / **Aunt Fanny's**	288
Twirls, coconut / **Aunt Fanny's**	na
Twirls, pecan / **Aunt Fanny's**	226
White Koo Koo / **Dolly Madison**	180
Zingers	
Creme / **Dolly Madison**	110
Devil's food / **Dolly Madison**	140
Raspberry / **Dolly Madison**	160
Yellow / **Dolly Madison**	140

Candy

CALORIES

Almond Joy bar / 1.76 oz	250
Baby Ruth / 2.2 oz / **Nestlé**	300
Bar None / bar / 1.5 oz	240
Bit-O-Honey / 1.7 oz / **Nestlé**	200
Bounty / dark chocolate bar / 1 oz	140

CALORIES

Bounty / milk chocolate bar / 1 oz	140
Breath candy / 1 piece	
Certs Clear	8
Certs Mini Mints Sugar Free	1
Certs Pressed	6
Certs Sugar Free	7
Clorets Mini Mints	2
Clorets Mints Clear	8
Clorets Mints Pressed	6
Butter mints / 1 piece / **Kraft**	8
Butterfinger / 2.1 oz / **Nestlé**	280
Caramel Nip / 1 oz / **Pearson**	120
Caramels / 1 piece / **Kraft**	30
Charleston Chew / 1 oz	120
Choclairs / 1 piece	200
Chocolate bars	
Golden Almond / 1.5 oz	240
Hershey's / 1.55 oz	240
Hershey's Special Dark / 1.45 oz	220
Hershey's Symphony / 1.4 oz	220
Nestlé / 1.45 oz	220
Chocolate bars w almonds / 1.45 oz / **Hershey's**	230
Chocolate bars w almonds / 1.45 oz. / **Nestlé**	220
Chocolate bars w almonds and toffee chips / 1.4 oz /	
Hershey's Symphony	220
Chocolate-covered nuts and fruit	
Golden Almond Solitaires / ½ bag	240
Harmony Maltballs / 1 oz	140
Peanuts / 1 oz / **Harmony**	150
Peanuts / 1-⅜ oz / **Nestlé** Goobers	200
Raisins / 1 oz / **Harmony**	110
Raisins / 1-⅜ oz / **Nestlé** Raisinets	180
Chocolate fudgies / 1 piece / **Kraft**	35
Chocolate Mint Nip / 1 oz / **Pearson**	120
Chocolate parfait / 1 oz / **Pearson**	120
Chunky / 1.4 oz / **Nestlé**	170
Coffee Nip / 1 oz / **Pearson**	120
Crunch / 1.4 oz / **Nestlé**	200
Fifth Avenue bar / 2 oz / **Fifth Avenue**	280
Fruit 'n Nut Mix / 1 oz / **Planters**	150
Grand bar / 1.5 oz / **Nestlé**	200

	CALORIES
Gummy bears / 1 oz / **Harmony**	80
Junior Mints / 12 pieces / **Life Savers**	120
Kisses / 9 pieces / **Hershey's**	220
Kisses w almonds / 6 pieces / **Hershey's**	160
Kit Kat bar / 1.5 oz	230
Krackel bar / 1.45 oz	220
Kudos / 1.30 oz	200
Laffy Taffy / 1 oz /**Beich**	
Banana flavor	120
Fruit punch flavor	120
Sour apple flavor	110
Sour cherry flavor	110
Sour grape flavor	110
Strawberry flavor	110
Vanilla flavor	110
Watermelon flavor	110
Licorice Nip / 1 oz / **Pearson**	120
M & M's, holidays chocolate candy / 1 oz	140
M & M's, peanut / 1.74 oz	250
M & M's, peanut butter chocolate / 1.63 oz	240
M & M's, plain / 1.69 oz	230
Mars Almond Bar / 1.76 oz	240
Marshmallows	
Campfire / 2 large or 24 mini	40
Kraft Funmallows / 1 piece	30
Kraft Jet Puffed / 1 piece	25
Marshmallows, miniature	
Kraft / 10 pieces	18
Kraft Funmallows / 10 pieces	18
Milky Way bar / 2.15 oz	280
Milky Way dark bar / 1.76 oz	220
Mounds bar / 1.9 oz	260
Mr. Goodbar bar / 1.65 oz	260
Munch bar 1.42 oz	220
Oh Henry / 2 oz / **Nestlé**	250
Original Peanut Bar / 1 bar / **Planters**	230
Party mints / 1 piece / **Kraft**	8
PB Max real peanut butter bars / 1.48 oz	240
Peanut brittle / 1 oz / **Kraft**	130
Peanut butter parfait / 1 oz / **Pearson**	120
Peanut candy / 1 oz / **Planters**	140

Pom Poms / ½ box	100
Reese's peanut butter cups, crunchy / 1.8 oz	280
Reese's peanut butter cups, plain / 1.6 oz	250
Reese's Pieces / 1.75 oz	240
Rolo / 8 pieces	270
Skittles bite size / 2.30 oz	270
Skor bar / 1.4 oz	220
Snickers bar / 2.07 oz	280
Snickers peanut butter bar / 1.76 oz	280
Sno Caps / 1 oz / **Nestlé**	140
Starburst fruit chews / 2.07 oz	240
Sugar Babies / 1 pkg	180
Sugar Daddy / 1 pop	150
Thin mints / 1 piece / **Nestlé** Rowntree	35
Three Musketeers bar / 2.13 oz	260
Turtles / 1 piece / **Demet**	90
Twix bar / 1 oz	140
Whatchamacallit bar / 1.7 oz	250
White bar / 1.25 oz / **Nestlé**	200
Y&S Cherry Nibs / 1.0 oz	100
Y&S Twizzlers / strawberry / 1.0 oz	100
Y&S Twizzlers Bites / cherry / 1.0 oz	100
York peppermint pattie / 1.5 oz	180

DIETETIC CANDY

Caramels / 1 piece / **Estee**	30
Chocolate coconut bar / 2 squares / **Estee**	60
Chocolate cream-filled wafers / 1 wafer / **Estee**	20
Chocolate milk almond bar / 2 squares / **Estee**	60
Chocolate milk crunch bar / 2 squares / **Estee**	45
Chocolate milk deluxe dark bar / 2 squares / **Estee**	60
Chocolate milk fruit and nut bar / 2 squares / **Estee**	60
Chocolate mint bar / 2 squares / **Estee**	60
Fruit nut mix / .25 oz / **Estee**	40
Gum drops / 4 pieces / **Estee**	25
Lollipops / 1 pop / **Estee**	25
Mint coolers / 2 pieces / **Estee**	25
Peanut brittle / .25 oz / **Estee**	35
Peanut butter cups / 1 piece / **Estee**	40

CALORIES

Tropical mix / 2 pieces / **Estee**	25
Vanilla cream-filled wafers / 1 wafer / **Estee**	20

Cereals

COLD

CALORIES

1 oz unless noted

Addam's Family / **Ralston Purina**	110
All-Bran / **Kellogg's**	70
All-Bran w extra fiber / **Kellogg's**	50
Almond raisin / **Kellogg's** Nutri-Grain	140
Alpha-Bits / **Post**	110
Amaranth Crunch w raisins / **Health Valley**	100
Amaranth w bananas / **Health Valley**	110
Apple Almond Muesli / ½ cup / **Ralston Purina**	150
Apple Cinnamon Squares / **Kellogg's**	90
Apple Corns / **Arrowhead Mills**	100
Apple Jacks / **Kellogg's**	110
Apple Raisin Crisp / **Kellogg's**	130
Arrowhead Crunch / **Arrowhead Mills**	120
Basic 4 / 1.3 oz / **General Mills**	130
Bill & Ted's / **Ralston Purina**	110
Blueberry Squares / **Kellogg's**	90
Body Buddies Natural Fruit / **General Mills**	110
Booberry / **General Mills**	110
Bran / **Health Valley**	90
Bran, 100% / **Nabisco**	70
Bran Buds / **Kellogg's**	70
Bran flakes	
Arrowhead Mills	100
Kellogg's	90
Malt-O-Meal	90
Bran w apples and cinnamon / **Health Valley**	90
Bran w raisin / **Health Valley** 100% Organic	90

CALORIES

Brown crisp rice / **Health Valley** 100% Organic	90
Brown rice, puffed / ½ cup / **Health Valley**	50
C. W. Post / **Post**	130
Cap'n Crunch / ¾ cup / **Quaker**	113
Cap'n Crunch Peanut Butter / ¾ cup / **Quaker**	119
Cap'n Crunch's Crunchberries / ¾ cup / **Quaker**	113
Cheerios Apple Cinnamon / **General Mills**	110
Cheerios Honey Nut / **General Mills**	110
Cheerios / **General Mills**	110
Cinnamon and Raisin / **Nature Valley**	120
Cinnamon Life / ⅔ cup / **Quaker**	101
Cinnamon mini buns / **Kellogg's**	110
Cinnamon Toast Crunch / **General Mills**	120
Clusters / **General Mills**	110
Cocoa Krispies / **Kellogg's**	110
Cocoa Pebbles / **Post**	110
Cocoa Puffs / **General Mills**	110
Cookie-Crisp Chocolate Chip / **Ralston Purina**	110
Corn Chex / **Ralston Purina**	110
Corn flakes	
Arrowhead Mills	110
Country Corn Flakes	110
Health Valley 100% Organic	90
Kellogg's	100
Malt-O-Meal	110
Post Toasties	110
Total	110
Corn flakes / apple cinnamon / **Wonder Ralston Purina**	110
Corn Pops / **Kellogg's**	110
Corn, puffed / .5 oz / **Arrowhead Mills**	50
Corn, puffed / ½ cup / **Health Valley**	50
Count Chocula / **General Mills**	110
Cracklin' Oat Bran / **Kellogg's**	110
Cranberry Walnut Muesli / ½ cup / **Ralston Purina**	150
Crispix / **Kellogg's**	110
Crispy Rice / **Malt-O-Meal**	110
Crispy Wheats 'N Raisin / **General Mills**	100
Crunchy Nut Ohs / 1 cup / **Quaker**	127
Date Almond Muesli / ½ cup / **Ralston Purina**	140
Double Dip Crunch / **Kellogg's**	120
Fiber One / **General Mills**	60

CALORIES

Fiber Seven Flakes / **Health Valley** 100% Organic	90
Fiber Seven Flakes w raisins / **Health Valley** 100% Organic	90
Fiberwise / **Kellogg's**	90
Frankenberry / **General Mills**	110
Froot Loops / **Kellogg's**	110
Frosted Flakes / **Kellogg's**	110
Frosted Krispies / **Kellogg's**	110
Frosted Mini-Wheats / **Kellogg's**	100
Frosted Mini-Wheats, bite size / **Kellogg's**	100
Fruit & Fibre / 1.25 oz / **Post**	
Dates	120
Peaches	120
Tropical	120
Fruit and Fitness / 2 oz / **Health Valley**	220
Fruit and Nut / **Nature Valley**	130
Fruit Lites / ½ cup / **Health Valley**	45
Fruit Wheats, apple / **Nabisco**	90
Fruitful Bran / **Kellogg's**	120
Fruity Marshmallow Krispies / **Kellogg's**	140
Fruity Pebbles / **Post**	110
Fruity Yummy Mummy / **General Mills**	110
Golden Grahams / **General Mills**	110
Graham oat rings / **Wonder Ralston Purina**	110
Granola / **Health Valley** Fat Free	90
Granola, maple nut / **Arrowhead Mills**	250
Granola w almonds / ¼ cup / **Sun Country Quaker**	130
Granola w raisins / ¼ cup / **Sun Country Quaker**	125
Granola w raisins and dates / ¼ cup / **Sun Country Quaker**	123
Grape-Nuts / **Post**	110
Grape-Nuts Flakes / **Post**	100
Grape-Nuts, raisin / **Post**	100
Healthy Crunch almond date / **Health Valley**	90
Healthy Crunch apple cinnamon / **Health Valley**	90
Healthy O's / **Health Valley**	90
Heartland, plain / ¼ cup	130
Heartland, raisin / ¼ cup	130
Honey Almond Delight / **Ralston Purina**	110
Honey and Nut / **Malt-O-Meal**	110
Honey bran / **Kellogg's** Oatbake	110

CALORIES

Honey Bunches of Oats, honey-roasted / **Post**	110
Honey Bunches of Oats w almonds / **Post**	120
Honey Graham Ohs / 1 cup / **Quaker**	122
Honey Nut Crispy Rice / **Wonder Ralston Purina**	110
Honeycomb / **Post**	110
I Love Double Chex / **Ralston Purina**	100
Jetsons / **Ralston Purina**	110
Just Right w fiber / **Kellogg's**	100
Just Right w raisins, dates and nuts / **Kellogg's**	140
Kaboom / **General Mills**	110
Kenmei Rice Bran / **Kellogg's**	110
King Vitamin / 1-½ cups / **Quaker**	110
Kix / **General Mills**	110
Life / ⅔ cup / **Quaker**	101
Lucky Charms / **General Mills**	110
Maple Corns / **Arrowhead Mills**	100
Millet, puffed / .5 oz / **Arrowhead Mills**	50
Mueslix Crispy Blend / **Kellogg's**	160
Mueslix Golden Crunch / **Kellogg's**	120
Multi Bran Chex / **Ralston Purina**	90
Natural Bran Flakes / **Post**	90
Nature O's / **Arrowhead Mills**	110
Nut and Honey Crunch / **Kellogg's**	110
Nut and Honey Crunch O's / **Kellogg's**	110
Oat bran / **Kellogg's** Common Sense	100
Oat bran / ¾ cup / **Quaker**	100
Oat bran flakes / **Arrowhead Mills**	110
Oat Bran Flakes / **Health Valley** 100% Organic	90
Oat Bran Flakes w almonds and dates / **Health Valley**	90
Oat Bran Flakes w raisins / **Health Valley** 100% Organic	90
Oat Bran O's / **Health Valley**	110
Oat Bran O's / **Health Valley** 100% Organic	90
Oat Bran w raisins / **Kellogg's** Common Sense	130
Oat Flakes / **Post**	110
Oatmeal Crisp / **General Mills**	110
Oatmeal Raisin Crisp / **General Mills**	130
Orangeola w almonds and dates / **Health Valley**	90
Orangeola w bananas and fruit / **Health Valley**	90
Organic Amaranth Flakes / **Health Valley**	90
Peach Pecan Muesli / ½ cup / **Ralston Purina**	150
Popeye Sweet Crunch / 1 cup / **Quaker**	113

Prince of Thieves / **Ralston Purina**	110
Product 19 / **Kellogg's**	100
Puffed rice / **Malt-O-Meal**	50
Puffed wheat / **Malt-O-Meal**	50
Quaker 100% Natural / ¼ cup / **Quaker**	127
Quaker 100% Natural Raisin & Date / ¼ cup / **Quaker**	123
Quaker 100% Natural w apples & cinnamon / ¼ cup / **Quaker**	126
Quaker Crunchy Bran / ⅔ cup / **Quaker**	89
Quaker Oat Squares / ½ cup / **Quaker**	105
Raisin bran	
Kellogg's	120
Kellogg's Nutri Grain	130
Post / 1.4 oz	120
Total	140
Raisin Bran Flakes / **Health Valley** 100% Organic	90
Raisin Bran Flakes / 1.4 oz / **Malt-O-Meal**	130
Raisin Nut / **Kellogg's** Oatbake	110
Raisin Nut Bran / **General Mills**	110
Raisin Squares / **Kellogg's**	90
Raspberry Almond Muesli / ½ cup / **Ralston Purina**	150
Real Almond Crunch / **Health Valley**	90
Real Hawaiian Fruit / **Health Valley**	100
Real Raisin / **Health Valley**	100
Rice bran w almonds and dates / **Health Valley**	110
Rice Chex / **Ralston Purina**	110
Rice Chex, Frosted / **Ralston Purina**	110
Rice Krispies / **Kellogg's**	110
Rice, puffed / .5 oz / **Arrowhead Mills**	50
Rice, puffed / 1 cup / **Quaker**	54
S'Mores Grahams / **General Mills**	120
Shredded Wheat / 1 biscuit / **Nabisco**	80
Shredded Wheat, spoon size / **Nabisco**	90
Shredded Wheat 'n Bran / **Nabisco**	90
Shredded Wheat w Oat Bran / **Nabisco**	100
Slimer And The Real Ghostbusters / **Ralston Purina**	110
Smacks / **Kellogg's**	110
Smurf Magic Berries / **Post**	120
Special K / **Kellogg's**	110
Sprouts Seven w bananas and fruit / **Health Valley**	90
Sprouts Seven w raisins / **Health Valley** 100% Organic	90

CALORIES

Strawberry Squares / **Kellogg's**	90
Sugar Frosted Flakes / **Malt-O-Meal**	110
Sugar Puffs / **Malt-O-Meal**	110
Sunflakes Multi Grain / **Ralston Purina**	100
Super Golden Crisp / **Post**	110
Swiss Breakfast, raisin / **Health Valley**	80
Swiss Breakfast, tropical fruit / **Health Valley**	80
Team Flakes / **Nabisco**	110
Teenage Mutant Ninja Turtles / **Ralston Purina**	110
Toasted Oat / **Nature Valley**	130
Toasty O's / **Malt-O-Meal**	110
Tootic Fruities / **Malt-O-Meal**	110
Total / **General Mills**	100
Triples / **General Mills**	110
Trix / **General Mills**	110
Wheat / **Kellogg's Nutri Grain**	90
Wheat bran / 2 oz / **Arrowhead Mills**	50
Wheat Chex, whole grain / **Ralston Purina**	100
Wheat flakes / **Arrowhead Mills**	110
Wheat, puffed	
Arrowhead Mills / .5 oz	50
Health Valley / ½ cup	50
Quaker / 1 cup	50
Wheat, shredded / 2 biscuits / **Quaker**	132
Wheaties / **General Mills**	100
Whole grain shredded wheat / **Kellogg's**	90

TO BE COOKED

Dry, uncooked, unless noted

Barley, pearled / ¼ cup / **Quaker** Scotch Brand Medium	172
Barley, pearled / ⅓ cup / **Quaker** Scotch Brand Quick	172
Bear Mush / 1 oz / **Arrowhead Mills**	100
Cracked wheat / 2 oz / **Arrowhead Mills**	180
Cream of Rice / 1 oz / **Nabisco**	100
Cream of Wheat	
Nabisco Instant / 1 oz	100
Nabisco Quick / 1 oz	100
Nabisco Regular / 1 oz	100
Cream of Wheat, apple and cinnamon / 1 oz / **Nabisco**	
Mix'n Eat	130

CALORIES

Cream of Wheat, brown sugar cinnamon / 1 oz / **Nabisco** Mix'n Eat	130
Cream of Wheat, maple brown sugar / 1 oz / **Nabisco** Mix'n Eat	130
Cream of Wheat, original / 1 oz / **Nabisco** Mix'n Eat	100
Farina / 1 oz / **Highspire**	100
Farina / ⅓ cup prepared / **Pillsbury**	80
Four grain cereal / 2 oz / **Arrowhead Mills**	94
Grits	
Corn, white / 2 oz / **Arrowhead Mills**	200
Corn, yellow / 2 oz / **Arrowhead Mills**	200
Hominy, white / 3 tbsp / **Aunt Jemima** Quick	101
Hominy, white / 3 tbsp / **Aunt Jemima** Regular	101
Hominy, white / 3 tbsp / **Quaker** Quick	101
Hominy, white / 3 tbsp / **Quaker** Regular	101
Hominy, yellow / 3 tbsp / **Quaker** Quick	101
Instant / 1 packet / **Quaker** Instant Grits Product	79
Instant w imitation bacon bits / 1 packet / **Quaker** Instant Grits Product	101
Instant w imitation ham bits / 1 packet / **Quaker** Instant Grits Product	99
Instant w real cheddar cheese flavor / 1 packet / **Quaker** Instant Grits Product	104
Malt-O-Meal, chocolate / 1 oz	100
Malt-O-Meal, oat bran / 1.3 oz	130
Malt-O-Meal, quick / 1 oz	100
Maltex / 1 oz / **Highspire**	105
Maypo 30 seconds / 1 oz / **Highspire**	100
Maypo Vermont style / 1 oz / **Highspire**	105
Oat bran	
Arrowhead Mills / 1 oz	110
Mother's / ⅔ cup cooked	92
Quaker / ⅔ cup cooked	92
Oat bran w apples and cinnamon / 1 oz / **Health Valley**	100
Oat bran w raisins and spice / 1 oz / **Health Valley**	100
Oatmeal, instant	
Arrowhead Mills Regular / 1 oz	100
Quaker Extra Fortified, regular flavor / 1 packet	95
Quaker Extra Fortified, raisins & cinnamon / 1 packet	129
Quaker Regular / 1 packet	94

CALORIES

w apple, date and almond / **Arrowhead Mills** / 1 oz	130
w apple spice / **Arrowhead Mills** / 1 oz	130
w apples and cinnamon / **Quaker** / 1 packet	118
w cinnamon and spice / **Quaker** / 1 packet	164
w cinnamon, raisin and almond / **Arrowhead Mills** / 1 oz	140
w maple and brown sugar / **Quaker** / 1 packet	152
w peaches and cream / **Quaker** / 1 packet	129
w raisins and spice / **Quaker** / 1 packet	149
w raisins, dates and walnuts / **Quaker** / 1 packet	141
w strawberries and cream / **Quaker** / 1 packet	129
Oats and oatmeal	
Arrowhead Mills steel cut / 1 oz	220
Quaker Old Fashioned / ⅔ cup cooked	99
Quaker Quick / ⅔ cup cooked	99
Ralston High Fiber / 1 oz / **Ralston Purina**	90
Rice and Shine / .25 oz / **Arrowhead Mills**	160
Seven grain cereal / 1 oz / **Arrowhead Mills**	100
Wheatena / 1 oz / **Highspire**	100
Whole wheat / ⅔ cup cooked / **Mother's**	92
Whole wheat / ⅔ cup cooked / **Quaker**	92

Cheese

CALORIES

Non-brand name

1 oz unless noted

American, pasteurized process	105
American, pasteurized process food	95
American, pasteurized process spread	80
Blue	100
Brick	105
Brie	95
Camembert / 1.3 oz	115
Caraway	107

CALORIES

Cheddar	115
Cheshire	110
Colby	112
Cottage, cream, large curd w 4% fat / ½ cup	118
Cottage, cream, small curd w 4% fat / ½ cup	108
Cottage, cream, lowfat 2% / ½ cup	103
Cottage, dry / ½ cup	63
Cream	100
Edam	101
Feta	75
Fontina	110
Gjetost	132
Goat, hard	128
Goat, semi-soft	103
Goat, soft	76
Gouda	101
Limburger	93
Monterey jack	105
Mozzarella, part skim	80
Mozzarella substitute	70
Mozzarella, whole milk	80
Muenster	105
Neufchatel	74
Parmesan	130
Port de salut	100
Provolone	100
Ricotta, part skim / ½ cup	170
Ricotta, whole milk / ½ cup	215
Romano	110
Roquefort	105
Swiss	105
Swiss, pasteurized process	95
Tilsit	96

Brand name

1 oz unless noted

American
    Borden Slices   110
    Weight Watchers Slices / colored   50

CALORIES

Weight Watchers Low Sodium Slices / colored	50
Weight Watchers Low Sodium Slices / white	50
Weight Watchers Slices / white	50
Blue / **Kraft**	100
Brick / **Kraft**	110
Casino / **Kraft** Harvarti	120
Cheddar	
Kraft	110
Kraft Cracker Barrel Light / sharp	80
Kraft Light Naturals / mild	80
Kraft Light Naturals / sharp	80
Weight Watchers / mild	80
Weight Watchers Low Sodium / mild	80
Weight Watchers / sharp	80
Weight Watchers Cup / sharp	70
Weight Watchers Shredded / mild	80
Colby	
Kraft	110
Kraft Light Naturals	80
Weight Watchers	80
Edam / **Kraft**	90
Farmer / **Friendship** / 4 oz	160
Farmer / **Friendship** No Salt Added / 4 oz	160
Gouda / **Kraft**	110
Hoop / **Friendship** No Salt Added / 4 oz	84
Limburger / **Mohawk Valley** Little Gem Size	90
Monterey jack	
Kraft	110
Kraft Light Naturals	80
Weight Watchers	80
w caraway seeds / **Kraft**	100
w jalapeno peppers / **Kraft**	110
w peppers / **Kraft** Light Naturals	80
Mozzarella	
Kraft Light Naturals	80
Low moisture / **Kraft**	90
Low moisture, part-skim / **Kraft**	80
Low moisture, part-skim w jalapeno peppers / **Kraft** String Cheese	80
Weight Watchers	70
Weight Watchers Shredded	80

CALORIES

Parmesan / **Kraft**	100
Port wine / **Weight Watchers**	70
Provolone / **Kraft**	100
Romano / **Kraft**	100
Swiss	
Borden	100
Kraft	110
Kraft Aged	110
Kraft Casino	110
Kraft Cracker Barrel Natural Baby	110
Kraft Light Naturals	90
Kraft Low Sodium	110
Weight Watchers	90

COTTAGE CHEESE

Creamed	
Borden / ½ cup	120
Borden Unsalted / ½ cup	120
Breakstone's Small Curd / 4 oz	110
Friendship California Style / ½ cup	120
Knudsen Large Curd / 4 oz	120
Knudsen Small Curd / 4 oz	120
w pineapple / **Breakstone's** / 4 oz	140
w pineapple / **Friendship** / ½ cup	140
Dry / No salt added / **Breakstone's** / 4 oz	90
Dry curd / **Borden** / ½ cup	80
Low fat	
Breakstone's / 4 oz	100
Friendship Lactose Reduced / ½ cup	90
Friendship No Salt Added / ½ cup	90
Friendship Pot Style / ½ cup	100
Friendship Whipped / ½ cup	90
Knudsen / 4 oz	100
Light n' Lively / 4 oz	80
Light n' Lively Garden Salad / 4 oz	80
Lite-Line / ½ cup	90
Sealtest / 4 oz	100
Weight Watchers 1% / ½ cup	90
Weight Watchers 2% / ½ cup	100
w fruit cocktail / **Knudsen** / 4 oz	130

w mandarin orange / **Knudsen** / 4 oz	110
w peach / **Knudsen** / 6 oz	170
w peach and pineapple / **Light n' Lively** / 4 oz	100
w pear / **Knudsen** / 4 oz	110
w pineapple / **Friendship** / ½ cup	110
w pineapple / **Knudsen** / 6 oz	170
w spiced apple / **Knudsen** / 6 oz	180
w strawberry / **Knudsen** / 6 oz	170

Nonfat
Friendship / ½ cup	70
Knudsen / 4 oz	70
Light n' Lively / 4 oz	90

CREAM AND NEUFCHATEL

1 oz

Cream cheese
Kraft Philadelphia Brand	100
Kraft Philadelphia Brand, Light	60
Kraft Philadelphia Brand, soft	100
Weight Watchers	35
w chives / **Kraft** Philadelphia Brand	90
w chives and onions / **Kraft** Philadelphia Brand, soft	100
w herb and garlic / **Kraft** Philadelphia Brand, soft	100
w olives and pimento / **Kraft** Philadelphia Brand, soft	90
w pimento / **Kraft** Philadelphia Brand	90
w pineapple / **Kraft** Philadelphia Brand, soft	90
w smoked salmon / **Kraft** Philadelphia Brand, soft	90
w strawberries / **Kraft** Philadelphia Brand, soft	90

Cream cheese, whipped
Kraft Philadelphia Brand	100
Temp-Tee	100
w chives / **Kraft** Philadelphia Brand	90
w onions / **Kraft** Philadelphia Brand	90
w smoked salmon / **Kraft** Philadelphia Brand	90

Neufchatel / **Kraft** Philadelphia Brand, Light	80

GRATED AND SHREDDED

Colby and Monterey Jack / **Kraft** Light Naturals / 1 oz	80
Parmesan / **Kraft** / 1 oz	130
Parmesan / **Progresso** / 1 tbsp	23
Romano / **Kraft** / 1 oz	130
Romano / **Progresso** / 1 tbsp	23
Taco / **Kraft** / 1 oz	110

CHEESE FOODS

1 oz unless noted

American	
Borden Singles	90
Borden Light Singles cheese product	70
Kraft Grated	130
Kraft Light Singles process cheese product	70
Kraft Light Singles, white process cheese product	70
Kraft Loaf	110
Kraft Singles	90
Kraft Singles, white	90
Kraft Slices	110
Kraft Old English Slices, sharp	110
Lite-Line Singles cheese product	50
Lite-Line Reduced Sodium Singles cheese product	70
Lite-Line Sodium Lite Singles cheese product	70
American, flavored	
Kraft Light n' Lively Singles process cheese product	70
Kraft Light n' Lively Singles, white process cheese product	70
Kraft Golden Image imitation process	90
Ched-O-Mate / shredded cheese substitute / **Fisher**	90
Cheddar	
Medium / **Kraft** Spreadery process cheese product	70
Mild / **Kraft** Golden Image Imitation	110
Sharp / **Kraft** Cracker Barrel	100

CALORIES

Sharp / **Kraft** Light n' Lively Singles process cheese product	70
Sharp / **Kraft** Light Singles process cheese product	70
Sharp / **Kraft** Spreadery process cheese product	70
Sharp / **Weight Watchers** Slices	50
Sharp, extra / **Kraft** Cracker Barrel	90
Sharp w almonds / **Kraft** Cracker Barrel Cheese Ball	100
Smokey w almonds / **Kraft** Cracker Barrel Cheese Log	90
Vermont white / **Kraft** Spreadery process cheese product	70
Sharp w almonds / **Kraft** Cracker Barrel Cheese Log	90
Cheese 'n Bacon **Kraft** Singles	90
Cheeztwin Singles cheese substitute	90
Colby / **Kraft** Golden Image Imitation	110
Monterey Jack / **Kraft** Singles	90
Mozzarella-flavor / **Lite-Line** cheese product	50
Nacho / **Kraft** Spreadery process cheese product	70
Neufchatel	
w french onion / **Kraft** Spreadery process cheese product	70
w garden vegetables / **Kraft** Spreadery process cheese product	70
w garlic and herb / **Kraft** Spreadery process cheese product	70
w ranch flavor / **Kraft** Spreadery process cheese product	70
w strawberries / **Kraft** Spreadery process cheese product	70
Pimento / **Kraft** Singles	90
Pimento / **Kraft** Slices	100
Pizza-Mate / shredded mozzarella substitute/ **Fisher**	90
Port wine / **Kraft** Cracker Barrel	100
Port wine / **Kraft** Spreadery process cheese product	70
Port wine cheddar w almonds / **Kraft** Cracker Barrel Cheese Log	90
Process	
Nippy	90
w garlic / **Kraft**	90

CALORIES

w jalapeno peppers / **Kraft**	90
Process cheese food w real bacon / **Kraft** Cracker Barrel	90
Process cheese product / **Harvest Moon**	70
Process cheese product / mild Mexican w jalapeno peppers / **Kraft** Spreadery	70
Process cheese substitute / **Lite-Line** Singles	90
Sandwich slices / **Kraft** Lunch Wagon	90
Sandwich-Mate cheese substitute / **Fisher** Singles	90
Sharp / **Kraft** Old English Loaf	110
Sharp / **Kraft** Singles	100
Sharp, cheddar flavor / **Lite-Line** cheese product	50
Swiss	
Kraft Singles	90
Kraft Slices	90
Weight Watchers Slices	50
Swiss flavor **Kraft** Light Singles process cheese product	70
Swiss flavor cheese product / **Lite-Line**	50
Swiss flavored / **Kraft** Light n' Lively Singles process cheese product	70
Velveeta / **Kraft** Light Singles process cheese product	70

CHEESE SPREADS

1 oz

American / **Kraft**	80
Blue / **Kraft** Roka	70
Cheez Whiz	80
Garlic flavor / **Kraft** Squeez-A-Snack	80
Hickory smoke flavor / **Kraft** Squeez-A-Snack	80
Jalapeno / **Kraft** Loaf	80
Jalapeno pepper / **Kraft**	70
Limburger / **Mohawk Valley**	70
Mexican, mild / **Cheez Whiz**	80
Olives and pimento / **Kraft**	60
Pimento / **Kraft**	70
Pineapple / **Kraft**	70
Sharp / **Kraft** Old English	80
Sharp / **Kraft** Squeez-A-Snack	80
Kraft	80
Kraft Shredded	100

CALORIES

Kraft Slices	90
Mexican hot / **Kraft**	80
Mexican mild / **Kraft**	80
Pimento / **Kraft**	80
Velveeta	
w bacon / **Kraft**	80
w bacon / **Kraft** Squeez-A-Snack	80
w jalapeno pepper / **Kraft** Hot Mexican Shredded	100
w jalapeno pepper / **Kraft** Mild Mexican Shredded	100
w jalapeno pepper / **Kraft** Squeez-A-Snack	80
w jalapeno pepper / **Cheez Whiz**	80

Chewing Gum

CALORIES

1 stick or piece

Big Red / **Wrigley's**	10
Bubble Gum / Classic / **Wrigley's** Extra Sugarfree	6
Bubble Gum / Original / **Wrigley's** Extra Sugarfree	7
Bubblicious	25
Chewels	8
Chiclets	6
Cinnamon / **Wrigley's** Extra Sugarfree	8
Clorets	6
Clorets Stick	9
Crystal Sugarless	5
Dentyne	6
Dentyne Cinn-A-Burst	9
Dentyne Sugar Free	5
Doublemint / **Wrigley's**	10
Freedent / all flavors / **Wrigley's**	10
Freshen-Up	13
Juicy Fruit / **Wrigley's**	10
Peppermint / **Wrigley's** Extra Sugarfree	8
Spearmint / **Wrigley's**	10
Spearmint / **Wrigley's** Extra Sugarfree	8

CALORIES

Trident Slab	5
Trident Soft Bubble Gum	9
Winter Fresh / **Wrigley's** Extra Sugarfree	8

Chinese Foods

CALORIES

Bamboo shoots / canned / ¼ cup / **La Choy**	6
Bean sprouts / canned / ⅔ cup / **La Choy**	8
Beef Oriental w vegetables and rice / frozen / 8-⅝ oz / **Stouffer's** Lean Cuisine Entree	290
Beef pepper / canned / ¾ cup / **La Choy** Bi-Pack	80
Beef pepper / canned / ¾ cup / **La Choy** Oriental	100
Beef pepper Oriental / frozen / 13 oz / **Chun King** Entree	310
Chicken	
Crunchy walnut / frozen / 13 oz / **Chun King** Entree	310
Imperial / frozen / 13 oz / **Chun King** Entree	300
Oriental / frozen / 10 oz / **Armour** Classics Lite	180
Chicken cashew in sauce w rice / frozen / 9.5 oz / **Stouffer's**	380
Chicken teriyaki / canned / ¾ cup / **La Choy**	90
Chicken teriyaki / canned / ¾ cup / **La Choy** Bi-Pack	85
Chop suey beef / frozen / 12 oz / **Stouffer's**	300
Chop suey vegetables / canned / ½ cup / **La Choy**	8
Chow mein	
Beef / canned / ¾ cup / **La Choy**	50
Beef / canned / ¾ cup / **La Choy** Bi-Pack	70
Chicken / canned / ¾ cup / **La Choy**	80
Chicken / canned / ¾ cup / **La Choy** Bi-Pack	80
Chicken / frozen / 13 oz / **Chun King** Entree	370
Chicken / frozen / 8.50 oz / **Healthy Choice** Entrees	220
Chicken / frozen / ½ package / **La Choy**	300
Chicken / frozen / 8 oz / **Stouffer's**	130
Chicken / frozen / 12 oz / **Ultra Slim-Fast** Entrees	320
Meatless / canned / ¾ cup / **La Choy**	25
Pork / canned / ¾ cup / **La Choy** Bi-Pack	80

	CALORIES
Shrimp / canned / ¾ cup / **La Choy**	35
Shrimp / canned / ¾ cup / **La Choy** Bi-Pack	70
Egg foo young / mix prepared / 2 pieces / **La Choy** Dinner Classics	170

Egg rolls

Almond chicken / frozen / 3 oz / **La Choy**	120
Chicken / frozen / 3.60 oz / **Chun King**	220
Chicken / frozen / 1.45 oz / **La Choy**	90
Chicken / frozen / 3 oz / **La Choy**	150
Lobster / frozen / 1.45 oz / **La Choy**	75
Meat and shrimp / frozen / 3.60 oz / **Chun King**	220
Meat and shrimp / frozen / 1.45 oz / **La Choy**	80
Pork / frozen / 3 oz / **Chun King** Restaurant Style	180
Pork / frozen / 3 oz / **La Choy** Restaurant Style	150
Shrimp / frozen / 3.60 oz / **Chun King**	200
Shrimp / frozen / 1.45 oz / **La Choy**	75
Shrimp / frozen / 3 oz / **La Choy** Restaurant Style	150
Fortune cookies / boxed / 1 piece / **La Choy**	15
Fried rice w chicken / frozen / 8 oz / **Chun King** Side Dishes	260
Fried rice w pork / frozen / 8 oz / **Chun King** Side Dishes	270

Noodles

Chow mein / canned / 1.5 oz / **China Boy** Thin	200
Chow mein / canned / 1.5 oz / **China Boy** Wide	200
Chow mein / canned / ½ cup / **La Choy**	150
Egg / canned / 2 oz / **Kame**	210
Lo mein, wide / canned / 2 oz / **Kame**	200
Ramen beef-flavored / canned / 1 cup / **La Choy**	225
Ramen chicken-flavored / canned / 1 cup / **La Choy**	200
Restaurant-style, wide / canned / ½ cup / **La Choy**	150
Rice / canned / ½ cup / **La Choy**	130
Rice sticks / canned / 2 oz / **Kame**	0
Pea pods / frozen / 1.50 oz / **Chun King**	20
Pepper steak / mix prepared / ¾ cup / **La Choy** Dinner Classics	180
Snow peas / frozen / 3 oz / **La Choy**	35

Sweet and sour

Chicken / canned / ¾ cup / **La Choy**	230
Chicken / mix prepared / ¾ cup / **La Choy**	310
Chicken / canned / ¾ cup / **La Choy** Bi-Pack	120
Chicken / frozen / 10.19 oz / **Weight Watchers**	240

CALORIES

Pork / frozen / 13 oz / **Chun King** Entree	400
Pork / canned / ¾ cup / **La Choy**	250
Vegetables, fancy mix / canned / ½ cup / **La Choy**	12
Water chestnuts, sliced / canned / ¼ cup / **La Choy**	18
Water chestnuts, whole / canned / 4 pieces / **La Choy**	14

Chips, Crisps, Bars and Similar Snacks

CALORIES

Breakfast bars: 1 bar unless noted	
Blueberry / **Kellogg's** Smart Start	180
Chocolate / **Carnation** Slender	135
Chocolate / **Figurines**	100
Chocolate caramel / **Figurines**	100
Chocolate chip / **Carnation** Breakfast Bar	200
Chocolate chip / **Carnation** Slender	135
Chocolate crunch / **Carnation** Breakfast Bar	190
Chocolate peanut butter / **Carnation** Slender	135
Chocolate peanut butter / **Figurines**	100
Corn flakes w berry / **Kellogg's** Smart Start	170
Oat bran w raspberry / **Kellogg's** Smart Start	170
Peanut butter crunch / **Carnation** Breakfast Bar	190
Peanut butter w chocolate chips / **Carnation** Breakfast Bar	200
Raisin bran / **Kellogg's** Smart Start	160
Rice Krispies w almonds / **Kellogg's** Smart Start	130
S'mores / **Figurines**	100
Strawberry / **Kellogg's** Smart Start	180
Vanilla / **Carnation** Slender	135
Vanilla / **Figurines**	100
Granola bars: 1 bar	
Blueberry apple / **Health Valley**	140
Caramel nut / **Quaker** Dipps	148
Chocolate chip / **Quaker** Chewy	128

CALORIES

Chocolate chip / **Quaker** Dipps	139
Chocolate fudge / **Quaker** Dipps	160
Cinnamon / **Nature Valley**	120
Date almond flavor / **Health Valley**	140
Honey and oats / **Quaker** Chewy	125
Nut and raisin / **Quaker** Chewy	131
Oat Bran Honey Graham / **Nature Valley**	110
Oats and honey / **Nature Valley**	120
Peanut butter / **Nature Valley**	120
Peanut butter / **Quaker** Chewy	128
Peanut butter / **Quaker** Dipps	170
Peanut butter chocolate chip / **Quaker** Chewy	131
Peanut butter chocolate chip / **Quaker** Dipps	174
Raisin cinnamon / **Quaker** Chewy	128
Raspberry / **Health Valley**	140
Rice bran cinnamon graham / **Nature Valley**	90
S'mores / **Quaker** Chewy	126

1 oz unless noted

Snacks

Bugles / **General Mills**	150
Bugles Nacho Cheese / **General Mills**	160
Bugles Ranch Flavor / **General Mills**	150
Cheddar Valley / **Frito-Lay**	160
Chee•tos, crunch / **Frito-Lay**	150
Chee•tos, curls / **Frito-Lay**	150
Chee•tos, light / **Frito-Lay**	140
Chee•tos, paws / **Frito-Lay**	160
Chee•tos, puffed balls / **Frito-Lay**	160
Chee•tos, puffs **Frito-Lay**	160
Cheez Doodles, puffed / **Wise**	150
Cheese Waffies / **Wise**	140
Cheez Balls / **Planters**	160
Cheez Balls, nacho / **Planters**	160
Cheez Curls, nacho / **Planters**	160
Cheez Curls / **Planters**	160
Cheez Doodles, crunchy / **Wise**	160
Chex Mix / **Ralston Purina**	120
Chex Mix, barbecue / **Ralston Purina**	130
Chex Mix, golden cheddar / **Ralston Purina**	130

CALORIES

Chex Mix, sour cream and onion / **Ralston Purina**	130
Combos / 1.80 oz	240
Corn crunchies / **Wise**	160

Corn chips

Fritos Bar-B-Q	150
Fritos Chili Cheese	160
Fritos Crisp 'n Thin	160
Fritos Dip Size	150
Fritos Nacho Cheese	150
Fritos Original	150
Fritos Wild 'n Mild	160
Planters	160
Wise	160
Pringles Fresh Roasted	140
Pringles Nacho Cheese	140
Pringles White Popcorn	140

Corn snackers, lightly salted / .5 oz / **Weight Watchers**	60
Corn snackers / nacho cheese flavor / .5 oz / **Weight Watchers**	60
Corn Spirals, nacho / **Wise**	160
Corn Spirals, toasted / **Wise**	160

Crunch Tators

Lay's Amazin' Cajun	150
Lay's Hoppin' Jalapeno	140
Lay's Mighty Mesquite	150
Lay's Original	150
Lay's Supreme Sour Cream	150

Onion-flavored rings / **Funyuns**	140
Pork skins, fried / **Baken-ets**	160
Pork skins, fried / **Baken-ets** Hot'n Spicy	150

Potato chips

Cottage Fries, No Salt Added	160
Lay's Bar-B-Q	150
Lay's Cheddar Cheese	150
Lay's Flamin' Hot	150
Lay's Kansas City Bar-B-Q	150
Lay's Original	150
Lay's Ranch	160
Lay's Salt & Vinegar	150
Lay's Sour Cream & Onion	160
Lay's Unsalted	150

CALORIES

Munchos	160
New York Deli	160
Pringles Cheez Ums	170
Pringles Crisps	160
Pringles Crisps Cheez Ums	160
Pringles Crisps, Sour Cream 'n Onion	160
Pringles Idaho Rippled	170
Pringles Idaho Rippled BBQ	170
Pringles Idaho Rippled Cheddar 'n Sour Cream	170
Pringles Light	150
Pringles Light, BBQ	150
Pringles Light Crisps / .9 oz	130
Pringles Light Crisps, BBQ / .9 oz	130
Pringles Light Crisps, cheddar / .9 oz	130
Pringles Light Crisps, ranch / .9 oz	130
Pringles Light, ranch	150
Pringles Original	170
Pringles Sour Cream 'n Onion	170
Ruffles Cheddar & Sour Cream	160
Ruffles Light	130
Ruffles Light Sour Cream & Onion	130
Ruffles Mesquite	160
Ruffles Monterey Jack	160
Ruffles Original	150
Ruffles Ranch	160
Ruffles Sour Cream & Onion	160
Wise	160
Wise Barbecue	150
Potato Sticks / **Planters**	160
Potato Sticks, BBQ / **Planters**	160
Snack chips, cheddar and jack / **Suprimos**	140
Snack chips, onion / **Suprimos**	140
Sunchips, multigrain, French onion / 12 chips	140
Sunchips, multigrain, original flavor / 12 chips	150
Tortilla chips	
Doritos Cool Ranch	140
Doritos Jumpin' Jack	140
Doritos Nacho Cheese	140
Doritos Salso Rio	140
Doritos Taco	140
Doritos Toasted Corn	140

CALORIES

LaFamous	140
LaFamous No Salt Added	140
Old El Paso / 9 chips	160
Planters	150
Planters Nacho Cheese	150
Santitas	140
Santitas Cantina Style	140
Santitas Fajita Flavored, Cantina Style	140
Santitas Strips	140
Tostitos	140
Tostitos Bite Size	150
Tostitos Lime 'n Chile	150
Tostitos White Corn	130
Tyson	140
Tyson Nacho Cheese	140
Tyson Ranch Flavor	140
Tyson Unsalted	140
Wise Nacho	150

Chocolate and Chips

CALORIES

For baking: 1 oz unless noted

Chips

Butterscotch / **Nestlé** Morsels	150
Chocolate, flavor, semi-sweet / ¼ cup / **Baker's**	200
Chocolate, milk / **Baker's**	140
Chocolate, milk / ¼ cup / **Baker's** Big Chip	240
Chocolate, milk / 1.5 oz / **Hershey's**	220
Chocolate, real, semi-sweet / ¼ cup / **Baker's**	200
Chocolate, semi-sweet / ¼ cup / **Baker's** Big Chip	220
Chocolate, semi-sweet / 1.5 oz / **Hershey's** regular and miniature	220
Chocolate, semi-sweet / **Nestlé** Morsels	140
Chocolate mint / 1.5 oz / **Hershey's**	230

CALORIES

Peanut butter-flavored / 1.5 oz / **Hershey's**	230
Vanilla / 1.5 oz / **Hershey's**	240
Choco Bake / **Nestlé**	180
Chocolate, solid Chunks, semi-sweet / **Hershey's**	140
Chunks / **Hershey's**	160
German sweet / **Baker's**	140
Semi-sweet / **Baker's**	140
Semi-sweet / **Hershey's**	140
Semi-sweet / **Nestlé**	160
Unswt / **Baker's**	140
Unswt / **Hershey's**	190
Unswt / **Nestlé**	180

Cocktails

NONALCOHOLIC MIXES, DRY

CALORIES

1 packet unless noted

Collins / **Bar-Tender's**	68
Collins / **Bar-Tender's** Lite	6
Daiquiri	
Bar-Tender's	67
Bar-Tender's Lite	6
Holland House / .56 oz	64
Mai Tai / .56 oz / **Holland House**	64
Margarita	
Bar-Tender's	55
Bar-Tender's Lite	6
Holland House / .56 oz	56
Margarita, strawberry / .56 oz / **Holland House**	64
Piña Colada / .56 oz / **Holland House**	75
Pussycat / **Bar-Tender's**	75
Tom Collins / .56 oz / **Holland House**	64
Whiskey Sour	
Bar-Tender's	67

CALORIES

Bar-Tender's Lite	6
Holland House / .56 oz	64

NONALCOHOLIC MIXES, LIQUID

Bloody Mary / 6 fl oz / **Libby's**	40
Collins / 6 fl oz / **Cragmont**	58
Collins Mixer / 6 fl oz / **Canada Dry**	60
Collins Mixer / 6 fl oz / **Schweppes**	70
Cream of Coconut / 2 fl oz / **Holland House**	144
Daiquiri / 3 fl oz / **Holland House**	108
Daiquiri, raspberry / 3 fl oz / **Holland House**	84
Daiquiri, strawberry / 3.5 fl oz / **Holland House**	98
Fuzzy Navel / 2 fl oz / **Holland House**	64
Mai Tai / 4.5 fl oz / **Holland House**	144
Manhattan / 1 fl oz / **Holland House**	28
Margarita / 3 fl oz / **Holland House**	72
Margarita, strawberry / 3.5 fl oz / **Holland House**	98
Old Fashioned / 1 fl oz / **Holland House**	32
Piña Colada / 4.5 fl oz / **Holland House**	144
Sour Mixer / 6 fl oz / **Canada Dry**	70
Sweet n Sour / 3 fl oz / **Holland House**	96
Tom Collins / 3 fl oz / **Holland House**	132
Whiskey Sour / 3 fl oz / **Holland House**	108

Cocoa

COCOA

CALORIES

Hershey's / 1 oz	110
Hershey's European / 1 oz	90

COCOA MIX

Instant / **Lucerne** Sugar Free / 1 env	50
Instant / **Ovaltine** / 1 oz	120

	CALORIES
Instant, milk chocolate / **Swiss Miss** / 1 oz	110
Instant, milk chocolate, sugar free / **Swiss Miss** / .53 oz	50
Instant, milk chocolate w marshmallows / **Swiss Miss** / 1 oz	120
Instant, mocha, sugar free / **Carnation** / 1 env	50
Instant, rich chocolate / **Carnation** / 1 env	70
Instant, rich chocolate, sugar free / **Carnation** / 1 env	50
Instant, sugar free / **Ovaltine** / 1 oz	40
Instant **Weight Watchers** / 1 env	60
Instant, white chocolate / **Swiss Miss** / 1 oz	110

Coconut

FRESH

	CALORIES
Meat / 1 piece (2x2x½ in)	160
Meat / shredded or grated / 1 cup	285

CANNED OR PACKAGED

⅓ cup unless noted

	CALORIES
Town House / 1 oz	150
Plain, bag / **Baker's** Angel Flake	120
Plain, can	
Baker's Angel Flake	110
Baker's Angel Flake, Toasted	200
Baker's Premium Shred	140

Coffee

All regular coffee has about:
    2 calories per cup for ground roasted
    4 calories per cup for instant and instant freeze-dried

	CALORIES
Flavored coffee, instant mixes, prepared; 6 fl oz	
Cafe Francais / **General Foods** International	60
Cafe Francais / **General Foods** International, Sugar Free	35
Cafe Irish Creme / **General Foods** International	50
Cafe Vienna / **General Foods** International	60
Cafe Vienna / **General Foods** International, Sugar Free	30
Double Dutch Chocolate / **General Foods** International	50
Dutch Chocolate Mint / **General Foods** International	50
Orange Cappuccino / **General Foods** International	60
Orange Cappuccino / **General Foods** International, Sugar Free	30
Suisse Mocha / **General Foods** International	50
Suisse Mocha / **General Foods** International, Sugar Free	30
Kava instant coffee / 1 tsp	2
Postum Instant coffee flavor / 6 fl oz	12
Postum Instant hot beverage / 6 fl oz	12

Condiments

	CALORIES
See also Sauces *and* Seasonings.	
Catsup	
Del Monte / ¼ cup	60
Del Monte No Salt / ¼ cup	60
Heinz / 1 tbsp	16
Heinz Hot / 1 tbsp	16
Heinz Lite / 1 tbsp	8
Hunt's / 1 tbsp	15
Hunt's No Added Salt / 1 tbsp	20
Smucker's / ¼ cup	8
Weight Watchers / 2 tsp	8
Chili Sauce / **Heinz** / 1 tbsp	16
Dips: 2 tbsp	
Bacon and horseradish	
Breakstone's	70
Kraft	60
Kraft Premium	50
Sealtest	70
Bacon and onion / **Breakstone's**	70
Bacon and onion / **Kraft** Premium	60
Blu cheese / **Kraft** Premium	50
Clam	
Breakstone's	50
Kraft	60
Kraft Premium	45
Sealtest	50
Creamy cucumber / **Kraft** Premium	50
Creamy onion / **Kraft** Premium	45
Cucumber and onion / **Breakstone's**	50
Cucumber and onion / **Sealtest**	50
French onion	
Breakstone's	50

CALORIES

Kraft	60
Kraft Premium	45
Sealtest	50
Green onion / **Kraft**	60
Jalapeno cheddar / **Breakstone's**	70
Mushroom and herb / **Breakstone's**	50
Toasted onion / **Breakstone's**	50
Horseradish	
Heinz / 1 tbsp	74
Kraft Cream Style / 1 tbsp	12
Kraft Sauceworks / 1 tbsp	14
Horseradish, mustard / 1 tbsp / **Kraft**	14
Horseradish, prepared / 1 tbsp / **Kraft**	10
Mustard: 1 tsp unless noted	
French's Bold & Spicy	6
French's Creamy Spread	8
French's Dijon	8
French's Horseradish	6
French's Sweet Onion	8
French's Yellow	4
Gulden's Spicy Brown / .25 oz	8
Heinz	3
Kraft / 1 tbsp	11
Diablo/ ¼ oz / **Gulden's**	8
Dijon / 1 tbsp / **Grey Poupon**	6
Dijon / 1 tbsp / **Grey Poupon** Country	6
Parisian / 1 tbsp / **Grey Poupon**	6
Sauce diable / 1 tbsp / **Escoffier**	20
Seafood cocktail / ¼ cup / **Del Monte**	70
Seafood cocktail / 1 tbsp / **Heinz**	17
Soy sauce / ½ tsp / **La Choy**	2
Soy sauce / ½ tsp / **La Choy** Lite	1
Steak sauce / 1 tbsp / **Heinz** 57	17
Steak sauce / 1 tbsp / **Heinz** Traditional	12
Tartar sauce	
Heinz / 1 tbsp	71
Kraft Sauceworks / 1 tbsp	50
Kraft Sauceworks lemon and herb flavor / 1 tbsp	70
Vinegar	
Apple cider / 1 tbsp / **Hain**	2
Apple cider / 1 fl oz / **Lucky Leaf**	4

CALORIES

Apple cider / 1 fl oz / **Musselman's**	4
Cider / 1 tbsp / **Hain**	2
Red wine / 1 fl oz / **Lucky Leaf**	4
Red wine / 1 fl oz / **Musselman's**	4
Red wine / 1 tbsp / **Progresso**	0
Red wine / 1 fl oz / **Regina**	4
White distilled / 1 fl oz / **Lucky Leaf**	4
White distilled / 1 fl oz / **Musselman's**	4
Wine, cooking / sherry / 4 oz / **Great Western** Cooking	160
Wine, cooking / sherry / 4 oz / **Taylor** Cooking	146
Worcestershire: 1 tbsp	
French's Hickory	8
French's Regular	8
Heinz	5

Cookies

CALORIES

1 piece unless noted

Almond and date bar / **Health Valley**	160
Almond date / **Health Valley**	70
Almond shortbread / **Archway**	60
Almond toast / **Stella D'Oro**	60
Amaranth / **Health Valley**	60
Angel bars / **Stella D'Oro**	80
Angel wings / **Stella D'Oro**	70
Angelica Goodies / **Stella D'Oro**	110
Anginetti / **Stella D'Oro**	30
Animal cookies, candied / 5 cookies / **Grandma's**	140
Animal crackers / 5 pieces / **Barnum's** Animal	60
Anisette sponge / **Stella D'Oro**	50
Anisette toast / **Stella D'Oro**	50
Anisette toast, jumbo / **Stella D'Oro**	110
Apple Bakes / **Health Valley**	100
Apple fruit bars / **Health Valley**	109
Apple, fruit centers / **Health Valley**	70

Apple newtons / **Nabisco**	70
Apple raisin / **Health Valley**	70
Apple raisin bar / **Weight Watchers**	100
Apple spice / 3 pieces / **Health Valley**	75
Apricot almond / 2 pieces / **Health Valley**	90
Apricot bakes / **Health Valley**	100
Apricot delights / 3 pieces / **Health Valley**	75
Apricot-filled / **Archway**	95
Apricot fruit bars / **Health Valley**	140
Apricot, fruit centers / **Health Valley**	70
Apricot-raspberry / **Pepperidge Farm**	50
Arrowroot biscuit / **National**	20
Black walnut ice box / **Archway**	120
Blueberry-filled / **Archway**	100
Blueberry nut fiber / **Health Valley**	100
Bordeaux / **Pepperidge Farm**	35
Breakfast Treat / **Stella D'Oro**	100
Brownie chocolate nut / **Pepperidge Farm**	55
Brussels / **Pepperidge Farm**	55
Brussels mint / **Pepperidge Farm**	65
Cappuccino / **Pepperidge Farm**	50
Capri / **Pepperidge Farm**	80
Castelets / **Stella D'Oro**	70
Castelets, chocolate / **Stella D'Oro**	60
Chantilly / **Pepperidge Farm**	80
Cherry-filled / **Archway**	100
Chessman / **Pepperidge Farm**	90
Chinese Dessert / **Stella D'Oro**	170
Chips Ahoy	
Nabisco Chewy	60
Nabisco Mini / 6 pieces	70
Nabisco Pure Chocolate Chips	50
Nabisco Selections / chocolate-chocolate chunk	90
Nabisco Selections / chocolate-chocolate walnut	95
Nabisco Selections / chocolate chunk pecan	100
Nabisco / sprinkled	50
Nabisco / striped	90
Chocolate / 3 pieces / **Weight Watchers**	80
Chocolate chip	
Archway	110
Archway Chocolate Drop	100

CALORIES

Archway Ice Box	130
Archway Supreme	130
Duncan Hines	55
Nabisco Almost Home	60
Nabisco Chips Ahoy Selections	90
Pepperidge Farm	50
Tastykake Soft 'n Chewy	170
Chocolate chip bar / **Tastykake**	190
Chocolate chip snaps / 3 pieces / **Nabisco**	70
Chocolate-chocolate chip / **Tastykake** Soft 'n Chewy	170
Chocolate chunk / **Pepperidge Farm**	120
Chocolate chunk pecan / **Pepperidge Farm**	120
Chocolate chunk pecan / **Pepperidge Farm** Special Collection	70
Chocolate middles / **Nabisco**	80
Chocolate snaps / 4 pieces / **Nabisco**	70
Chocolate toffee chip / **Pepperidge Farm**	50
Chocolate walnut / **Pepperidge Farm**	120
Cinnamon / 2 oz / **Health Valley**	100
Cinnamon apple / **Archway**	110
Cinnamon raisin nut newton / **Nabisco**	60
Cinnamon snaps / **Archway**	40
Coconut / **Stella D'Oro** Dietetic	50
Coconut macaroon / **Archway**	90
Coconut macaroon / **Stella D'Oro**	60
Coconut squares / **Archway**	105
Como Delights / **Stella D'Oro**	150
Date and almond fruit bar / **Health Valley**	140
Date Bakes / **Health Valley**	100
Date Delights / 3 pieces / **Health Valley**	75
Date fruit bars / **Health Valley**	140
Date, fruit centers / **Health Valley**	70
Date pecan / 2 pieces / **Health Valley**	90
Deep Night fudge / **Stella D'Oro**	65
Devil's food cakes / **Nabisco**	70
Dutch apple bar / **Stella D'Oro**	110
Dutch cocoa / **Archway**	100
Egg biscuit / **Stella D'Oro** Dietetic	45
Egg biscuits, sugared / **Stella D'Oro**	80
Egg, jumbo / **Stella D'Oro**	50
Frosty lemon / **Archway**	120

Fruit and Fitness Bars / **Health Valley**	100
Fruit and nut bar / **Health Valley**	140
Fruit 'n honey / **Archway**	100
Fruit slices / **Stella D'Oro**	60
Fudge bar / **Tastykake**	200
Fudge chocolate chip / **Grandma's**	175
Fudge chocolate chip / **Nabisco** Almost Home	70
Geneva / **Pepperidge Farm**	65
Ginger snaps / **Nabisco**	30
Gingerman / **Pepperidge Farm**	35
Gingersnaps / **Archway**	35
Golden bars / **Stella D'Oro**	110
Grab Cookie Bites	
Vanilla / 8 cookies / **Grandma's**	140
Chocolate / 8 cookies / **Grandma's**	140
Peanut butter / 8 cookies / **Grandma's**	140
Graham crackers	
Amaranth / **Health Valley** / 1.2 oz	120
Apple cinnamon / **Honey Maid** Graham Bites / 11 pieces	60
Brown sugar 'n spice / **Honey Maid** Graham Bites / 11 pieces	60
Chocolate / **Nabisco**	30
Cinnamon / **Health Valley** / 1 oz	110
Cinnamon / **Honey Maid**	30
Cookies 'n fudge / **Nabisco** Party Grahams	45
Ginger / **Health Valley** / 1 oz	110
Honey / **Health Valley** / 1 oz	130
Honey / **Honey Maid**	30
Honey 'n oat bran / **Honey Maid** Graham Bites / 11 pieces	60
Nabisco	30
Nabisco Bugs Bunny / 5 pieces	60
Oat bran / **Health Valley** / 1.16 oz	120
Oat bran and honey / **Health Valley** / 1 oz	110
Hawaiian fruit / 3 pieces / **Health Valley**	75
Hazelnut / **Pepperidge Farm**	55
Heyday bars / **Nabisco**	110
Holiday Trinkets / **Stella D'Oro**	40
Hostess assortment / **Stella D'Oro**	40
Iced molasses / **Archway**	130

	CALORIES
Ideal bars / **Nabisco**	90
Irish oatmeal / **Pepperidge Farm**	45
Kichel / **Stella D'Oro** Dietetic	8
Lady Stella assortment / **Stella D'Oro**	40
Lemon drop / **Archway**	85
Lemon nut crunch / **Pepperidge Farm**	55
Lemon snaps / **Archway**	35
Lido / **Pepperidge Farm**	90
Linzer / **Pepperidge Farm**	120
Lorna Doone / 3 pieces / **Nabisco**	70
Love cookies / **Stella D'Oro**	110
Mallomars / **Nabisco**	60
Margherite, chocolate / **Stella D'Oro**	70
Margherite, vanilla / **Stella D'Oro**	70
Marshmallow puffs / **Nabisco**	90
Marshmallow twirls / **Nabisco**	140
Milano / **Pepperidge Farm**	60
Milk chocolate chip / **Duncan Hines**	55
Milk chocolate, macadamia / **Pepperidge Farm**	120
Milk chocolate, macadamia / **Pepperidge Farm** Special Collection	70
Milk chocolate, oatmeal / **Pepperidge Farm**	110
Mint Milano / **Pepperidge Farm**	75
Molasses	
Archway	110
Grandma's / 2 pieces	320
Nabisco Pantry	80
Molasses crisp / **Pepperidge Farm**	35
Mud pie / **Archway**	110
Mystic mint / **Nabisco**	90
Nassau / **Pepperidge Farm**	80
Newtons / **Nabisco**	60
Nutter Butter / **Nabisco**	70
Nutter Butter Patties / **Nabisco**	40
Nutty fudge / **Archway**	69
Oat bran / 2 oz / **Health Valley**	120
Oat bran fruit / 2 oz / **Health Valley**	120
Oat bran fruit and nut / 1 oz / **Health Valley**	110
Oatmeal	
Archway	110
Archway apple-filled	100

CALORIES

Nabisco Baker's Bonus	
and raisin / **Archway**	80
Apple bran / **Archway**	120
Apple spice / **Grandma's**	120
Chocolate chunk / **Nabisco** Selections	165
Date-filled / **Archway**	95
Golden / **Archway**	100
Iced / **Archway**	120
Raisin	140
Archway	50
Duncan Hines	55
Nabisco Almost Home	70
Pepperidge Farm	100
Pepperidge Farm Old Fashioned / 2 pieces	110
Tastykake Soft 'n Chewy	160
Raisin bar / **Tastykake**	210
Raisin bran / **Archway**	110
Ruth's / **Archway**	120
Spice / **Weight Watchers** / 3 pieces	80
Old-fashioned molasses / **Archway**	120
Old-fashioned peanut butter / **Archway**	120
Old-fashioned sugar / **Nabisco** Almost Home	70
Orange Milano / **Pepperidge Farm**	75
Oreo	
Nabisco	50
Big Stuff / **Nabisco**	250
Double Stuff / **Nabisco**	70
Fudge-covered / **Nabisco**	110
White fudge-covered / **Nabisco**	110
Orleans / 3 pieces / **Pepperidge Farm**	90
Orleans sandwich / **Pepperidge Farm**	60
Peanut butter / **Grandma's**	205
Peanut butter / 2 oz / **Health Valley**	140
Peanut butter, milk chocolate / **Pepperidge Farm**	110
Peanut chunks / **Health Valley**	45
Peanut jumble / **Archway**	110
Pecan crunch / **Archway**	65
Pecan fiber chunky / **Health Valley**	100
Pecan ice box / **Archway**	125
Pecan shortbread / **Nabisco**	80
Pecan shortbread / **Pepperidge Farm**	70

Pfeffernusse / **Stella D'Oro**	40
Pinwheels / **Nabisco**	130
Pirouettes / **Pepperidge Farm**	35
Pirouettes, chocolate laced / **Pepperidge Farm**	35
Raisin / **Grandma's**	160
Raisin and cinnamon fruit bar / **Health Valley**	140
Raisin apple, fruit centers / **Health Valley**	70
Raisin Bakes / **Health Valley**	100
Raisin fruit bars / **Health Valley**	140
Raisin nut / **Health Valley**	70
Raisin nut fiber / 1 oz / **Health Valley**	100
Raisin oat bran / **Health Valley**	45
Raisin oatmeal / **Health Valley**	25
Raisin raisin / **Health Valley**	70
Raspberry / **Health Valley**	70
Raspberry-filled / **Archway**	100
Raspberry, fruit centers / **Health Valley**	70
Raspberry newtons / **Nabisco**	70
Rocky road / **Archway**	130
Roman egg biscuit / **Stella D'Oro**	140
Round toast peanut butter sandwiches / 6 sandwiches / **Planters**	200
Royal nuggets / **Stella D'Oro**	2
Sandwich creme / **Nabisco** Cameo	70
Sandwich creme / vanilla / **Nabisco** Cookie Break	50
Sandwich creme / vanilla / **Nabisco** Giggles	60
Select assortment / **Archway**	50
Sesame / **Stella D'Oro**	50
Shortbread	
Pepperidge Farm	75
Weight Watchers / 3 pieces	80
Nabisco Cookies 'n Fudge / striped	60
Social tea biscuits / **Nabisco**	20
Soft sugar drop / **Archway**	90
Strawberry / **Pepperidge Farm**	50
Strawberry-filled / **Archway**	100
Strawberry newtons / **Nabisco**	70
Suddenly S'mores / **Nabisco**	100
Sugar / **Archway**	100
Sugar / **Pepperidge Farm**	50
Swiss fudge / **Stella D'Oro**	70

Tahiti / **Pepperidge Farm**	90
Teddy grahams	
Chocolate / 11 pieces / **Nabisco**	60
Chocolate w vanilla creme / 4 pieces / **Nabisco**	
Bearwiches	70
Cinnamon / 11 pieces / **Nabisco**	60
Cinnamon w vanilla creme / 4 pieces / **Nabisco**	
Bearwiches	70
Honey / 11 pieces / **Nabisco**	60
Vanilla / 11 pieces / **Nabisco**	60
Vanilla w chocolate creme / 4 pieces / **Nabisco**	
Bearwiches	70
Tofu / 2 oz / **Health Valley**	90
Tropical fruit / **Health Valley**	45
Tropical fruit / **Health Valley**	70
Tropical, fruit centers / **Health Valley**	70
Vanilla shortbread / **Tastykake**	60
Wafers	
Vanilla / **Archway**	30
Brown-edge / 2-½ pieces / **Nabisco**	70
Chocolate / 2-½ pieces **Nabisco** Famous	70
Cinnamon / 3-½ pieces / **Nilla**	60
Nilla / 3-½ pieces /	60
Striped / **Nabisco** Cookies 'n Fudge	70
Sugar / **Nabisco** Biscos / 4 pieces	70
Waffle creams / 2 pieces / **Nabisco** Biscos	70
Wheat free / 2 oz / **Health Valley**	80
Windmill / **Archway**	140
Zurich / **Pepperidge Farm**	60

COOKIE MIXES

Prepared according to package directions

Brownies	
Betty Crocker Fudge, Family Size / ¼₄ pkg	140
Betty Crocker Fudge Light / 1 brownie	100
Betty Crocker Fudge, Regular Size / ¼₄ pkg	150
Betty Crocker MicroRave Frosted / 1 brownie	180
Betty Crocker MicroRave Fudge / 1 brownie	150
Betty Crocker Supreme, Frosted / ¼₄ pkg	160

CALORIES

Betty Crocker Supreme, Original / ¼₄ pkg	140
Betty Crocker Supreme Party / ¼₄ pkg	160
Duncan Hines Double Fudge / ¼₄ pkg	150
Duncan Hines Fudge / ⅟₁₆ pkg	130
Duncan Hines Gourmet Turtle / ⅟₁₆ pkg	200
Gold Medal Pouch Mixes / ⅟₁₆ mix	100
Pillsbury Double Chocolate / 2-in sq	140
Pillsbury Double Chocolate / 2-in sq prepared w egg whites	130
Pillsbury Fudge / 2-in sq	140
Pillsbury Fudge / 2-in sq prepared w egg whites	140
Pillsbury Fudge Family Size / 2-in sq	150
Pillsbury Fudge Family Size / 2-in sq prepared w egg whites	150
Pillsbury Fudge Lovin' Lites / ¼₄ pkg prepared w egg whites	100
Pillsbury Fudge Lovin' Lites / ¼₄ pkg	100
Pillsbury Fudge Microwave / ⅑ pkg	190
Pillsbury Fudge w Frosting, Microwave / ⅑ pkg	240
Pillsbury Funfetti Frosted / 2-in sq	160
Pillsbury Funfetti Frosted / 2-in sq prepared w egg whites	150
Caramel / **Betty Crocker** Supreme / ¼₄ pkg	120
Chocolate chip / **Betty Crocker** Supreme / ¼₄ pkg	140
German chocolate / **Betty Crocker** Supreme / ¼₄ pkg	160
Milk chocolate / **Duncan Hines** / ¼₄ pkg	160
Peanut butter / **Duncan Hines** / ¼₄ pkg	150
w hot fudge frosting / **Betty Crocker** MicroRave Singles / 1 serv	350
Walnut	
Betty Crocker MicroRave / 1 brownie	160
Betty Crocker Supreme / ¼₄ pkg	140
Duncan Hines / ¼₄ pkg	150
Pillsbury / 2-in sq	140
Pillsbury / 2-in sq prepared w egg whites	130
Chocolate chip / **Betty Crocker** Big Batch / ⅟₃₆ mix (2 cookies)	120
Date bar / 1 bar / **Betty Crocker**	60

CALORIES

REFRIGERATED DOUGH

1 piece

Candy / **Pillsbury** Oven Lovin	70
Candy cookie w chocolate candy / **Pillsbury** Oven Lovin	70
Candy cookie w Reese's pieces / **Pillsbury** Oven Lovin	70
Chocolate chip	
Pillsbury	70
Pillsbury Oven Lovin	70
Pillsbury's Best	70
Chocolate chocolate chip / **Pillsbury's** Best	70
Oatmeal raisin / **Pillsbury's** Best	60
Peanut butter / **Pillsbury's** Best	70
Reese's Pieces / **Pillsbury** Oven Lovin	70
Sugar / **Pillsbury's** Best	70

Crackers

CALORIES

Barbecue flavor / ½ oz / **Weight Watchers** Great Snackers	60
Cheddar cheese flavor / ½ oz / **Weight Watchers** Great Snackers	60
Cheddar cracker snacks / 13–16 pieces / **Frito-Lay**	70
Cheddar wedges / 31 pieces / **Nabisco**	70
Cheddars / 10 pieces / **Nabisco** Better	70
Cheddars / 10 pieces / **Nabisco** Better, Low Salt	70
Cheese / 6 pieces / **Hain**	70
Cheese 'n crackers / 1 pkg / **Kraft** Handi-Snacks	120
Cheese 'n crackers, bacon / 1 pkg / **Kraft** Handi-Snacks	130
Cheese-filled / 6 pieces / **Frito-Lay**	210
Cheese Nips / 13 pieces / **Nabisco**	70
Cheese Tidbits / 16 pieces / **Nabisco**	7
Chicken in a Biskit / 7 pieces / **Nabisco**	80
Cool Ranch / 1 oz / **Doritos**	140
Country Butter / 1 oz / **McCrakens**	140

CALORIES

Cracked wheat / 4 pieces / **Nabisco**	70
Cracked wheat / 3 pieces / **Pepperidge Farm**	100
Crispbread	
Garlic flavor / 2 pieces / **Weight Watchers**	30
Golden wheat / 2 pieces / **Weight Watchers**	30
Harvest rice / 2 pieces / **Weight Watchers**	30
Crown Pilot / 1 piece / **Nabisco**	70
Dairy butter / 4 pieces / **Nabisco**	70
English Water Biscuits / 4 pieces / **Pepperidge Farm**	70
Escort / 3 pieces / **Nabisco**	70
Flutters	
Butter / ¾ oz / **Pepperidge Farm**	100
Garden herb / ¾ oz / **Pepperidge Farm**	100
Golden sesame / ¾ oz / **Pepperidge Farm**	110
Toasted wheat / ¾ oz / **Pepperidge Farm**	110
Goldfish	
Cheddar cheese / 1 oz / **Pepperidge Farm**	120
Cheddar cheese, low salt / 1 oz / **Pepperidge Farm**	120
Original / 1 oz / **Pepperidge Farm**	130
Parmesan cheese / 1 oz / **Pepperidge Farm**	120
Pizza-flavored / 1 oz / **Pepperidge Farm**	130
Pretzel / 1 oz / **Pepperidge Farm**	110
Harvest crisps / 6 pieces / **Nabisco** 5 Grain	60
Harvest crisps / 6 pieces / **Nabisco** Oat	60
Hearty Wheat / 4 pieces / **Pepperidge Farm**	100
Matzos	
American / 1 sheet / **Manischewitz**	115
Egg n' Onion / 1 sheet / **Manischewitz**	112
Egg Passover / 1 sheet / **Manischewitz**	132
Egg Passover / 10 pieces / **Manischewitz**	108
Miniatures / 10 pieces / **Manischewitz**	80
Passover / 1 sheet / **Manischewitz**	129
Thin Dietetic / 1 sheet / **Manischewitz**	91
Thin Salted / 1 sheet / **Manischewitz**	100
Thin Tea / 1 sheet / **Manischewitz**	103
Unsalted / 1 sheet / **Manischewitz**	110
Whole Wheat w bran / 1 sheet / **Manischewitz**	110
Meal Mates / 3 pieces / **Nabisco** Sesame Bread Wafers	70
Nacho cheese / 1 oz / **Doritos**	140
Oat Krisp / ½ oz / **Ralston Purina**	50

CALORIES

Onion
    Hain / 6 pieces 70
    Hain No Salt / 6 pieces 70
    Nabisco / 4 pieces 70
Peanut butter 'n cheese / 1 pkg / **Kraft** Handi-Snacks 190
Peanut butter-filled / 6 pieces / **Frito-Lay** 210
Rice bran / 1 oz / **Health Valley** 100
Rich / 4 pieces / **Hain** 70
Rich / 4 pieces / **Hain** No Salt 70
Ritz
    Nabisco / 4 pieces 70
    Nabisco Bits / 22 pieces 70
    Nabisco Cheese Bits / 22 pieces 70
    Nabisco Low Salt / 4 pieces 70
    Nabisco Low Salt Bits / 22 pieces 70
    Nabisco Bits Sandwiches, cheese / 6 pieces 80
    Nabisco Bits Sandwiches, peanut butter/ 6 pieces 80
    Nabisco Royal Lunch / 1 piece 60
Rye / 6 pieces / **Hain** 70
Rye / 6 pieces / **Hain** No Salt 60
Rykrisp **Ralston Purina** / ½ oz 40
    Seasoned / **Ralston Purina** / ½ oz 45
    Sesame / **Ralston Purina** / ½ oz 50
Saltines and soda crackers, premium
    Nabisco / 5 pieces 60
    Nabisco Bits / 16 pieces 70
    Nabisco Fat Free / 5 pieces 50
    Nabisco Low Salt / 5 pieces 60
    Nabisco Unsalted Tops / 5 pieces 60
    Nabisco Whole Wheat Plus / 5 pieces 60
Sesame
    Hain / 6 pieces 70
    Hain No Salt / 6 pieces 70
    Nabisco / 4 pieces 70
    Pepperidge Farm / 4 pieces 80
Snack Mix: 1 oz
    Classic / **Pepperidge Farm** 140
    Lightly smoked / **Pepperidge Farm** 150
    Spicy / **Pepperidge Farm** 140
Snack Sticks: 8 pieces
    Pretzel / **Pepperidge Farm** 120

CALORIES

Pumpernickel / **Pepperidge Farm**	140
Sesame / **Pepperidge Farm**	140
Three cheese / **Pepperidge Farm**	130
Sociables / 6 pieces / **Nabisco**	70
Soup and oyster / 20 pieces / **Nabisco** Dandy	60
Soup and oyster / 18 pieces / **Nabisco** Oysterettes	60
Sour cream and chives / 1 oz / **McCrakens**	140
Sour cream and chives / 5 pieces / **Hain**	60
Sour cream and chives / 5 pieces / **Hain** No Salt	70
Sourdough / 6 pieces / **Hain**	70
Sourdough / 6 pieces / **Hain** No Salt	70
Swiss cheese / 7 pieces / **Nabisco**	70
Tam Tams / 10 pieces / **Manischewitz**	147
Tam Tams, no salt / 10 pieces / **Manischewitz**	138
Tams: 10 pieces	
Garlic / **Manischewitz**	153
Onion / **Manischewitz**	150
Wheat / **Manischewitz**	150
Tangy Cheddar / 1 oz / **McCrakens**	140
Thins	
Bacon Flavored / **Nabisco** / 7 pieces	70
Butter Flavored / **Pepperidge Farm** / 4 pieces	70
Goldfish, cheese / **Pepperidge Farm** / 4 pieces	50
Oat / **Nabisco** / 8 pieces	70
Toasted bran / **Nabisco** / 7 pieces	60
Vegetable / **Nabisco** / 7 pieces	70
Wheat / **Nabisco** / 8 pieces	70
Wheat / **Nabisco** Low Salt / 8 pieces	70
Wheat / **Nabisco** Nutty / 7 pieces	70
Toasted onion flavor / ½ oz / **Weight Watchers** Great Snackers	60
Toasted poppy / 4 pieces / **Nabisco**	70
Toasted wheat / 1 oz / **McCrakens**	140
Toasted wheat / 4 pieces / **Pepperidge Farm**	80
Triscuit	
Nabisco / 3 pieces	60
Nabisco Bits / 8 pieces	60
Nabisco Low Salt / 3 pieces	60
Nabisco Wheat 'n Bran / 3 pieces	60
Twigs / 5 pieces / **Nabisco**	70
Uneeda biscuits / 2 pieces / **Nabisco**	60

	CALORIES
Vegetable / 6 pieces / **Hain**	60
Vegetable / 6 pieces / **Hain** No Salt	70
Waverly / 4 pieces / **Nabisco**	70
Waverly / 4 pieces / **Nabisco** Low Salt	70
Wheat / ½ oz / **Health Valley**	40
Wheat / 10 pieces / **Manischewitz**	80
Wheat, stoned / ½ oz / **Health Valley** No Salt	55
Wheat, stoned, 7 grain / ½ oz / **Health Valley** No Salt	55
Wheat, stoned, herb / ½ oz / **Health Valley** No Salt	55
Wheat, stoned, sesame / ½ oz / **Health Valley** No Salt	55
Wheat w cheese flavor / ½ oz / **Health Valley**	40
Wheat w herbs / ½ oz / **Health Valley**	40
Wheat w onion / ½ oz / **Health Valley**	40
Wheat w vegetables / ½ oz / **Health Valley** No Salt	40
Wheatsworth / 4 pieces / **Nabisco**	70
Zesty Italian / 13–16 pieces / **Frito-Lay**	70
Zwieback / 2 pieces / **Nabisco**	60

Cream

	CALORIES
Half and half (cream and milk) / 1 cup	315
Half and half (cream and milk) / 1 tbsp	20
Light, coffee or table / 1 cup	470
Light, coffee or table / 1 tbsp	30
Light whipping / 1 cup (about 2 cups whipped)	700
Light whipping / 1 tbsp	45
Heavy whipping / 1 cup (about 2 cups whipped)	820
Heavy whipping / 1 tbsp	50

SOUR CREAM

	CALORIES
1 cup	495
1 tbsp	25
Sour cream	
Breakstone's / 1 tbsp	30

CALORIES

Knudsen Hampshire / 1 oz	60
Sealtest / 1 tbsp	30
Imitation sour cream / 1 tbsp / **Pet**/Dairymate	25
Imitation sour cream alternative / 1 tbsp / **Light n' Lively** Nonfat	10
Sour cream, half and half / 1 tbsp / **Breakstone**'s Light Choice	25
Sour cream, half and half / 1 tbsp / **Sealtest** Light Cultured	25
Sour cream, light / 1 oz / **Knudsen** Light n' Lively	40

Dinners

FROZEN

1 Dinner	CALORIES
Beans	
and frankfurters / 10 oz / **Banquet**	350
and franks / 8.5 oz / **Morton**	300
and franks / 10-½ oz **Swanson**	440
Beef	
Banquet / 9 oz	230
Banquet Extra Helping / 15.5 oz	430
Swanson / 11.25 oz	310
Tyson Champignon / 10.5 oz	370
Tyson Wile E. Coyote Hamburger Pizza / 6 oz	310
in barbecue sauce / 11 oz / **Swanson**	460
Chopped sirloin	
Le Menu / 12-¼ oz	430
Swanson / 10-¾ oz	340
Chopped steak / 16-¾ oz / **Swanson** Hungry Man	640
Pattie w gravy / 9 oz / **Banquet**	250
Patty sandwich w cheese / 6.25 oz / **Kid Cuisine**	430
Patty sandwich w cheese / 9.1 oz / **Kid Cuisine** Mega Meal	480
Patty w gravy / 9 oz / **Morton**	270
Pepper steak / 11 oz / **Healthy Choice**	290
Pepper steak / 11-½ oz / **Le Menu**	370

83

Ribs / 11 oz / **Healthy Choice**	330
Short ribs / 11 oz / **Tyson**	470
Sirloin tips / 11.75 oz / **Healthy Choice**	280
Sirloin tips / 11-½ oz / **Le Menu**	400
Sirloin w barbecue sauce / 11 oz / **Healthy Choice**	300
Sliced / 15-¼ oz / **Swanson** Hungry Man	450
Stroganoff / 10 oz / **Le Menu**	430
Yankee pot roast / 11 oz / **Healthy Choice**	250
Yankee pot roast / 10 oz / **Le Menu**	330
Broccoli and cheddar baked potato / 10-⅜ oz / **Stouffer's** Lean Cuisine	290
Broccoli and cheese baked potato / 10.5 oz / **Weight Watchers**	290
Burrito, beef and bean / 9.5 oz / **Banquet**	390
Chicken	
À l'orange / 9.5 oz / **Tyson**	300
À la king / 9 oz / **Banquet** Dining Light	240
À la king / 9 oz / **Chun King** Dining Light	240
À la king / 10-¼ oz / **Le Menu**	330
and dumplings / 10 oz / **Banquet**	270
Boneless	
Banquet Drumsnacker Platter / 7 oz	290
Banquet Meals and Platters / 7 oz	290
Bugs Bunny / 7.7 oz / **Tyson**	290
Boneless nuggets / 6 oz / **Banquet** Meals and Platters	340
Boneless pattie / 6.75 oz / **Banquet** Meals and Platters	310
Cacciatore / 12.5 oz / **Healthy Choice**	310
Cordon bleu / 11 oz / **Le Menu**	460
Dijon / 11 oz / **Healthy Choice**	260
Francais / 9.5 oz / **Tyson**	280
Fried	
Banquet Extra Helping / 14.25 oz	790
Banquet Meals and Platters / 9 oz	520
Kid Cuisine / 7.5 oz	430
Kid Cuisine Mega Meal / 10.8 oz	720
Fried, barbecue / 10 oz / **Swanson**	540
Fried, dark meat / 9-¾ oz / **Swanson**	560
Fried, southern / 13.25 oz / **Banquet** Extra Helping	790

CALORIES

Fried, white meat / 14.25 oz / **Banquet** Extra Helping	760
Fried, white meat / 10-¼ oz / **Swanson**	550
Glazed / 9.25 oz / **Tyson**	240
Glazed BBQ / 7 oz / **Tyson** Yosemite Sam	230
Glazed breast / 10 oz / **Le Menu** Light	230
Grilled / 7.75 oz / **Tyson**	220
Herb roasted / 12.3 oz / **Healthy Choice**	290
Herb roasted / 10 oz / **Le Menu** Light	240
Kiev / 9.25 oz / **Tyson**	520
Marsala / 9 oz / **Tyson**	200
Mesquite / 10.5 oz / **Healthy Choice**	340
Mesquite / 9.5 oz / **Tyson**	320
Nuggets	
Kid Cuisine / 6.8 oz	360
Kid Cuisine Mega Meal / 9.7 oz	470
Swanson / 8-¾ oz	470
Nuggets w barbecue sauce / 10 oz / **Banquet** Extra Helping	540
Nuggets w sweet and sour sauce / 10 oz / **Banquet** Extra Helping	540
Oriental / 11.25 oz / **Healthy Choice**	230
Parmigiana / 11.5 oz / **Healthy Choice**	270
Parmigiana / 11.25 oz / **Tyson**	380
Picatta / 9 oz / **Tyson**	240
Salsa / 11.25 oz / **Healthy Choice**	240
Sandwich / 6.7 oz / **Tyson** Road Runner	300
Sandwich / 8.2 oz / **Kid Cuisine**	470
Sweet and sour	
Healthy Choice / 11.5 oz	280
Le Menu / 11-¼ oz	400
Le Menu Light / 10 oz	250
Tyson / 11 oz	440
w gravy / 9 oz / **Tyson**	230
w noodles / 9 oz / **Chun King** Dining Light	240
w wine sauce / 10 oz / **Le Menu**	280
Chicken and pasta divan / 10.5 oz / **Healthy Choice**	310
Chicken chow mein / 9 oz / **Banquet** Dining Light	180
Chimichanga / 9.5 oz / **Banquet**	480
Enchilada	
Beef / 11 oz / **Banquet**	370
Beef / 12.75 oz / **Healthy Choice**	350
Beef / 10 oz / **Morton**	300

CALORIES

Beef / 13-¾ oz / **Swanson**	480
Chicken / 11 oz / **Banquet**	340
Chicken / 12.75 oz / **Healthy Choice**	330
Fettucini w vegetables / 12.5 oz / **Healthy Choice**	350
Fiesta / 12 oz / **Patio**	460
Fish	
Banquet / 8 oz	270
and chips / 10 oz / **Swanson**	500
Lemon pepper / 10.7 oz / **Healthy Choice**	300
Sticks / 7 oz / **Kid Cuisine**	360
Sticks / 7.5 oz / **Tyson** Sylvester	290
w mashed potatoes and carrots / 9.25 oz / **Morton**	350
Frankfurter w bun / 6.7 oz / **Kid Cuisine**	450
Ham	
Banquet / 8.25 oz	200
Glazed / 8 oz / **Morton**	230
Lorraine baked potato / 11 oz / **Weight Watchers**	250
Steak / 10 oz / **Le Menu**	300
Italian style / 9 oz / **Banquet** Meals and Platters	180
Lasagna / 9 oz / **Banquet** Dining Light	240
Lasagna, cheese / 9 oz / **Banquet** Dining Light	260
Macaroni and beef / 12 oz / **Swanson**	370
Macaroni and cheese	
Banquet / 9 oz	240
Banquet / 6.5 oz	290
Kid Cuisine Mega Meal / 12.45 oz	470
Morton / 6.5 oz	290
Swanson / 12-¼ oz	370
Tyson Tweety / 8 oz	340
w mini franks / 9 oz / **Kid Cuisine**	360
Meat loaf	
Banquet Extra Helping / 16.25 oz	640
Banquet / 9.5 oz	340
Swanson / 11 oz	360
and tomato sauce / 9 oz / **Morton**	280
Mexican style	
Banquet / 11 oz	410
Banquet Extra Helping / 19 oz	680
Kid Cuisine / 5.7 oz	290
Patio / 13.25 oz	540
Swanson / 14.25 oz	490

CALORIES

Swanson Hungry Man / 20.25 oz 820
Mexican style combination / 11 oz / **Banquet** 360
Noodles and chicken / 10 oz / **Banquet** Meals and Platters 170
Noodles and chicken / 10-½ oz / **Swanson** 280
Pasta
    Tyson Bugs Bunny and Tasmanian Devil / 8 oz 290
    Tyson Daffy Duck and Elmer Fudd / 8 oz 270
    Tyson Foghorn Leghorn / 8 oz 230
    Tyson Sylvester and Tweety / 8 oz 250
Pasta primavera / 11 oz / **Healthy Choice** 280
Pasta shells in tomato sauce, stuffed / 12 oz / **Healthy
  Choice** 380
Pasta w shrimp / 12.5 oz / **Healthy Choice** 270
Pasta, teriyaki w chicken / 12.6 oz / **Healthy Choice** 350
Pepperoni pizza / 6.35 oz / **Tyson** Foghorn Leghorn 400
Pork, loin / 10-¾ oz / **Swanson** 280
Pork, pattie / 6.5 oz / **Tyson** Porky Pig 370
Ravioli, mini / 8.75 oz / **Kid Cuisine** 290
Rigatoni w chicken / 12.5 oz / **Healthy Choice** 360
Salisbury steak
    Banquet / 9 oz 280
    Banquet Dining Light / 9 oz 200
    Banquet Extra Helping / 16.25 oz 590
    Healthy Choice / 11.5 oz 300
    Le Menu / 10.5 oz 370
    Le Menu Light / 10 oz 280
    Swanson / 10.75 oz 400
    Swanson Hungry Man / 16.5 oz 680
    Tyson / 10 oz 430
    w gravy / 9 oz / **Morton** 270
    w mushroom gravy / 11 oz / **Healthy Choice** 280
Spaghetti / 9 oz / **Banquet** Dining Light 220
Spaghetti and meatballs / 12-½ oz / **Swanson** 390
Spaghetti and meatballs / 8.65 oz / **Tyson** Daffy Duck 340
Spaghetti and meat sauce / 8.75 oz / **Banquet** 160
Spaghetti and meat sauce / 8.5 oz / **Morton** 170
Spaghetti w meat sauce / 9.25 oz / **Kid Cuisine** 310
Swedish meatballs and sauce / 9 oz / **Banquet** Dining
  Light 280
Swiss steak / 10 oz / **Swanson** 350
Tamale, beef / 11 oz / **Banquet** 420

CALORIES

Turkey

	CALORIES
Healthy Choice / 10 oz	290
Swanson / 11.5 oz	350
Tyson / 11.5 oz	380
Divan / 10 oz / **Le Menu** Light	260
Sliced / 10 oz / **Le Menu** Light	210
Sliced w gravy / 10 oz / **Healthy Choice**	270
Tetrazzini / 12.6 oz / **Healthy Choice**	340
w dressing / 6.5 oz / **Tyson** Elmer Fudd	260
w mushroom gravy / 10-½ oz / **Le Menu**	300
Veal parmigiana / 8.75 oz / **Morton**	230
Veal parmigiana / 12-¼ oz / **Swanson**	430
Western style / 11-½ oz / **Swanson**	430

DINNER MIXES

Beef / ½ cup as packaged / **Lipton** Noodles and Sauce	120
Beef vegetable / 11 oz as packaged / **Lipton** Hearty Ones	229
Broccoli and mushroom / ½ cup prepared / **Golden Grain** Noodle Roni	240
Broccoli and vegetables / ½ cup prepared / **Kraft** Pasta Salad	210
Broccoli au gratin / ½ cup prepared / **Golden Grain** Noodle Roni	190
Broccoli, creamy / ½ cup as packaged / **Lipton** Pasta Salad	120
Butter noodles / ½ cup as packaged / **Lipton** Noodles and Sauce	142
Butter and herb noodles / ½ cup as packaged / **Lipton** Noodles and Sauce	136
Cajun beans and sauce / ½ cup as packaged / **Lipton**	125
Carbonara Alfredo / ½ cup as packaged / **Lipton** Noodles and Sauce	126
Cheddar broccoli / ½ cup prepared / **Kraft** Pasta and Cheese	180
Cheddar broccoli / ½ cup prepared / **Lipton** Pasta and Sauce	131
Cheddar, mild / ½ cup prepared / **Golden Grain** Noodle Roni	190
Cheese noodles / ½ cup as packaged / **Lipton** Noodles and Sauce	136

CALORIES

Chicken

Chicken Helper Cheesy Broccoli / ⅕ mix dry	160
Chicken Helper Cheesy Broccoli / ⅕ serv prepared	270
Chicken Helper Creamy Chicken / ⅕ mix dry	170
Chicken Helper Creamy Chicken / ⅕ serv prepared	290
Chicken Helper Creamy Mushroom / ⅕ mix dry	170
Chicken Helper Creamy Mushroom / ⅕ serv prepared	280
Chicken Helper Fettucine Alfredo / ⅕ mix dry	170
Chicken Helper Fettucine Alfredo / ⅕ serv prepared	270
Chicken Helper Stir Fried Chicken / ⅕ mix dry	170
Chicken Helper Stir Fried Chicken / ⅕ serv prepared	330
Chicken and mushroom / 1.2 oz dry / **Golden Grain** Noodle Roni	134
Chicken and mushroom / ½ cup prepared / **Golden Grain** Noodle Roni	180
Chicken, beans and sauce / ½ cup as packaged / **Lipton**	125
Chicken broccoli / ½ cup as packaged / **Lipton** Noodles and Sauce	124
Chicken noodles, creamy / ½ cup as packaged / **Lipton** Noodles and Sauce	125

Chicken-flavored noodles

Lipton Noodles and Sauce / ½ cup as packaged	125
Lipton Hearty Ones / 11 oz as packaged	227
Minute Family Size Microwave / ½ cup prepared	160
Minute Single Size Microwave / ½ cup prepared	160
Chicken w herbs / ½ cup prepared / **Kraft** Pasta and Cheese	170
Creamy chicken / ½ cup prepared / **Golden Grain** Noodle Roni	180
Creamy garlic / 1.5 oz dry / **Golden Grain** Noodle Roni	172
Creamy garlic / ½ cup prepared / **Golden Grain** Noodle Roni	240
Egg noodle and cheese / ¾ cup prepared / **Kraft**	340
Egg noodle w chicken / ¾ cup prepared / **Kraft**	240
Egg noodles / 2 oz dry / **Golden Grain**	210
Fettuccini / 1.5 oz dry / **Golden Grain** Noodle Roni	181
Fettuccini / ½ cup prepared / **Golden Grain** Noodle Roni	250

Fettuccini Alfredo / ½ cup prepared / **Kraft** Pasta and Cheese	180
Garden medley / 11 oz as packaged / **Lipton** Hearty Ones	322
Garden primavera / ½ cup prepared / **Kraft** Pasta Salad	170
Garlic, creamy / ½ cup as packaged / **Lipton** Pasta and Sauce	145
Hamburger	
Hamburger Helper Beef Noodle / ⅕ mix dry	150
Hamburger Helper Beef Noodle / ⅕ serv prepared	330
Hamburger Helper Beef Romanoff / ⅕ mix dry	180
Hamburger Helper Beef Romanoff / ⅕ serv prepared	350
Hamburger Helper Beef Taco / ⅕ mix dry	160
Hamburger Helper Beef Taco / ⅕ serv prepared	330
Hamburger Helper Cheddar 'n Bacon / ⅕ mix dry	190
Hamburger Helper Cheddar 'n Bacon / ⅕ serv prepared	380
Hamburger Helper Cheeseburger Macaroni / ⅕ mix dry	190
Hamburger Helper Cheeseburger Macaroni / ⅕ serv prepared	370
Hamburger Helper Cheesy Italian / ⅕ mix dry	170
Hamburger Helper Cheesy Italian / ⅕ serv prepared	370
Hamburger Helper Chili Macaroni / ⅕ mix dry	150
Hamburger Helper Chili Macaroni / ⅕ serv prepared	330
Hamburger Helper Hamburger Hash / ⅕ mix dry	140
Hamburger Helper Hamburger Hash / ⅕ serv prepared	320
Hamburger Helper Hamburger Pizza / ⅕ mix dry	180
Hamburger Helper Hamburger Pizza / ⅕ serv prepared	360
Hamburger Helper Hamburger Stew / ⅕ mix dry	120
Hamburger Helper Hamburger Stew / ⅕ serv prepared	300
Hamburger Helper Lasagna / ⅕ mix dry	160
Hamburger Helper Lasagna / ⅕ serv prepared	340
Hamburger Helper Nacho Cheese / ⅕ mix dry	160

CALORIES

Hamburger Helper Nacho Cheese / ⅕ serv prepared	360
Hamburger Helper Pizzabake / ⅕ mix dry	150
Hamburger Helper Pizzabake / ⅕ serv prepared	320
Hamburger Helper Potato Stroganoff / ⅕ mix dry	140
Hamburger Helper Potato Stroganoff / ⅕ serv prepared	330
Hamburger Helper Potatoes Au Gratin / ⅕ mix dry	140
Hamburger Helper Potatoes Au Gratin / ⅕ serv prepared	350
Hamburger Helper Rice Oriental / ⅕ mix dry	180
Hamburger Helper Rice Oriental / ⅕ serv prepared	340
Hamburger Helper Stroganoff / ⅕ mix dry	190
Hamburger Helper Stroganoff / ⅕ serv prepared	390
Hamburger Helper Zesty Italian / ⅕ mix dry	170
Hamburger Helper Zesty Italian / ⅕ serv prepared	340
Herb and butter / 1 oz dry / **Golden Grain** Noodle Roni	114
Herb and butter / ½ cup prepared / **Golden Grain** Noodle Roni	240
Herb tomato / ½ cup as packaged / **Lipton** Pasta and Sauce	130
Homestyle / ½ cup prepared / **Kraft** Pasta Salad	240
Italian / ½ cup prepared / **Kraft** Light Pasta Salad	130
Italian, Robust / ½ cup as packaged / **Lipton** Pasta Salad	126
Italiano / 11 oz as packaged / **Lipton** Hearty Ones	327
Macaroni and cheese Mix: ¾ cup prepared	
Kraft	290
Kraft Deluxe	260
Kraft Dinomac	310
Kraft Family Size	290
Kraft Spirals	340
Kraft Teddy Bears	310
Kraft Wild Wheels	310
Meatloaf / ⅕ mix dry / **Hamburger Helper** Meat Loaf	70
Meatloaf / ⅕ serv prepared / **Hamburger Helper** Meat Loaf	360
Minestrone / 11 oz as packaged / **Lipton** Hearty Ones	189

Mushroom, creamy / ½ cup as packaged / **Lipton** Pasta and Sauce	143
Noodles Alfredo / ½ cup prepared / **Minute** Family Size Microwave	170
Noodles Alfredo / ½ cup prepared / **Minute** Single Size	160
Noodles and sauce Alfredo / ½ cup as packaged / **Lipton**	130
Noodles and sauce, chicken flavor / ½ cup as packaged / **Lipton**	125
Noodles and sauce, Parmesan / ½ cup as packaged / **Lipton**	138
Noodles and sauce, Stroganoff / ½ cup as packaged / **Lipton**	110
Noodles Parmesan / ½ cup prepared / **Minute** Family Size	170
Noodles Parmesan / ½ cup prepared / **Minute** Single Size	160
Noodles w chicken / 10.5 oz microwave prepared / **Chef Boyardee**	170
Parmesan / ½ cup prepared / **Kraft** Pasta and Cheese	180
Parmesano / 1.2 oz dry / **Golden Grain** Noodle Roni	135
Parmesano / ½ cup prepared / **Golden Grain** Noodle Roni	250
Pasta / 2 oz dry / **Golden Grain**	203
Pasta and cheddar cheese / ½ cup prepared / **Minute** Family Size	160
Pasta and cheddar cheese / ½ cup prepared / **Minute** Single Size	160
Rancher's Choice / ½ cup prepared / **Kraft** Light Pasta Salad	170
Rancher's Choice w bacon / ½ cup prepared / **Kraft** Pasta Salad	250
Romanoff	
Golden Grain Noodle Roni / 1.5 oz dry	168
Golden Grain Noodle Roni / ½ cup prepared	200
Lipton Noodles and Sauce / ½ cup dry	135
Shells and cheddar / 11 oz as packaged / **Lipton** Hearty Ones	367
Shells and cheese / prepared	
Mix: ½ cup / **Kraft** Velveeta	210
Mix: ½ cup / **Kraft** Velveeta Bits of Bacon	240
Mix: ½ cup / **Kraft** Velveeta Touch of Mexico	210

CALORIES

Shells in mushroom sauce / 7.5 oz microwave prepared /
    Chef Boyardee   170
Sloppy Joe / ⅙ mix dry / **Hamburger Helper** Sloppy Joe
    Bake   180
Sloppy Joe / ⅙ serv prepared / **Hamburger Helper**
    Sloppy Joe Bake   340
Sour cream and chives
    Lipton Noodles and Sauce / ½ cup as packaged   141
    Golden Grain Noodle Roni / ½ cup prepared   240
    Kraft Pasta and Cheese / ½ cup prepared   180
Spaghetti / ⅕ mix dry / **Hamburger Helper**   160
Spaghetti / ⅕ serv prepared / **Hamburger Helper**   340
Stroganoff / 2 oz dry / **Golden Grain** Noodle Roni   225
Stroganoff / ½ cup prepared / **Golden Grain** Noodle Roni   200
Taco / ⅙ mix dry / **Hamburger Helper** Tacobake   170
Taco / ⅙ serv prepared / **Hamburger Helper** Tacobake   320
Three cheeses w vegetables / ½ cup prepared / **Kraft**
    Pasta and Cheese   180
Tomato Alfredo / ½ cup as packaged / **Lipton** Noodles
    and Sauce   126
Tuna
    Tuna Helper Au Gratin / ⅕ mix dry   180
    Tuna Helper Au Gratin / ⅕ serv prepared   280
    Tuna Helper Buttery Rice / ⅕ mix dry   160
    Tuna Helper Buttery Rice / ⅕ serv prepared   280
    Tuna Helper Cheesy Noodles / ⅕ mix dry   160
    Tuna Helper Cheesy Noodles / ⅕ serv prepared   240
    Tuna Helper Creamy Mushroom / ⅕ mix dry   140
    Tuna Helper Creamy Mushroom / ⅕ serv prepared   220
    Tuna Helper Creamy Noodles / ⅕ mix dry   220
    Tuna Helper Creamy Noodles / ⅕ serv prepared   300
    Tuna Helper Fettucine Alfredo / ⅕ mix dry   160
    Tuna Helper Fettucine Alfredo / ⅕ serv prepared   300
    Tuna Helper Romanoff / ⅕ mix dry   210
    Tuna Helper Romanoff / ⅕ serv prepared   290
    Tuna Helper Tetrazzini / ⅕ mix dry   160
    Tuna Helper Tetrazzini / ⅕ serv prepared   240
    Tuna Helper Tuna Pot Pie / ⅙ mix dry   290
    Tuna Helper Tuna Pot Pie / ⅙ serv prepared   420
    Tuna Helper Tuna Salad / ⅕ mix dry   140
    Tuna Helper Tuna Salad / ⅕ serv prepared   420

CALORIES

Vegetable Alfredo / ½ cup prepared / **Golden Grain**
Noodle Roni   240

Doughnuts

CALORIES

1 doughnut unless noted

Chocolate-coated / **Dolly Madison**	130
Chocolate-iced, jumbo / **Dolly Madison**	200
Cinnamon / **Tastykake**	180
Cinnamon sugar, jumbo / **Dolly Madison**	190
Coconut crunch / **Dolly Madison**	140
Donut gems, chocolate-coated / 2 doughnuts / **Dolly Madison**	130
Donut gems, coconut crunch / 2 doughnuts / **Dolly Madison**	120
Donut gems, powdered sugar / 2 doughnuts / **Dolly Madison**	120
Dunkin'n stix / 1 stick / **Dolly Madison**	210
Honey wheat / **Tastykake**	210
Mini, cinnamon / **Tastykake**	50
Mini, honey wheat / **Tastykake**	40
Mini, powdered sugar / **Tastykake**	40
Mini, rich frosted / **Tastykake**	60
Old fashioned, chocolate-glazed / **Dolly Madison**	260
Old fashioned, chocolate-iced / **Dolly Madison**	300
Old fashioned, glazed / **Dolly Madison**	280
Old fashioned, white-iced / **Dolly Madison**	300
Orange-glazed / **Tastykake**	220
Plain / **Dolly Madison**	120
Plain / **Tastykake**	190
Plain, jumbo / **Dolly Madison**	190
Powdered sugar / **Dolly Madison**	120
Powdered sugar / **Tastykake**	180
Rich frosted / **Tastykake**	260
Sugar, jumbo / **Dolly Madison**	210

Eggs and Egg Dishes

EGGS

Chicken: raw, large
Whole, without shell / 1 egg	75
1 white	15
1 yolk	60

EGG DISHES, FROZEN

Egg, beefsteak and cheese / 4-9/10 oz / **Swanson** Great Starts	360
Egg, Canadian bacon and cheese / 5-1/5 oz / **Swanson** Great Starts	420
Egg, Canadian bacon and cheese / 4-1/10 oz / **Swanson** Great Starts	290
Egg, sausage and cheese / 5-1/2 oz / **Swanson** Great Starts	460
Eggs w mini oatbran muffins / 4-3/4 oz / **Swanson** Great Starts Reduced Chol	250
Omelet w cheese sauce and ham / 7 oz / **Swanson** Great Starts	390
Scrambled eggs w bacon and home fries / 5-3/5 oz / **Swanson** Great Starts	340
Scrambled eggs w cheese and pancakes / 3-2/5 oz / **Swanson** Great Starts	290
Scrambled eggs w home fries / 4-3/5 oz / **Swanson** Great Starts	260

CALORIES

Scrambled eggs w sausage and hash browns / 6-½ oz /
Swanson Great Starts 430
Scrambler and cheese / 3-½ oz / **Morningstar Farms** 220
Scrambler and pattie / 4-½ oz / **Morningstar Farms** 300
Scrambler, pattie and cheese / 5 oz / **Morningstar Farms** 350
Scramblers / ¼ cup / **Morningstar Farms** 60
Scramblers, cheese and home fries / 5 oz / **Morningstar
Farms** 210
Scramblers, links and hash browns / 5 oz / **Morningstar
Farms** 240
Scramblers, links and muffins / 4 oz / **Morningstar
Farms** 220

EGG MIXES

Egg, imitation
    Fleischmann's Egg Beaters / ¼ cup 25
    Healthy Choice Chol Free / 1-⁹⁄₁₀ oz 30
    Morningstar Farms Better'n Eggs / ¼ cup frozen 30
    Morningstar Farms Better'n Eggs / ¼ cup 25
Omelette mix, cheese / ½ pkg / **Fleischmann's** Egg
Beaters 110
Omelette mix, vegetable / ½ cup / **Fleischmann's** Egg
Beaters 50

Fish and Seafood

FRESH

3 oz raw unless noted

	CALORIES
Abalone	89
Bass, mixed species	97
Bass, striped	82
Bluefish	105
Butterfish	47
Carp	108
Cod	70
Crab Queen	76
Crayfish	76
Croaker	83
Cuttlefish	67
Dolphinfish	73
Drum	101
Herring	166
Ling	74
Lingcod	72
Lobster, spiny	95
Mackerel, Atlantic	174
Mackerel, King	89
Mackerel, Pacific and Jack	133
Milkfish	126
Monkfish	64
Mussels	73
Oysters, Pacific / 1 medium	41

CALORIES

Pike and walleye	79
Pollock	78
Pout	67
Rockfish	80
Roe	173
Roughy, orange	59
Sablefish	166
Salmon, Chinook	153
Seatrout	88
Scallops / 2 large	26
Shad	167
Spot	105
Sturgeon	90
Sucker, white	79
Sunfish, Pumpkinseed	76
Tuna, Skipjack	88
Tuna, yellowfin	92
Whitefish	114
Wolffish	82
Yellowtail	124

CANNED AND FROZEN

CALORIES

Clams	
Chopped / canned / 6-½ oz / **Doxsee**	90
Chopped / canned / 2 oz / **S & W**	28
Fried / frozen / 2-½ oz / **Mrs. Paul's**	200
Juice / canned / 3 fl oz / **Doxsee**	4
Juice / canned / 6 fl oz / **Mott's Clamato**	96
Minced / canned / 2 oz / **S & W**	28
Minced / canned / 6-½ oz / **Snow's**	90
Minced / canned, drained / ½ cup / **Progresso**	90
Minced / canned, undrained / ½ cup / **Progresso**	40
Whole baby, chowder / canned / 2 oz / **S & W**	33
Cod	
Frozen / 1 fillet / **Mrs. Paul's Light**	240
Light fillets / frozen / 1 fillet / **Van de Kamp's**	250
Natural fillets / frozen / 4 oz / **Van de Kamp's**	90
Crab	
Deviled / frozen / 1 cake / **Mrs. Paul's**	180
Deviled / frozen / 3-½ oz / **Mrs. Paul's** Miniatures	240
Dungeness / canned / 3-¼ oz / **S & W**	81

CALORIES

Fish, frozen

Cakes / 2 cakes / **Mrs. Paul's**	190
Fillets / 2 fillets / **Mrs. Paul's**	220
Fillets / batter-dipped / 2 fillets / **Mrs. Paul's**	330
Fillets / battered / 2 fillets / **Mrs. Paul's**	280
Fillets / battered / 1 fillet / **Van de Kamp's**	170
Fillets / breaded / 2 fillets / **Van de Kamp's**	280
Fillets, large / 1 fillet / **Van de Kamp's** Microwave	290
Fillets / light in butter sauce / 1 fillet / **Mrs. Paul's**	140
Fillets, small / 1 fillet / **Van de Kamp's** Microwave	140
Portion / battered / 2 portions / **Mrs. Paul's**	300
Portion / breaded / 2 portions / **Mrs. Paul's**	230
Sticks	
Mrs. Paul's / 4 sticks	190
Battered / 4 sticks / **Mrs. Paul's**	210
Breaded / 4 sticks / **Mrs. Paul's**	140
Van de Kamp's Microwave / 3 sticks	130
Battered / 4 sticks / **Van de Kamp's**	160
Breaded / 4 sticks / **Van de Kamp's**	200
Fishlets / can or jar / 1 piece / **Manischewitz**	8

Flounder, frozen

Mrs. Paul's Light / 1 fillet	240
Battered / 2 fillets / **Mrs. Paul's**	220
Light fillets / 1 fillet / **Van de Kamp's**	260
Natural fillets / 4 oz / **Van de Kamp's**	100

Gefilte fish, canned or in jars: 1 piece unless noted

Manischewitz (4-piece, 12-oz jar)	53
Manischewitz (8-piece, 24-oz jar)	53
Manischewitz (24-piece, 4-lb jar)	48
Manischewitz, homestyle (4-piece, 12-oz jar)	55
Manischewitz, homestyle (8-piece, 24-oz jar)	55
Manischewitz, homestyle (24-piece, 4-lb jar)	50
Manischewitz, sweet (4-piece, 12-oz jar)	65
Manischewitz, sweet (8-piece, 24-oz jar)	65
Manischewitz, sweet (24-piece, 4-lb jar)	59
Whitefish and pike	
Manischewitz / (4-piece, 11-oz jar)	49
Manischewitz (8-piece, 24-oz jar)	49
Manischewitz (24-piece, 4-lb jar)	44
Whitefish and pike, sweet	
Manischewitz (4-piece, 12-oz jar)	64
Manischewitz (8-piece, 24-oz jar)	64

CALORIES

Manischewitz (24-piece, 4-lb jar)	58
Haddock, frozen	
Mrs. Paul's Light / 1 fillet	220
Battered / 2 fillets / **Mrs. Paul's**	190
Fillets / battered / 2 fillets / **Van de Kamp's**	250
Fillets / breaded / 2 fillets / **Van de Kamp's**	270
Light fillets / 1 fillet / **Van de Kamp's**	240
Natural fillets / 4 oz / **Van de Kamp's**	90
Halibut, frozen fillets / battered / 2 fillets / **Van de Kamp's**	150
Oysters wo shell / canned / ½ cup / **Bumble Bee**	100
Oysters, whole / canned / 2 oz / **S & W**	95
Perch, frozen fillets / battered / 2 fillets / **Van de Kamp's**	310
Light fillets / 1 fillet / **Van de Kamp's**	280
Natural fillets / 4 oz / **Van de Kamp's**	130
Salmon, canned	
Keta / ½ can (3-⁷/₁₀ oz) / **Libby's**	130
Keta, regular / 3-½ oz / **Bumble Bee**	160
Pink	
Chicken of the Sea / 2 oz	60
Del Monte / ½ cup	160
Libby's / 7-¾ oz	310
Bumble Bee regular / 3-½ oz	160
Bumble Bee skinless, boneless / 3-½ oz	120
Red	
Del Monte / ½ cup	180
Bumble Bee regular / 3-½ oz	180
Bumble Bee skinless, boneless / 3-½ oz	130
Red sockeye	
Chicken of the Sea / 2 oz	60
Libby's / 7-¾ oz	380
S & W / 2 oz	190
Sardines, canned	
in mustard sauce / 3-¾ oz / **Underwood**	220
in oil / 3-¾ oz / **Underwood**	460
in olive oil / 1.5 oz / **S & W**	130
in olive oil / 3-¾ oz / **Underwood**	260
in soy oil / 3-¾ oz / **Underwood**	230
in tomato sauce / ½ cup / **Del Monte**	360
in tomato sauce / 3-¾ oz / **Underwood**	220
w Tabasco brand pepper sauce / 3-¾ oz / **Underwood**	220
Scallops, frozen / fried / 3 oz / **Mrs. Paul's**	160

CALORIES

Shrimp, canned / deveined whole / 2 oz / **S & W**	65
Sole, frozen	
Mrs. Paul's Light / 1 fillet	240
Light fillets / 1 fillet / **Van de Kamp's**	250
Natural fillets / 4 oz / **Van de Kamp's**	100
Tuna, canned: 2 oz unless noted	
Light, solid / ⅓ cup / **Progresso**	150
Light, chunk in oil	
Bumble Bee	160
Chicken of the Sea	170
S & W	140
StarKist	150
Light, chunk in water	
Bumble Bee	60
Chicken of the Sea	60
Chicken of the Sea Less Salt	60
S & W	60
StarKist Diet	65
StarKist Hickory Smoke	50
StarKist Select, Less Salt	65
Weight Watchers No Salt Added	60
Light, chunk in water / **Chicken of the Sea** Lite	70
Light, solid in oil / **Chicken of the Sea**	120
Light, solid in oil / **StarKist** Prime Catch	150
Light, solid in water / **StarKist**	60
Light, solid in water / **StarKist** Prime Catch	60
White, chunk in oil / **Bumble Bee**	160
White, chunk in oil / **StarKist**	140
White, chunk in water	
Bumble Bee	70
Chicken of the Sea Dietetic	60
StarKist	70
StarKist Diet	70
StarKist Select, Less Salt	70
White, solid in oil	
Bumble Bee	130
Chicken of the Sea	120
S & W	160
StarKist	140
White, solid in water	
Bumble Bee	70
Chicken of the Sea	60

StarKist	70
StarKist Hickory Smoke	60
Weight Watchers, No Salt Added	70

FISH AND SEAFOOD ENTREES, FROZEN

Fillet of fish au gratin / 9-¼ oz / **Weight Watchers**	200
Fish and fries / 6-½ oz / **Swanson** Homestyle	340
Fish Dijon / 8-¾ oz / **Mrs. Paul's** Light	200
Fish Divan / 10-⅜ oz / **Stouffer's** Lean Cuisine	210
Fish Florentine / 8 oz / **Mrs. Paul's** Light	220
Fish Florentine / 9-⅝ oz / **Stouffer's** Lean Cuisine	220
Fish Mornay / 9 oz / **Mrs. Paul's** Light	230
Lobster Newberg / 6-½ oz / **Stouffer's**	380
Oven-fried fish / 7 oz / **Weight Watchers**	240
Seafood Creole w rice / 9 oz / **Swanson** Homestyle	240
Seafood Lasagna / 9-½ oz / **Mrs. Paul's** Light	290
Seafood Newburg / 8 oz / **Healthy Choice**	200
Seafood Rotini / 9 oz / **Mrs. Paul's** Light	240
Shrimp and clams w linguini / 10 oz / **Mrs. Paul's** Light	240
Shrimp Creole	
Armour Classics Lite / 11-¼ oz	260
Healthy Choice / 11 oz	230
UltraSlim-Fast / 12 oz	240
Shrimp Marinara / 10-½ oz / **Healthy Choice**	260
Sole w lemon and butter sauce / 8-¼ oz / **Healthy Choice**	230
Sole au Gratin / 11 oz / **Healthy Choice**	270
Tuna noodle casserole / 10 oz / **Stouffer's**	310

Flavorings, Sweet

CALORIES

1 tsp

Almond extract, pure / **McCormick/Schilling**	10
Anise extract, pure / **McCormick/Schilling**	23
Banana extract, imitation / **McCormick/Schilling**	11

CALORIES

Black walnut extract, imitation / **McCormick/Schilling**	12
Brandy extract, imitation / **McCormick/Schilling**	20
Chocolate extract, imitation / **McCormick/Schilling**	8
Coconut extract, imitation / **McCormick/Schilling**	7
Lemon extract, pure / **McCormick/Schilling**	35
Maple flavor, imitation / **McCormick/Shilling**	8
Mint extract, pure / **McCormick/Schilling**	20
Orange extract, pure / **McCormick/Schilling**	23
Pineapple extract, imitation / **McCormick/Schilling**	12
Rum extract, imitation / **McCormick/Schilling**	19
Sherry extract, pure / **McCormick/Schilling**	14
Strawberry extract, imitation / **McCormick/Schilling**	7
Vanilla butter and nut flavor / **McCormick/Schilling**	na
Vanilla extract, pure / **McCormick/Schilling**	12

Flour and Meal

FLOUR

CALORIES

1 cup unless noted

Biscuit mix / **Bisquick**	240
Buckwheat, dark, sifted	326
Buckwheat, light, sifted	340
Carob	250
Lima bean, sifted	432
Oat flour blend / **Gold Medal**	390
Peanut, defatted	224
Rye	
Light	314
Medium / **Pillsbury's Best**	400
Dark	
Stone ground / **Robin Hood**	360
Wheat	
Pillsbury's Best	400

CALORIES

All purpose	500
Bread	500
Bread / **Pillsbury's Best**	400
Cake or pastry	430
Gluten	530
Self-rising	440
Whole wheat	400
Whole wheat / **Gold Medal**	350
Whole wheat / **Pillsbury's Best**	400
Whole wheat blend / **Gold Medal**	380
White	
Aunt Jemima Self-Rising / ¼ cup	109
Ballard All Purpose	400
Drifted Snow	400
Gold Medal All Purpose	400
Gold Medal Self-Rising	380
Gold Medal Unbleached	400
La Pina	400
Pillsbury's Best Bleached	400
Pillsbury's Best Self-Rising	380
Pillsbury's Best Shake and Blend	50
Pillsbury's Best Unbleached	400
Red Band All Purpose	390
Red Band Self-Rising	380
Robin Hood All Purpose	400
Robin Hood Self-Rising	380
Robin Hood Unbleached	400
Softasilk / ¼ cup	100
White Deer All Purpose	400
Wondra	400
High protein / **Gold Medal** Better for Bread	400

MEAL

Almond, partially defatted / 1 oz	116
Corn	
White / 1 oz uncooked / **Albers**	100
White / 3 tbsp / **Aunt Jemima**	102
White / 3 tbsp / **Aunt Jemima** Bolted	99
White / 3 tbsp / **Aunt Jemima** Buttermilk Self-Rising	101
White / 3 tbsp / **Aunt Jemima** Self-Rising	98

CALORIES

White / 3 tbsp / **Quaker**	102
White, enriched / 3 tbsp / **Aunt Jemima** Bolted Self-Rising	99
Yellow / 1 oz uncooked / **Albers**	100
Yellow / 3 tbsp / **Aunt Jemima**	102
Yellow / 3 tbsp / **Aunt Jemima** Self-Rising	100
Yellow / 3 tbsp / **Quaker**	102
Matzo farfel / 1 cup / **Manischewitz**	180
Matzo meal / 1 cup / **Manischewitz**	514

Frostings

READY TO SPREAD

CALORIES

¹⁄₁₂ can unless noted

Butter fudge / **Pillsbury**	140
Butter pecan / **Betty Crocker**	170
Caramel pecan / **Pillsbury**	150
Cherry / **Betty Crocker**	160
Chocolate / **Betty Crocker**	160
Chocolate / **Betty Crocker** Light	130
Chocolate / **Duncan Hines**	160
Chocolate chip / **Betty Crocker**	170
Chocolate chip / **Pillsbury**	150
Chocolate fudge / **Pillsbury**	150
Chocolate fudge / **Pillsbury** Frosting Supreme Funfetti	140
Chocolate fudge / **Pillsbury** Lovin' Lites	130
Chocolate w choc chips / **Betty Crocker** Party Frostings	160
Chocolate w dinosaurs / **Betty Crocker** Party Frostings	160
Chocolate w racers / **Betty Crocker** Party Frostings	160
Coconut almond / **Pillsbury**	150
Coconut pecan / **Betty Crocker**	160
Coconut pecan / **Pillsbury**	160
Cream cheese	
Betty Crocker	170

Duncan Hines	160
Pillsbury	160
Dark Dutch fudge / **Betty Crocker**	160
Double Dutch / **Pillsbury**	140
Dutch fudge / **Duncan Hines**	160
Icing, cake and cookie / **Pillsbury** Decorator Icing	60
Lemon	
Betty Crocker	170
Duncan Hines	60
Pillsbury	160
Milk chocolate	
Betty Crocker	160
Betty Crocker Light	140
Duncan Hines	160
Pillsbury	150
Pillsbury Lovin' Lites	130
Milk chocolate w fudge swirl / **Pillsbury**	150
Pink vanilla / **Pillsbury** Frosting Supreme Funfetti	150
Rainbow chip / **Betty Crocker**	170
Sour cream, chocolate / **Betty Crocker**	160
Sour cream, white / **Betty Crocker**	160
Strawberry / **Pillsbury**	160
Sunshine vanilla / **Pillsbury** Frosting Supreme Funfetti	150
Vanilla	
Betty Crocker	160
Betty Crocker Light	140
Duncan Hines	160
Pillsbury	160
Pillsbury Frosting Supreme Funfetti	150
Pillsbury Lovin' Lites	130
Vanilla w bears / **Betty Crocker** Party Frostings	160
Vanilla w fudge swirl / **Pillsbury**	150

MIXES

¹⁄₁₂ package prepared, unless noted

Chocolate fudge / **Betty Crocker**	140
Coconut pecan / **Betty Crocker**	110
Fudge / ¾ oz dry / **Jiffy**	90
Milk chocolate / **Betty Crocker**	140

CALORIES

Vanilla / **Betty Crocker**	150
White / **Betty Crocker**	70
White / ¾ oz dry / **Jiffy**	100

Fruit

FRESH

	CALORIES
Acerola cherries / 1 fruit	2
Apples	
w skin / 1 small (about 4 per lb)	61
w skin / 1 medium (about 3 per lb)	80
w skin / 1 large (about 2 per lb)	125
Peeled / sliced, 1 cup	65
Dried, sulfured / 10 rings	155
Apricots / raw, wo pits / 3 fruits (about 12 per lb)	50
Avocados, California / raw, whole, wo skin and seed / 1 fruit (about 2 per lb)	305
Avocados, Florida / raw, whole, wo skin and seed / 1 fruit (about 1 per lb)	340
Bananas / raw, wo peel / 1 fruit (about 2-½ per lb)	105
Bananas / raw / 1 cup (sliced)	140
Blackberries / raw / 1 cup	75
Blueberries / raw / 1 cup	80
Cherries	
Raw, sour, red, wo pits / 1 cup	77
Raw, sweet wo pits / 10 fruits	50
Cranberries	
Raw, chopped / 1 cup	54
Raw, whole / 1 cup	46
Dates	
Chopped / 1 cup	490
Whole wo pits / 10 fruits	230
Elderberries / raw / 1 cup	105

CALORIES

Figs	
Dried / 10 fruits	475
Raw / 1 medium	37
Raw / 1 large	47
Gooseberries / raw / 1 cup	67
Grapefruit / 3-¾-in diam / half	40
Grapefruit sections / 1 cup w juice	74
Grapes	
Raw, American (slip skin) / 10 fruits	15
Raw, European, (adherent skin)	
Thompson seedless / 10 fruits	35
Tokay and Emperor, seeded / 10 fruits	40
Kiwifruit / raw, wo skin / 1 fruit (about 5 per lb)	45
Lemons	
Raw, wo peel / 1 fruit (about 4 per lb)	15
Raw, w peel / 1 medium	22
Raw, w peel / 1 wedge	5
Limes / raw / 1 fruit	20
Logans / raw / 1 fruit	2
Loquats / raw / 1 fruit	5
Lychees / raw / 1 fruit	6
Mangos / raw, wo skin / 1 fruit (about 1-½ per lb)	135
Melons	
Canteloupe, 5-½-in diam / ½ fruit (2-⅓ lb whole)	95
Casaba, cubed / 1 cup	45
Honeydew, 6-½-in diam /¹⁄₁₀ fruit (5-¼ lb whole)	45
Mulberries / raw / 1 cup	61
Nectarines / raw / 1 fruit (about 3 per lb)	65
Oranges	
Whole, wo peel, 2-⅝-in diam / 1 fruit (about 2-½ per lb)	60
Sections, wo membranes / 1 cup	85
Papayas / raw, ½-in cubes / 1 cup	65
Peaches	
Raw, whole, peeled / 1 fruit (about 4 per lb)	35
Raw, sliced, peeled / 1 cup	75
Pears	
Raw, whole, Asian / 1 small fruit	51
Raw, whole, Asian / 1 large fruit	115
Raw, w skin, cored, Bartlett / 1 fruit (about 2-½ per lb)	100
Raw, w skin, cored, Bosc / 1 fruit (about 3 per lb)	85

CALORIES

Raw, w skin, cored, D'Anjou / 1 fruit (about 2 per lb)	120
Persimmons	
Raw, Japanese / 1 fruit	118
Raw, Native / 1 fruit	32
Pineapple / raw, diced / 1 cup	75
Plantains / raw, wo peel / 1 fruit	220
Plums	
Raw, wo pits, 2-½-in diam / 1 fruit (about 6-½ per lb)	35
Raw, wo pits, 1-½-in diam / 1 fruit (about 15 per lb)	15
Pomegranates / raw, 3-⅜-in diam / 1 fruit	104
Raspberries / raw / 1 cup	60
Rhubarb	
Cooked, w sugar / 1 cup	280
Raw, diced / 1 cup	26
Strawberries / raw, whole / 1 cup	45
Tangerines / raw, wo peel, 2-⅜-in diam / 1 fruit (about 4 per lb)	35
Watermelon	
Raw, wo rind, diced / 1 cup	50
Raw, wo rind, wedge / 1 piece, 4 in x 8 in	155

CANNED AND FROZEN

CALORIES

Apples, sliced, canned: 4 oz unless noted	
Luck's fried / 8 oz	200
Luck's fried w raisins / 8 oz	230
Lucky Leaf Chipped	50
Lucky Leaf Diced	50
Lucky Leaf Syrup Pack	50
Lucky Leaf Water Pack	50
Lucky Leaf unpeeled	90
Musselman's Chipped	50
Musselman's Diced	50
Musselman's Syrup Pack	50
Musselman's Water Pack	50
Musselman's unpeeled	90
Apple slices, frozen / **Lucky Leaf** / 4 oz	70
Apple slices, frozen / **Musselman's** / 4 oz	70
Apples, whole, peeled, canned	
Lucky Leaf / 1 apple	90

Lucky Leaf apple rings, spiced / 4 oz	100
Musselman's / 1 apple	90
Musselman's apple rings, spiced / 4 oz	100
Apples, whole, baked, canned / 1 apple / **Lucky Leaf**	110
Apples, whole, baked, canned / 1 apple / **Musselman's**	110
Applesauce in cans or jars: 4 oz unless noted	
Del Monte / ½ cup	90
Del Monte Lite / ½ cup	50
Lucky Leaf w Prune	100
Lucky Leaf Chunky	80
Lucky Leaf Chunky Cranberry	80
Lucky Leaf Grapefruit	90
Lucky Leaf Juice Pack	50
Lucky Leaf Natural Cinnamon	50
Lucky Leaf Sweetened	80
Lucky Leaf Unsweetened	50
Lucky Leaf w Apricot	90
Lucky Leaf w Cherry	100
Lucky Leaf w Cranberry	100
Lucky Leaf w Orange	90
Lucky Leaf w Papaya	100
Lucky Leaf w Peach	90
Lucky Leaf w Pineapple	110
Lucky Leaf w Raspberry	100
Lucky Leaf w Strawberry	100
Mott's Cherry Fruit Pak / 3-¾ oz	72
Mott's Chunky	88
Mott's Cinnamon	92
Mott's Dutch Apple Spice	84
Mott's Mixed Fruit Pak / 3-¾ oz	80
Mott's Natural	48
Mott's Peach Fruit Pak / 3-¾ oz	75
Mott's Pineapple Fruit Pak / 3-¾ oz	86
Mott's Strawberry Fruit Pak / 3-¾ oz	76
Mott's Sweetened	88
Musselman's Chunky	80
Musselman's Chunky Cranberry	80
Musselman's Homestyle Chunky	90
Musselman's Juice Pack	50
Musselman's Natural Cinnamon	50
Musselman's Sweetened	80

Musselman's Unsweetened	50
Musselman's w Apricot	90
Musselman's w Cherry	100
Musselman's w Cranberry	100
Musselman's w Grapefruit	90
Musselman's w Orange	90
Musselman's w Papaya	100
Musselman's w Peach	90
Musselman's w Pineapple	110
Musselman's w Prune	100
Musselman's w Raspberry	100
Musselman's w Strawberry	100
Seneca / ½ cup	90
Seneca Cinnamon / ½ cup	90
Seneca Golden Delicious / ½ cup	90
Seneca McIntosh / ½ cup	90
Seneca Natural / ½ cup	50
Apricots, canned: ½ cup	
Halves, unpeeled / **Del Monte**	100
Halves, unpeeled / **Del Monte** Lite	60
Whole, peeled / **Del Monte**	100
Blueberries, canned: 4 oz	
Lucky Leaf Water Pack	40
Musselman's Water Pack	40
Cherries, canned	
Dark, sweet, pitted / ½ cup / **Del Monte**	90
Dark, sweet w pits / ½ cup / **Del Monte**	90
Red, tart, pitted / 4 oz / **Lucky Leaf**	50
Red, tart, pitted / 4 oz / **Musselman's**	50
Sweet w pits / ½ cup / **Del Monte** Lite	100
Crabapples, canned / spiced / 4 oz / **Lucky Leaf**	110
Crabapples, canned / spiced /4 oz / **Musselman's**	110
Figs, canned / ½ cup / **Del Monte**	100
Fruit cocktail, canned	
Del Monte / ½ cup	80
Del Monte Lite / ½ cup	50
Hunt's	90
Fruit salad, canned / ½ cup / **Del Monte** Tropical	90
Fruit salad, canned / tropical in light syrup / ½ cup / **Queen's Pride**	70
Fruits for salad, canned / ½ cup / **Del Monte**	90

CALORIES

Mandarin orange segments / canned / ½ cup / **Dole**	70
Mixed, canned	
Del Monte Chunky / ½ cup	80
Del Monte Fruit Cup / 5 oz	100
Del Monte Lite Chunky / ½ cup	50
Mixed, frozen in syrup / 5 oz / **Birds Eye** Quick Thaw	120
Oranges, Mandarin, canned / 5-½ oz / **Del Monte**	100
Peaches, canned	
Cling, diced / 5 oz / **Del Monte** Fruit Cup	110
Cling, halves / ½ cup / **Del Monte**	80
Cling, halves / ½ cup / **Del Monte** Lite	50
Cling, halves / 4 oz / **Hunt's**	90
Cling, slices / ½ cup / **Del Monte**	80
Cling, slices / ½ cup / **Del Monte** Lite	50
Cling, slices / 4 oz / **Hunt's**	90
Freestone / ½ cup / **Del Monte** Lite	60
Freestone, halves / ½ cup / **Del Monte**	90
Freestone, slices / ½ cup / **Del Monte**	90
Spiced w pits / 3-½ oz / **Del Monte**	80
Pears, canned	
Halves / 4 oz / **Hunt's**	90
Bartlett, halves / ½ cup / **Del Monte**	80
Bartlett, halves / ½ cup / **Del Monte** Lite	50
Bartlett, slices / ½ cup / **Del Monte**	80
Bartlett, slices / ½ cup / **Del Monte** Lite	50
Pineapple, canned	
All cuts in juice / ½ cup / **Del Monte**	70
All cuts in juice / ½ cup / **Dole**	70
All cuts in syrup / ½ cup / **Del Monte**	90
All cuts in syrup / ½ cup / **Dole**	90
All cuts in unsweetened juice / 1 cup / **Libby's**	140
Pineapple-Mandarin orange segments / ½ cup / **Dole**	60
Spears / 2 spears / **Del Monte**	50
Raspberries, red, frozen in lite syrup / 5 oz / **Birds Eye** Quick Thaw	100
Strawberries, frozen	
Halves in lite syrup / **Birds Eye** Quick Thaw	90
Halves in syrup / 5 oz / **Birds Eye** Quick Thaw	120
Tropical fruit salad, canned / ½ cup / **Dole**	70

DRIED UNCOOKED

Apple, slices / 2 oz / **Del Monte**	140
Apricots / 2 oz / **Del Monte**	140
Berries / 6-¾ oz / **Betty Crocker** Squeezit	90
Cherries	
Betty Crocker Squeezit / 6-¾ oz	90
Sunkist Fruit Flippits / ⅘ oz	107
Currants, Zante / ½ cup / **Del Monte**	200
Dates, chopped / ½ cup / **Dole**	280
Dates, pitted / ½ cup / **Dole**	280
Fruit rolls	
Cherry Apricot / 1 roll / **Sunkist**	76
Betty Crocker Fruit By The Foot / 1 roll	80
Betty Crocker Fruit Roll-Ups / ½-oz roll	50
Sunkist / 1 roll	75
Crazy Colors / ½-oz roll / **Betty Crocker** Fruit Roll-Ups	50
Fruit Punch / ½-oz roll / **Betty Crocker** Fruit Roll-Ups	50
Grape	
Betty Crocker Fruit By The Foot / 1 roll	80
Betty Crocker Fruit Roll-Ups / ½-oz roll	50
Sunkist / 1 roll	76
Punch / 1 roll / **Sunkist**	74
Raspberry / ½-oz roll / **Betty Crocker** Fruit Roll-Ups	50
Raspberry / 1 roll / **Sunkist**	75
Strawberry	
Betty Crocker Fruit By The Foot / 1 roll	80
Betty Crocker Fruit Roll-Ups / ½-oz roll	50
Sunkist / 1 roll	74
Fruit snacks, apple / ½ oz / **Weight Watchers**	50
Fruit snacks, cinnamon flavor / ½ oz / **Weight Watchers**	50
Fruit snacks, peach flavor / ½ oz / **Weight Watchers**	50
Fruit snacks, strawberry flavor / ½ oz / **Weight Watchers**	50
Grapes / 6-¾ oz / **Betty Crocker** Squeezit	90
Mixed: 1 pouch unless noted	
Betty Crocker Berry Bears, Ass't Fruit	100
Betty Crocker Berry Bears, Fruit Punch	100
Betty Crocker Garfield and Friends 1-2 Punch	100
Betty Crocker Garfield and Friends Cat Cooler	100
Betty Crocker Garfield and Friends Fat Cat	50

CALORIES

Betty Crocker Garfield and Friends Fruit Party	50
Betty Crocker Shark Bites, Ass't Fruit	100
Betty Crocker Shark Bites, Fruit Punch	100
Betty Crocker Surf's Up, Sun Splash	100
Betty Crocker Surf's Up, Tutti Frutti	100
Betty Crocker Thunder Jets, Ass't Fruit	100
Betty Crocker Thunder Jets, Mach 1	100
Del Monte / 2 oz	130
Del Monte Orchard Fruit Snacks / 1 oz	80
Del Monte Sierra Fruit Snacks / 1 oz	150
Del Monte Tropical Fruit Snacks / 1 oz	90
Sunkist Fun Fruit, All Shapes / 9 oz	100
Sunkist Fun Fruit, Wacky Players / 9 oz	100
Oranges / 6-¾ oz / **Betty Crocker** Squeezit	90
Peaches / 2 oz / **Del Monte**	140
Prunes	
Del Monte Moist Pak / 2 oz	120
Pitted / **Del Monte** / 2 oz	140
w pits / **Del Monte** / 2 oz	120
Punch / 6-¾ oz / **Betty Crocker** Squeezit	90
Raisins, Golden / 3 oz / **Del Monte**	260
Raisins, Golden / ½ cup / **Dole**	260
Raisins, Natural / 3 oz / **Del Monte**	250
Raisins, Seedless / ½ cup / **Dole**	260
Raisins, strawberry yogurt / 1 oz / **Del Monte** Fruit Snacks	130
Raisins, yogurt / 1 oz / **Del Monte** Fruit Snacks	130
Strawberries	
Betty Crocker Garfield and Friends / 1 pouch	100
Betty Crocker Squeezit / 6-¾ oz	90

Fruit Drinks and Fruit-Flavored Beverages

CALORIES

In bottles, cans, cartons, pouches, boxes, frozen or as a mix: 6 fl oz unless noted

Apple-cranberry / 11.5 fl oz / **Mott's**	188
Apple-cranberry juice cocktail / **Welch's**	110
Apple-grape-cherry juice blend cocktail	
Frozen, reconstituted / **Welch's** Orchard	110
Welch's bottled	120
Welch's Orchard / 8.45 oz box	150
Apple-grape cocktail / frozen, reconstituted / **Welch's** Orchard	110
Apple-grape juice cocktail / bottled / **Welch's** Orchard	110
Apple-grape juice cocktail / 8.45 oz box / **Welch's** Orchard	150
Apple-grape-raspberry juice blend cocktail / frozen, reconstituted / **Welch's** Orchard	110
Apple-grape-raspberry juice cocktail / **Welch's**	120
Apple-grape-raspberry juice cocktail / 8.45 oz box / **Welch's** Orchard	150
Apple-orange-pineapple / bottled / **Welch's** Orchard	110
Apple-orange-pineapple juice cocktail / **Welch's**	110
Apple-orange-pineapple juice cocktail / frozen, reconstituted / **Welch's**	110
Apple-orange-pineapple juice cocktail / 8.45 fl oz box / **Welch's** Orchard	150
Apple-orange-pineapple juice cocktail / frozen, reconstituted **Welch's** Orchard	110
Apple-raspberry / 11.5 fl oz / **Mott's**	172

CALORIES

Berry / mix, prepared / 8 fl oz / **Wylers**, Sweetened Bunch 'O Berries	81
Berry / mix, prepared / 8 fl oz / **Wylers** Unsweetened, Berry Burst	2
Berry / mix, prepared / 8 fl oz / **Wylers** Unsweetened Bunch 'O Berries	2
Berry blue / mix, prepared / 8 fl oz / **Kool-Aid**	100
Berry blue / mix, prepared / 8 fl oz / **Kool-Aid** Sugar Free	4
Berry blue / mix, prepared / 8 fl oz / **Kool-Aid** Sugar Sweetened	80
Black cherry / 2 tbsp, reconstituted / **Hain**	70
Black cherry / mix, prepared / 8 fl oz / **Kool-Aid**	100
Cherry	
Tang / 8.45 fl oz	120
Crystal Light / mix, prepared / 8 fl oz	4
Kool-Aid / mix, prepared / 8 fl oz	100
Kool-Aid Koolers / as pkgd / 8.45 fl oz	140
Kool-Aid, Sugar Free / mix, prepared / 8 fl oz	4
Kool-Aid, Sugar Sweetened / mix, prepared / 8 fl oz	80
Wylers Sweetened Wild / mix, prepared / 8 fl oz	81
Wylers Unsweetened / mix, prepared / 8 fl oz	2
Wylers Unsweetened Black / mix, prepared / 8 fl oz	2
Citrus / mix, prepared / 8 fl oz / **Crystal Light**	4
Cranberry / 2 tbsp, reconstituted / **Hain**	40
Cranberry-apple juice cocktail / bottled or canned / **Seneca**	110
Cranberry-apple juice cocktail / frozen, reconstituted / **Seneca**	110
Cranberry-apple juice cocktail / frozen, reconstituted / **Welch's**	120
Cranberry-cherry juice cocktail / frozen, reconstituted / **Welch's**	110
Cranberry juice cocktail	
Seneca / bottled or canned	110
Seneca / frozen, reconstituted	110
Welch's / frozen, reconstituted	100
Welch's Juice Cocktail, No Sugar Added / frozen, reconstituted	40
Cranberry-orange juice cocktail / frozen, reconstituted / **Welch's**	110

Cranberry-raspberry juice cocktail / frozen, reconstituted / **Welch's**	110
Cranberry-raspberry juice cocktail / frozen, reconstituted / **Welch's** Juice Cocktail, No Sugar Added	40
Fruit punch / mix, prepared / 8 fl oz / **Crystal Light**	4
Fruit punch / 11.5 fl oz / **Mott's**	188
Grape	
Bama / 8.45 fl oz	120
Shasta Plus / 12 fl oz	176
Tang / 8.45 fl oz	130
Welch's	110
Kool-Aid / mix, prepared / 8 fl oz	100
Kool-Aid Koolers / as pkgd / 8.45 fl oz	140
Kool-Aid, Sugar Free / mix, prepared / 8 fl oz	4
Kool-Aid, Sugar Sweetened / mix, prepared / 8 fl oz	80
Welch's Juice Cocktail, No Sugar Added / frozen, reconstituted	40
Welch's Orchard / bottled	110
Welch's Orchard Juice Cocktail / 8.45 fl oz box	150
Wylers, Unsweetened / mix, prepared / 8 fl oz	2
Wylers Wild, Sweetened / mix, prepared / 8 fl oz	81
Grape-apple / 11.5 fl oz / **Mott's**	176
Grape-cranberry juice cocktail / bottled or canned / **Seneca**	110
Grape-cranberry juice cocktail / frozen, reconstituted / **Seneca**	110
Grapefruit, pink, juice cocktail / **Welch's**	90
Guava juice cocktail / frozen, reconstituted / **Welch's** Orchard Tropicals	100
Harvest Blend juice cocktail / as pkgd / 8.48 fl oz box / **Welch's** Orchard	150
Harvest Blend juice cocktail / frozen, reconstituted / **Welch's** Orchard	110
Harvest Blend juice cocktail / bottled / **Welch's** Orchard	110
Lemon-lime / mix, prepared / 8 fl oz / **Crystal Light**	4
Lemon lime / mix, prepared / 8 fl oz / **Kool-Aid**	100
Lemonade	
Mott's / 11.5 fl oz	140
Shasta Non Carb / 12 fl oz	168
Shasta Plus / 12 fl oz	172
Welch's Juice Cocktail	100

CALORIES

Wylers	64
Wylers / 8 fl oz	110.1
Country Time / mix, prepared / 8 fl oz	80
Country Time Sugar Free / mix, prepared / 8 fl oz	4
Crystal Light / mix, prepared / 8 fl oz	4
Kool-Aid / mix, prepared / 8 fl oz	100
Kool-Aid Pink / mix, prepared / 8 fl oz	100
Kool-Aid, Sugar Free / mix, prepared / 8 fl oz	4
Kool-Aid, Sugar Sweetened / mix, prepared / 8 fl oz	80
Wylers Crystals / mix, prepared / 8 fl oz	78
Wylers Sweetened, Pink / mix, prepared / 8 fl oz	78
Wylers Unsweetened / mix, prepared / 8 fl oz	3
Wylers Unsweetened, Pink / mix, prepared / 8 fl oz	3
Mixed fruit / 8.45 fl oz / **Tang**	140

Orange

Bama / 8.45 fl oz	120
Mott's Orange-Fruit Juice Blend / 11.5 fl oz	124
Shasta Plus / 12 fl oz	184
Tang / 8.45 fl oz	130
Tang Tropical / 8.45 fl oz	150
Kool-Aid / mix, prepared / 8 fl oz	100
Kool-Aid Koolers / 8.45 fl oz	110
Kool-Aid, Sugar Sweetened / mix, prepared / 8 fl oz	80
Tang Breakfast Crystals / mix, prepared	90
Tang Sugar Free Breakfast Crystals / mix, prepared	6
Wylers Unsweetened / mix, prepared / 8 fl oz	2
Orange-apricot / **Musselman's** Breakfast Cocktail	90
Orange-pineapple / **Musselman's** Breakfast Cocktail	90
Passion fruit / **Welch's** Orchard	100
Passion fruit / 8.45 fl oz box / **Welch's** Orchard	140
Passion fruit juice cocktail / frozen, reconstituted / **Welch's** Orchard Tropicals	100
Pineapple-banana / 8.45 fl oz box / **Welch's**	140
Pineapple-banana / **Welch's** Orchard	100
Pineapple-banana juice cocktail / frozen, reconstituted / **Welch's** Orchard Tropicals	100
Pineapple-grapefruit / **Del Monte**	90
Pineapple-orange / **Del Monte**	90
Pineapple-pink grapefruit / **Del Monte**	90

Punch

Bama / 8.45 fl oz	130

CALORIES

Kool-Aid Koolers, Mountain Berry / 8.45 fl oz	140
Kool-Aid Koolers, Rainbow / 8.45 fl oz	130
Kool-Aid Koolers, Tropical / 8.45 fl oz	130
Shasta Non Carb / 12 fl oz	196
Shasta Plus / 12 fl oz	168
Welch's Juice Cocktail	110
Welch's Orchard Juice Cocktail / box / 8.45 fl oz	150
Wylers Fruit / 8 fl oz	125.9
Kool-Aid Mountain Berry / mix, prepared / 8 fl oz	100
Kool-Aid Rainbow / mix, prepared / 8 fl oz	100
Kool-Aid, Sugar Free, Mountain Berry / mix, prepared / 8 fl oz	4
Kool-Aid, Sugar Free, Surfin' Berry / mix, prepared / 8 fl oz	4
Kool-Aid, Sugar Free, Tropical / mix, prepared / 8 fl oz	4
Kool-Aid, Sugar Sweetened, Mountain Berry / mix, prepared / 8 fl oz	80
Kool-Aid, Sugar Sweetened, Rainbow / mix, prepared / 8 fl oz	80
Kool-Aid, Sugar Sweetened, Tropical / mix, prepared / 8 fl oz	80
Kool-Aid Surfin' Berry / mix, prepared / 8 fl oz	100
Kool-Aid Tropical / mix, prepared / 8 fl oz	100
Welch's Orchard / frozen, reconstituted	110
Wylers Tropical / canned	82
Wylers Tropical Crystals / mix, prepared / 8 fl oz	80
Wylers Unsweetened / mix, prepared / 8 fl oz	2
Purplesaurus rex	
Kool-Aid / mix, prepared / 8 fl oz	100
Kool-Aid, Sugar Free / mix, prepared / 8 fl oz	4
Kool-Aid, Sugar Sweetened / mix, prepared / 8 fl oz	80
Raspberry	
Kool-Aid / mix, prepared / 8 fl oz	100
Kool-Aid, Sugar Sweetened / mix, prepared / 8 fl oz	80
Wylers, Unsweetened / mix, prepared / 8 fl oz	2
Raspberry-cranberry juice cocktail / bottled or canned / **Seneca**	110
Raspberry-cranberry juice cocktail / frozen, reconstituted / **Seneca**	110

CALORIES

Sharkleberry fin
Kool-Aid, Sugar Free / mix, prepared / 8 fl oz   4
Kool-Aid, Sugar Sweetened / mix, prepared / 8 fl oz   80
Kool-Aid / mix, prepared / 8 fl oz   100
Strawberry
Tang / 8.45 fl oz   120
Kool-Aid / mix, prepared / 8 fl oz   100
Kool-Aid, Sugar Sweetened / mix, prepared / 8 fl oz   80
Tang / 8.45 fl oz   120
Wylers Artificial, Wild / mix, prepared / 8 fl oz   85
Wylers Unsweetened / mix, prepared / 8 fl oz   2
Wylers Unsweetened, Wild / mix, prepared / 8 fl oz   2
Tropical juice cocktail / **Welch's**   110

Fruit Juices

FRESH

CALORIES

1 cup unless noted

Acerola cherry   51
Grapefruit   95
Lemon   60
Lime   65
Orange, all varieties   110
Passion, purple   126
Passion, yellow   149
Tangerine   106

BOTTLED, CANNED AND FROZEN

CALORIES

6 fl oz unless noted

Apple
Lucky Leaf	90
Mott's	88
Mott's Natural	76
Musselman's	90
Sippin' Pak / 8.45 fl oz	110
Seneca / bottled or canned	90
Welch's / bottled	80
Seneca / frozen, reconstituted	90
Seneca Granny-Smith / frozen, reconstituted	90
Seneca Natural / frozen, reconstituted	90

Apple cherry / **Del Monte** — 100
Apple cider / **Lucky Leaf** — 90
Apple cider / **Musselman's** — 90
Apple cider, sparkling
Lucky Leaf / bottled	80
Musselman's	80
Welch's	100

Apple-cranberry
Lucky Leaf	130
Mott's	83
Musselman's	130
Smucker's Naturally 100% / 8 fl oz	120

Apple-grape
Libby's Juicy Juice	90
Libby's Juicy Juice / 8.45 fl oz	120
Mott's	86

Apple nectar / **Libby's** — 100
Apple-raspberry / **Mott's** — 83
Apricot / **Fruition** 100% Juice Blend — 90
Apricot nectar
Del Monte	100
Kern's	100
Libby's	110

Apricot-orange / **Fruition** 100% Juice Blend — 90

CALORIES

Apricot-orange nectar / **Kern's**	112
Apricot-passion fruit / **Fruition** 100% Juice Blend	100
Apricot-pineapple / **Fruition** 100% Juice Blend	90
Apricot-pineapple nectar / **Kern's**	110
Banana nectar / **Libby's**	110
Banana-pineapple nectar / **Kern's**	120
Berry / **Libby's** Juicy Juice	90
Berry / 8.45 fl oz / **Libby's** Juicy Juice	130
Black cherry / 10 fl oz / **Smucker's** Fruit Juice Sparklers	120
Black cherry / 8 fl oz / **Smucker's** Naturally 100%	130
Boysenberry / 10 fl oz / **Smucker's** Fruit Juice Sparklers	130
Boysenberry / 8 fl oz / **Smucker's** Naturally 100%	120
Cherry	
Dole / bottled	90
Libby's Juicy Juice	90
Libby's Juicy Juice / 8.45 fl oz	130
Cinnamon-apple nectar / **Kern's**	110
Coconut-pineapple nectar / **Kern's**	120
Cranberry	
Lucky Leaf	110
Musselman's	110
Smucker's Fruit Juice Sparklers / 10 fl oz	140
Grape	
Libby's Juicy Juice	90
Libby's Juicy Juice / 7.1 fl oz	110
Libby's Juicy Juice / 8.45 fl oz	130
Lucky Leaf	130
Musselman's	130
Sippin' Pak / 8.45 fl oz	130
Welch's White / box / 8.45 fl oz	160
Seneca / bottled or canned	115
Welch's / bottled or canned	120
Welch's Red and White / bottled	120
Seneca Natural / frozen, reconstituted	115
Seneca Sweetened / frozen, reconstituted	100
Seneca White, Sweetened / frozen, reconstituted	110
Welch's / frozen, reconstituted	100
Welch's 100% Unsweetened / frozen, reconstituted	120
Welch's White, Sweetened / frozen, reconstituted	100
Grape, sparkling, red / **Welch's** / bottled	128
Grape, sparkling, white / **Welch's** / bottled	120

CALORIES

Grapefruit
    Citrus Hill Plus Calcium   70
    Del Monte, Unsweetened   70
    Libby's   70
    Mott's / 11.5 oz   130
    Welch's / bottled   70
Guava nectar / **Kern's**   110
Guava nectar / **Libby's**   110
Lemon
    Lucky Leaf   30
    Musselman's   30
    Realemon, Natural Strength / 1 fl oz   6
    Realemon Pure Lemon Juice / 1 fl oz   6
    Seneca / bottled or canned   6
Lime / 1 fl oz / **Realime**   6
Mango nectar / **Kern's**   110
Mango nectar / **Libby's**   110
Orange
    Citrus Hill Lite   60
    Citrus Hill Plus Calcium   90
    Citrus Hill Select   90
    Del Monte, Unsweetened   80
    Libby's, Unsweetened   80
    Mott's / 11.5 oz   204
    Sippin' Pak / 8.45 fl oz   110
Orange blend / bottled / **Welch's**   90
Papaya nectar / **Kern's**   110
Papaya nectar / **Libby's**   110
Passion fruit-orange nectar / **Kern's**   110
Peach / bottled / **Dole**   100
Peach / 8 fl oz / **Smucker's** Naturally 100%   120
Peach nectar / **Kern's**   110
Peach nectar / **Libby's**   100
Pear nectar / **Kern's**   110
Pear nectar / **Libby's**   110
Pine-orange-banana / canned / **Dole**   90
Pine-orange-guava / canned / **Dole** New Breakfast   100
Pine-passion-banana / canned / **Dole** New Breakfast   100
Pineapple
    Del Monte, Unsweetened   100
    Dole / canned   100

	CALORIES
Dole New Breakfast / canned	100
Libby's, Unsweetened	100
Mott's / 11.5 oz	148
Pineapple-grapefruit / canned / **Dole**	90
Pineapple-mandarin / **Del Monte**	90
Pineapple nectar / **Libby's**	110
Pineapple-orange / canned / **Dole**	90
Pineapple-orange / canned / **Dole** New Breakfast	90
Pineapple-orange-banana / canned / **Dole** New Breakfast	90
Pineapple-pink grapefruit / canned / **Dole**	100
Plum nectar / **Kern's**	110
Prune	
Del Monte, Unsweetened	120
Lucky Leaf	150
Mott's	130
Musselman's	150
Seneca / bottled or canned	140
Punch / **Libby's** Juicy Juice	100
Punch / 8.45 fl oz / **Libby's** Juicy Juice	140
Raspberry / bottled / **Dole**	90
Red raspberry / 10 fl oz / **Smucker's** Fruit Juice Sparklers	130
Red raspberry / 8 fl oz / **Smucker's** Naturally 100%	120
Ripe guava nectar / 8 fl oz / **Libby's**	140
Ripe passion fruit-orange nectar / 8 fl oz / **Libby's**	150
Ripe peach nectar / 8 fl oz / **Libby's**	130
Ripe strawberry-banana nectar / 8 fl oz / **Libby's**	150
Ripe strawberry nectar / 8 oz / **Libby's**	150
Strawberry / **Del Monte** Country	100
Strawberry-banana nectar / **Kern's**	100
Strawberry nectar / **Kern's**	110
Strawberry nectar / **Libby's**	110
Tangerine / bottled / **Dole**	100
Tropical / **Libby's** Juicy Juice	110
Tropical / 8.45 fl oz / **Libby's** Juicy Juice	150
Tropical nectar / **Kern's**	112

Gelatin

CALORIES

All flavors, mix, prepared / ½ cup unless noted
    D-Zerta — 8
    Jell-O — 80
    Jell-O 1-2-3 / ⅔ cup — 130
    Jell-O Sugar Free — 8
    Royal — 80
    Royal Sugar Free — 8
Orange flavor, mix / 1 envelope / **Knox** — 39

Gravies

CALORIES

Au jus
    Franco-American / canned / 2 fl oz — 10
    Heinz / canned / ¼ cup — 18
    Durkee / mix, prepared / ⅛ cup — 8
    Durkee Roastin' Bag / mix w roasting bag / 1 pkg — 64
    French's / mix, prepared / ¼ pkg — 10
    French's Roastin' Bag / mix w roasting bag / ⅛ pkg — 10
    McCormick/Schilling / mix, prepared / ¼ cup — 20
Beef / canned / 2 fl oz / **Franco-American** — 25

	CALORIES
Brown	
La Choy / bottled / ½ tsp	15
Heinz / canned / ¼ cup	25
Durkee / mix, prepared / ¼ cup	15
French's / mix, prepared / ¼ pkg	20
McCormick/Schilling / mix, prepared / ¼ cup	23
McCormick/Schilling Lite / mix, prepared / ¼ cup	10
Pillsbury / mix, prepared / ¼ cup	16
w mushrooms / mix, prepared / ¼ cup / **Durkee**	15
w onion / canned / ¼ cup / **Heinz**	25
w onion / mix, prepared / ¼ cup / **Durkee**	17
Chicken	
Franco-American / canned / 2 fl oz	45
Heinz / canned / ¼ cup	35
Durkee / mix, prepared / ¼ cup	23
French's / mix, prepared / ¼ pkg	25
McCormick/Schilling / mix, prepared / ¼ cup	22
McCormick/Schilling Lite / mix, prepared / ¼ cup	12
Pillsbury / mix, prepared / ¼ cup	25
Durkee Roastin' Bag / mix w roasting bag / 1 pkg	122
French's Roastin' Bag / mix w roasting bag / ⅕ pkg	25
Chicken, creamy / mix, prepared / ¼ cup / **Durkee**	39
Chicken, creamy / mix w roasting bag / 1 pkg / **Durkee** Roastin' Bag	242
Chicken giblet / canned / 2 fl oz / **Franco-American**	30
Chicken, Italian style / mix w roasting bag / 1 pkg / **Durkee** Roastin' Bag	144
Country, regular / mix, prepared / ¼ cup / **McCormick/Schilling**	40
Country, sausage / mix, prepared / ¼ cup / **McCormick/Schilling**	41
Cream / canned / 2 fl oz / **Franco-American**	35
Herb / mix, prepared / ¼ cup / **McCormick/Schilling**	20
Homestyle	
Durkee / mix, prepared / ¼ cup	18
French's / mix, prepared / ¼ pkg	20
McCormick/Schilling / mix, prepared / ¼ cup	24
Pillsbury / mix, prepared / ¼ cup	16
Lemon butter, fish / mix w roasting bag / ¼ pkg / **French's** Roastin' Bag	25
Meatloaf / mix w roasting bag / 1 pkg / **Durkee** Roastin' Bag	129

Meatloaf / mix w roasting bag / ⅙ pkg / **French's** Roastin'
  Bag   25
Mushroom
    Franco-American / canned / 2 fl oz   25
    Heinz / canned / ¼ cup   25
    Durkee / mix, prepared / ¼ cup   15
    French's / mix, prepared / ¼ pkg   20
    McCormick/Schilling / mix, prepared / ¼ cup   19
Onion
    Durkee / mix, prepared / ¼ cup   21
    French's / mix, prepared / ¼ pkg   25
    McCormick/Schilling / mix, prepared / ¼ cup   22
Pork
    Franco-American / canned / 2 fl oz   40
    Heinz / canned / ¼ cup   25
    Durkee / mix, prepared / ¼ cup   18
    French's / mix, prepared / ¼ pkg   20
    French's Roastin' Bag / mix w roasting bag / ⅙ pkg   25
    McCormick/Schilling / mix, prepared / ¼ cup   20
Pot roast / mix w roasting bag / ⅛ pkg / **French's** Roastin'
  Bag   18
Pot roast and stew / mix w roasting bag / 1 pkg **Durkee**
  Roastin' Bag   125
Pot roast, onion / mix w roasting bag / 1 pkg **Durkee**
  Roastin' Bag   124
Pot roast, onion / mix w roasting bag / ⅛ pkg / **French's**
  Roastin' Bag   18
Swiss steak
    Durkee / mix, prepared / 1-½ cup   68
    Durkee Roastin' Bag / mix w roasting bag / 1 pkg   115
    French's Roastin' Bag / mix w roasting bag / ⅙ pkg   20
Turkey
    Franco-American / canned / 2 fl oz   30
    Heinz / canned / ¼ cup   25
    Durkee / mix, prepared / ¼ cup   22
    French's / mix, prepared / ¼ pkg   25
    McCormick/Schilling / mix, prepared / ¼ cup   22

Health and "Natural" Foods

CALORIES

Flour, Grains, Meal, Rice, Yeast

Alfalfa seeds / 1 cup / **Arrowhead Mills**	40
Amaranth / 2 oz / **Arrowhead Mills**	200
Amaranth pasta / 2 oz / **Health Valley**	170
Baking mix	
Brown rice / ½ cup dry / **Fearn**	215
Rice / ½ cup dry / **Fearn**	260
Whole wheat / ⅓ cup dry / **Hain**	150
Whole wheat / ½ cup dry / **Fearn**	210
Barley / 2 oz / **Arrowhead Mills**	200
Barley flakes / 2 oz / **Arrowhead Mills**	200
Brown rice, long / 2 oz / **Arrowhead Mills**	200
Brown rice, long Basmati / 2 oz / **Arrowhead Mills**	200
Brown rice, medium / 2 oz / **Arrowhead Mills**	200
Brown rice, short / 2 oz / **Arrowhead Mills**	200
Buckwheat groats, brown or white / 2 oz / **Arrowhead Mills**	190
Corn, blue / 2 oz / **Arrowhead Mills**	210
Corn, yellow / 2 oz / **Arrowhead Mills**	210
Corn germ / ¼ cup / **Fearn** Naturfresh	130
Flax seeds / 1 oz / **Arrowhead Mills**	140
Flour: 2 oz (equals about ½ cup)	
Amaranth / **Arrowhead Mills**	200
Barley / **Arrowhead Mills**	200
Brown rice / **Arrowhead Mills**	200
Buckwheat / **Arrowhead Mills**	190

129

CALORIES

Cornmeal, blue / **Arrowhead Mills**	210
Cornmeal hi-lysine / **Arrowhead Mills**	210
Cornmeal, yellow / **Arrowhead Mills**	210
Garbanzo / **Arrowhead Mills**	200
Millet / **Arrowhead Mills**	185
Oat / **Arrowhead Mills**	200
Pastry / **Arrowhead Mills**	180
Rye / **Arrowhead Mills**	190
Soy / **Arrowhead Mills**	250
Teff / **Arrowhead Mills**	200
Vital wheat gluten / **Arrowhead Mills**	100
White, unbleached / **Arrowhead Mills**	200
Whole wheat, stone ground / **Arrowhead Mills**	200
Grain side dishes: ½ cup prepared	
Chicken / **Hain**	130
Herb / **Hain**	120
Rice almondine / **Hain**	130
Rice oriental / **Hain**	130
Millet, hulled / 1 oz / **Arrowhead Mills**	90
Oat flakes / 2 oz / **Arrowhead Mills**	220
Oat groats / 2 oz / **Arrowhead Mills**	220
Popcorn, yellow / 2 oz / **Arrowhead Mills**	210
Potato flakes / 2 oz / **Arrowhead Mills**	140
Quick brown rice, original / 2 oz / **Arrowhead Mills**	200
Spanish style / 2 oz / **Arrowhead Mills**	150
Vegetable herb / 2 oz / **Arrowhead Mills**	150
Wild rice and herb / 2 oz / **Arrowhead Mills**	140
Quinoa / 2 oz / **Arrowhead Mills**	200
Rice / ½ cup / **Fearn**	270
Rye, whole / 2 oz / **Arrowhead Mills**	190
Rye flakes / 2 oz / **Arrowhead Mills**	190
Sesame seeds, whole / 1 oz / **Arrowhead Mills**	160
Spaghetti pasta / 2 oz / **Health Valley**	170
Spinach spaghetti pasta / 2 oz / **Health Valley**	170
Teff / 2 oz / **Arrowhead Mills**	200
Whole wheat lasagna pasta w wheat germ / 2 oz / **Health Valley**	170

Seasonings and Gravy

Brown / mix, prepared / 2 tbsp / **La Loma** Gravy Quik	45

CALORIES

Brown gravy / mix / ¼ pkg / **Hain**	16
Catsup, natural / 1 tbsp / **Hain**	16
Catsup, natural / 1 tbsp / **Hain**, No Salt	16
Chicken / mix, prepared / 2 tbsp / **La Loma** Gravy Quik	45
Chili / mix / ¼ pkg / **Hain** Medium	30
Country / mix, prepared / 2 tbsp / **La Loma** Gravy Quik	10
Mushroom / mix, prepared / 2 tbsp / **La Loma** Gravy Quik	10
Mustard, stone ground / 1 tbsp / **Hain**	14
Mustard, stone ground / 1 tbsp / **Hain**, No Salt	14
Onion / mix, prepared / 2 tbsp / **La Loma** Gravy Quik	10
Salt, iodized sea / 1 tsp / **Hain**	0
Salt, sea / 1 tsp / **Hain**	0
Stroganoff mix / prepared / 4 oz / **Natural Touch**	90
Taco / mix / ¹⁄₁₀ pkg / **Hain**	10
Taco mix / prepared / 2 tbsp / **Natural Touch**	90

Soy Milk and Beverage Mixes

Kafree Roma / dry / 1 tsp brewed / **Natural Touch**	6
Liquid lecithen / 1 tbsp / **Fearn**	130
Liquid soya lecithin, mint / 1 tbsp / **Fearn**	113
Soy Moo / 1 cup dry / **Health Valley**	160
Soya granules / ¼ cup / **Fearn**	140
Soya lecithin granules / 2 tbsp / **Fearn**	100
Soya powder / ¼ cup / **Fearn**	100
Soya protein isolate / ¼ cup / **Fearn**	60
Soyagen, all purpose / ¼ cup dry / **La Loma**	130
Soyagen, carob / ¼ cup dry / **La Loma**	140
Soyagen, no sucrose / ¼ cup dry / **La Loma**	130
Soyamel, fortified / 1 oz dry / **Worthington**	130

Soybeans and legumes

Beans

Adzuki / 2 oz dry / **Arrowhead Mills**	190
Anasazi / 2 oz dry / **Arrowhead Mills**	200
Baked beans w tofu wieners / canned / 7-½ oz / **Health Valley**	140
Black beans w tofu wieners / canned / 7-½ oz / **Health Valley**	160
Black turtle / 2 oz dry / **Arrowhead Mills**	190

CALORIES

Black w vegetables / canned / 7-½ oz / **Health Valley**	150
Garbanzos / **Arrowhead Mills**	200
Kidney red / 2 oz dry / **Arrowhead Mills**	190
Lentils w tofu wieners / canned / 7-½ oz / **Health Valley**	170
Mung / 2 oz dry / **Arrowhead Mills**	50
Pinto / 2 oz dry / **Arrowhead Mills**	200
Soybean flakes / 2 oz / **Arrowhead Mills**	250
Soybeans / 2 oz dry / **Arrowhead Mills**	230
Blackbean crealo mix / 1.87 oz dry / **Fearn**	180
Lentil and garden vegetables / canned / 7-½ oz / **Health Valley**	150
Lentils, green / 2 oz dry / **Arrowhead Mills**	190
Lentils, red / 2 oz dry / **Arrowhead Mills**	195
Peas, split / 2 oz dry / **Arrowhead Mills**	200
Tri bean casserole mix / 1.62 oz dry / **Fearn**	160

Spreads and Sandwich Fillings: 2 tbsp unless noted

Almond butter, raw / **Hain**	190
Almond butter, toasted, blanched / **Hain**	220
Cashew butter, raw / **Hain**	190
Cashew butter, raw, unsalted / **Hain**	210
Cashew butter, toasted / **Hain**	210
Peanut butter, creamy / **Arrowhead Mills**	190
Peanut butter, creamy / **Health Valley**	170
Peanut butter, crunchy / **Arrowhead Mills**	190
Safflower margarine	
Hain / 1 tbsp	100
Hain Soft / 1 tbsp	100
Hain Unsalted / 1 tbsp	100
Sandwich spread / canned / 3 tbsp / **La Loma**	70
Sesame tahini / 1 oz / **Arrowhead Mills**	170

Sweets, Nuts and Snacks: 1 oz unless noted

Caramel corn puffs / **Health Valley**	100
Caramel corn puffs, apple cinnamon / **Health Valley**	100
Caramel corn puffs, peanut flavor / **Health Valley**	100
Carob peanut clusters / **Harmony**	150

CALORIES

Carob raisins / **Harmony**	110
Caroby almond bar / 4 sections / **Natural Touch**	150
Caroby milk bar / 4 sections / **Natural Touch**	150
Caroby milk-free bar / 4 sections / **Natural Touch**	160
Caroby mint bar / 4 sections / **Natural Touch**	150
Carrot chips / **Hain**	150
Carrot chips , barbecue / **Hain**	140
Carrot chips, no salt added / **Hain**	150
Carrot Lites / ½ oz / **Health Valley**	75
Cheddar Lites / ¼ oz / **Health Valley**	40
Cheddar Lites w green onion / ¼ oz / **Health Valley**	40
Cheese flavor puffs / **Health Valley**	100
Cheese flavor puffs w green onion / **Health Valley**	100
Cheese flavor puffs, zesty chili / **Health Valley**	100
Corn chips / ¾ oz / **Arrowhead Mills**	90
Corn chips w cheese / ¾ oz / **Arrowhead Mills**	90
Corn curls, unsalted / **Arrowhead Mills**	120
Corn curls, salted / **Arrowhead Mills**	120
Deluxe super trail mix / **Harmony**	110
Oriental party mix / **Harmony**	160
Pastamore party mix / **Harmony**	130
Raw trail mix / **Harmony**	120
Rice cakes: 5 cakes unless noted	
Apple-cinnamon / **Hain** Mini Cakes	60
Barbecue / **Hain** Mini Cakes	70
Cheese / **Hain** Mini Cakes	60
Five grain / 1 cake / **Hain**	40
Honey nut / **Hain** Mini Cakes	60
Nacho cheese / **Hain** Mini Cakes	70
Plain / 1 cake / **Hain**	40
Plain / **Hain** Mini Cakes	50
Plain, no salt / 1 cake / **Hain**	40
Plain, no salt / **Hain** Mini Cakes	50
Popcorn / **Hain** Mini Cakes	60
Popcorn, butter flavor / **Hain** Mini Cakes	70
Popcorn, white cheddar / **Hain** Mini Cakes	60
Ranch / **Hain** Mini Cakes	70
Sesame / 1 cake / **Hain**	40
Sesame, no salt / 1 cake / **Hain**	40
Teriyaki / **Hain** Mini Cakes	50
Ruskets biscuits / 2 biscuits / **La Loma**	110

CALORIES

Seeds, sunflower / **Arrowhead Mills**	160
Swiss trail mix / **Harmony**	130
Tortilla chips, sesame / **Hain**	140
Tortilla chips, sesame cheese / **Hain**	160
Tortilla chips, sesame, no salt added / **Hain**	140
Tortilla chips, taco style / **Hain**	160
Tropical trail mix / **Harmony**	110
Yogurt almonds / **Harmony**	150
Yogurt pretzels / **Harmony**	130
Yogurt raisins / **Harmony**	120

Vegetarian Meat Substitutes

Bean-barley stew mix / 1.75 oz dry / **Fearn**	180
Beef slices, smoked, frozen / 6 slices / **Worthington**	120
Beef style, frozen / **Worthington**	130
Bita-Burger granule, dry / 3 tbsp / **La Loma**	70
Bolono, frozen / 2 slices / **Worthington**	60
Brazil nut burger mix / ¼ cup dry / **Fearn**	100
Breakfast links, frozen / 2 links / **Morningstar Farms**	90
Breakfast patties, frozen / 2 patties / **Morningstar Farms**	190
Breakfast patty mix / ⅛ mix dry / **Fearn**	110
Breakfast strips, frozen / 3 strips / **Morningstar Farms**	80
Chicken style	
La Loma Chicken Supreme / ¼ cup dry	50
Worthington Diced Chik / canned / ¼ cup	90
Worthington Sliced Chik / canned / 2 slices	90
La Loma / fried, canned w gravy / 2 pieces	140
La Loma / fried, frozen / 1 piece	180
La Loma Chik Nuggets / frozen / 5 pieces	270
Worthington / frozen / 2 slices	130
Worthington Chic-ketts / frozen / ½ cup	160
Worthington ChikStiks / frozen / 1 piece	110
Worthington CrispyChik Nuggets / frozen / 6 pieces	280
Worthington CrispyChik Patties / frozen / 1 patty	220
Worthington Diced Chik Meatless / frozen / ½ cup	190
Worthington Golden Croquettes / frozen / 5 pieces	280
Chicken style, fried / canned / 2 pieces / **Worthington** FriChik	180
Chicken style, fried, frozen / 1 piece / **Worthington** FriPats	180

Chicken wieners / 1 frank / **Health Valley**	96
Chili / canned / ⅔ cup / **Worthington**	190
Chili, vegetarian / canned / ⅔ cup / **Natural Touch**	230
Choplets / canned / 2 slices / **Worthington**	100
Corn dogs / frozen / 1 corn dog / **La Loma**	190
Corned beef / frozen / 4 slices / **Worthington**	120
Country crisp patties / frozen / 1 patty / **Morningstar Farms**	220
Country stew / canned / 9.5 oz / **Worthington**	220
Cutlet, breaded / frozen / 1 patty / **Morningstar Farms**	230
Cutlet, multigrain / canned / 2 slices / **Worthington**	90
Cutlets / canned / 1.5 slices / **Worthington**	100
Dinner cuts / canned / 2 pieces / **La Loma**	110
Dinner entree / frozen / 1 patty / **Natural Touch**	230
Dinner roast / frozen / 2 oz / **Worthington**	120
Falafel mix / ⅑ mix dry / **Fearn**	80
Fillets / frozen / 2 pieces / **Worthington**	180
Frankfurters / canned / 1 frank / **La Loma**	110
Frankfurters / canned / 2 links / **La Loma** Sizzle Franks	170
Frankfurters / frozen / 1 link / **Morningstar Farms Deli Franks**	90
Garden pattie / frozen / 1 patty / **Natural Touch**	120
Granburger / dry / 6 tbsp / **Worthington**	110
Griddle steaks / frozen / 1 piece / **La Loma**	140
Grillers / frozen / 4 oz / **Morningstar Farms**	180
Leanies / frozen / 1 link / **Worthington**	100
Lentil rice loaf / frozen / 2-½-in slice / **Natural Touch**	200
Linketts / canned / 2 links / **La Loma**	140
Little links / canned / 2 links / **La Loma**	90
Loaf mix / dry / 4 oz prepared / **Natural Touch**	180
Nomeat balls / canned / 3 pieces / **Worthington**	100
Numete / canned / ½-in slice / **Worthington**	150
Nuteena peanut butter base / canned / ½-in slice / **La Loma**	160
Ocean platter / ¼ cup dry / **La Loma**	50
Okra patty / frozen / 1 patty / **Natural Touch**	160
Pancakes and links / frozen / 4 oz / **Morningstar Farms**	240
Patty mix / ¼ cup dry / **La Loma**	50
Prime stakes / canned / 1 piece / **Worthington**	160
Prosage links / frozen / 2 links / **Worthington**	130
Prosage patties / frozen / 2 patties / **Worthington**	210

CALORIES

Prosage roll / frozen / 2-⅜-in slice / **Worthington**	180
Protose / canned / ½-in slice / **Worthington**	180
Redi-Burger / canned / ½-in slice / **La Loma**	130
Salami, meatless / frozen / 2 slices / **Worthington**	70
Saucettes / canned / 2 links / **Worthington**	150
Savory dinner loaf / ¼ cup dry / **La Loma**	50
Savory meatballs / frozen / 7 pieces / **La Loma**	190
Savory slices / canned / 2 slices / **Worthington**	100
Sesame burger mix / ¼ cup dry / **Fearn**	130
Sizzle burger / frozen / 1 patty / **La Loma**	220
Stakelets / frozen / 1 piece / **Worthington**	150
Stripples / frozen / 4 strips / **Worthington**	120
Sunflower burger mix / ¼ cup dry / **Fearn**	120
Super links / canned / 1 link / **Worthington**	100
Swiss steak / canned / 1 piece / **La Loma**	170
Tender Bits / canned / 4 pieces / **La Loma**	80
Tender Rounds / canned / 6 pieces / **La Loma**	120
Tuno / frozen / 2 oz / **Worthington**	100
Turkee slices / canned / 2 slices / **Worthington**	130
Turkey slices, smoked / frozen / 4 slices / **Worthington**	180
Turkey wieners / 1 frank / **Health Valley**	96
Veelets / frozen / 1 patty / **Worthington**	230
Vege-Burger / canned / ½ cup / **La Loma**	110
Vegetable skallops / canned / ½ cup / **Worthington**	90
Vegetable skallops / canned / ½ cup / **Worthington** No Salt Added	80
Vegetable steaks / canned / 2-½ pieces / **Worthington**	110
Vegetarian beef pie / frozen / 1 pie / **Worthington**	360
Vegetarian burger / canned / ½ cup / **Worthington**	150
Vegetarian burger / canned / ½ cup / **Worthington** No Salt Added	150
Vegetarian chicken pie / frozen / 1 pie / **Worthington**	380
Vegetarian chili, mild w beans / 5 oz / **Health Valley**	140
Vegetarian chili, mild w black beans / 5 oz / **Health Valley**	140
Vegetarian chili, mild w lentils / 5 oz / **Health Valley**	140
Vegetarian chili, mild w three beans / 5 oz / **Health Valley**	90
Vegetarian chili, spicy w black beans / 5 oz / **Health Valley**	140
Vegetarian egg roll / frozen / 1 roll / **Worthington**	160

CALORIES

Veja-links / canned / 2 links / **Worthington**	140
Vita-Burger chunk / ¼ cup dry / **La Loma**	70
Wham / frozen / 3 slices / **Worthington**	120

Wheat and Wheat Germ

Bran, unprocessed / 2 tbsp / **Quaker**	8
Bulgur / 2 oz / **Arrowhead Mills**	200
Wheat, hard red spring / 2 oz / **Arrowhead Mills**	190
Wheat, hard red winter / 2 oz / **Arrowhead Mills**	190
Wheat, soft red for pastry / 2 oz / **Arrowhead Mills**	190
Wheat bran, toasted / ⅓ cup / **Kretschmer**	57
Wheat flakes / 2 oz / **Arrowhead Mills**	210
Wheat germ	
Arrowhead Mills / 2 oz	210
Fearn Naturfresh / ¼ cup	100
Kretschmer / ¼ cup	103
Wheat germ, honey crunch / ¼ cup / **Kretschmer**	105

Ice Cream and Similar Frozen Products

FROZEN DESSERTS

	CALORIES
½ cup unless noted	
Black cherry / **Sealtest** Free Nonfat	100
Bordeaux cherry / **Healthy Choice**	120
Chocolate	
Healthy Choice	130
Simple Pleasure	130
Simple Pleasure Fat Free	80
Weight Watchers Fat Free	80
Chocolate caramel sundae / **Simple Pleasure**	90
Chocolate chip / **Simple Pleasure**	140
Chocolate-flavored / **Sealtest** Free Nonfat	100
Chocolate fudge-flavored swirl / 1 bar / **Sealtest** Free Dessert Bars	90
Chocolate swirl / **Weight Watchers** Fat Free	90
Coffee / **Simple Pleasure**	120
Cookies 'n cream / **Simple Pleasure**	150
Cookies n' cream / **Healthy Choice**	130
Eskimo Pie / **Eskimo Pie** Sugar Free	140
Frozen dairy dessert / 2.5 fl oz / **Nestlé** Crunch Lite	140
Mint chocolate chip / **Simple Pleasure**	140
Neapolitan / **Healthy Choice**	120
Neapolitan / **Weight Watchers** Fat Free	89
Old-fashioned vanilla / **Healthy Choice**	120
Peach / **Sealtest** Free Nonfat	100

CALORIES

Peach / **Simple Pleasure**	120
Pecan praline / **Simple Pleasure**	140
Praline and caramel / **Healthy Choice**	130
Rocky road / **Healthy Choice**	160
Rum raisin / **Simple Pleasure**	130
Strawberry	
Healthy Choice	120
Sealtest Free Nonfat	100
Simple Pleasure	110
Toffee crunch / **Simple Pleasure**	130
Vanilla	
Healthy Choice	120
Simple Pleasure	120
Weight Watchers Fat Free	80
Vanilla-flavored / **Sealtest** Free Nonfat	100
Vanilla-flavored, chocolate, strawberry / **Sealtest** Free Nonfat	100
Vanilla-flavored fudge royale / **Sealtest** Free Nonfat	100
Vanilla-flavored strawberry royale / **Sealtest** Free Nonfat	100
Vanilla fudge-flavored swirl / 1 bar / **Sealtest** Free Dessert Bars	80
Vanilla fudge swirl / **Simple Pleasure**	90
Vanilla sandwich / 3.2 fl oz / **Eskimo Pie**	170
Vanilla-strawberry swirl / 1 bar / **Sealtest** Free Dessert Bars	80
Wild berry swirl / **Healthy Choice**	120

ICE CREAM

½ cup unless noted

Almond buttercrunch / **Baskin-Robbins** Light	130
Almond fudge jamoca / 1 scoop / **Baskin-Robbins**	270
Banana chunky / **Baskin-Robbins** Sugar Free	80
Butter almond / **Breyers**	170
Butter crunch / **Sealtest**	150
Butter pecan	
Baskin-Robbins / 1 scoop	280
Breyers	180
Frusen Glädjé	280

CALORIES

Häagen-Dazs	390
Lady Borden	180
Sealtest	160
Cafe mocha / **Baskin-Robbins** Truly Free	70
Caramel nut sundae / **Häagen-Dazs**	310
Cherries jubilee / 1 scoop / **Baskin-Robbins**	240
Cherry cordial / **Baskin-Robbins** Sugar Free	100
Cherry vanilla / **Breyers**	150
Chocolate	
Baskin-Robbins / 1 scoop	270
Breyers	160
Frusen Glädjé	240
Häagen-Dazs	270
Sealtest	140
Chocolate almond / 1 scoop / **Baskin-Robbins**	300
Chocolate caramel nut / **Baskin-Robbins** Light	130
Chocolate chip	
Baskin-Robbins / 1 scoop	260
Baskin-Robbins Sugar Free	100
Breyers	170
Sealtest	150
Chocolate-chocolate chip / **Frusen Glädjé**	270
Chocolate-chocolate chip / **Häagen-Dazs**	290
Chocolate-chocolate mint / **Häagen-Dazs**	300
Chocolate fudge / 1 scoop / **Baskin-Robbins**	290
Chocolate marshmallow sundae / **Sealtest**	150
Chocolate mousse / 1 scoop / **Baskin-Robbins**	320
Chocolate raspberry truffle / 1 scoop / **Baskin-Robbins**	310
Chocolate swirl / **Borden**	130
Chocolate world class / 1 scoop / **Baskin-Robbins**	280
Coffee	
Breyers	150
Frusen Glädjé	260
Häagen-Dazs	270
Sealtest	140
Cookies 'n cream	
Baskin-Robbins / 1 scoop	280
Breyers	170
Sealtest	150
Deep chocolate / **Häagen-Dazs**	290
Deep chocolate fudge / **Häagen-Dazs**	290

CALORIES

Deep chocolate peanut butter / **Häagen-Dazs**	330
Dutch chocolate / **Borden**	130
Espresso 'n cream / **Baskin-Robbins** Light	120
French vanilla / 1 scoop / **Baskin-Robbins**	280
French vanilla-flavored / **Sealtest**	140
Fudge brownie / 1 scoop / **Baskin-Robbins**	320
Fudge royale / **Sealtest**	140
German chocolate cake / 1 scoop / **Baskin-Robbins**	310
Heavenly hash / **Sealtest**	150
Honey vanilla / **Häagen-Dazs**	250
Jamoca / 1 scoop / **Baskin-Robbins**	240
Kahlua 'n cream / 1 scoop / **Baskin-Robbins**	270
Macadamia brittle / **Häagen-Dazs**	280
Maple walnut / **Sealtest**	160
Mint chocolate / **Breyers**	170
Mint chocolate chip / 1 scoop / **Baskin-Robbins**	260
Mint thin / **Baskin-Robbins** Sugar Free	90
Mocha chip / **Frusen Glädjé**	280
Peach / **Baskin-Robbins** Fat Free	100
Peach / **Breyers**	130
Peanut fudge sundae / **Sealtest**	140
Pineapple coconut / **Baskin-Robbins** Sugar Free	90
Pistachio almond / 1 scoop / **Baskin-Robbins**	290
Praline / **Baskin-Robbins** Light	130
Pralines 'n cream / 1 scoop / **Baskin-Robbins**	280
Pralines and cream / **Frusen Glädjé**	280
Rocky road / 1 scoop / **Baskin-Robbins**	300
Rum raisin / **Häagen-Dazs**	250
Strawberries 'n cream / **Borden**	130
Strawberry	
Baskin-Robbins Light	110
Baskin-Robbins Sugar Free	80
Borden	130
Breyers	130
Frusen Glädjé	230
Häagen-Dazs	250
Sealtest	130
Swiss almond Jamoca / **Baskin-Robbins** Sugar Free	90
Swiss chocolate candy almond / **Frusen Glädjé**	270
Tiny toon crunch / 1 scoop / **Baskin-Robbins**	250
Toffee chunk / **Frusen Glädjé**	270

CALORIES

Triple chocolate stripes / **Sealtest**	140
Twist, chocolate vanilla / **Baskin-Robbins** Fat Free	100
Vanilla	
Baskin-Robbins / 1 scoop	240
Borden	130
Borden Eagle Brand	150
Breyers	150
Frusen Glädjé	230
Häagen-Dazs	260
Sealtest	140
Vanilla and chocolate **Breyers**	160
Vanilla-chocolate / **Sealtest** Cubic Scoops	140
Vanilla, chocolate and strawberry / **Breyers**	150
Vanilla-flavored chocolate, strawberry / **Sealtest**	140
Vanilla-flavored chocolate, strawberry / **Sealtest** Cubic Scoops	130
Vanilla-flavored w orange sherbet / **Sealtest** Cubic Scoops	130
Vanilla-flavored w red raspberry sherbet / **Sealtest** Cubic Scoops	130
Vanilla fudge / **Baskin-Robbins** Light	110
Vanilla fudge / 4 fl oz / **Häagen-Dazs**	270
Vanilla fudge twirl / **Breyers**	160
Vanilla peanut butter swirl / **Häagen-Dazs**	280
Vanilla-red raspberry / **Frusen Glädjé**	230
Vanilla-Swiss almond / **Frusen Glädjé**	270
Vanilla-Swiss almond / **Häagen-Dazs**	290
Very berry / 1 scoop / **Baskin-Robbins**	220
Wild cherry / 4 fl oz / **Baskin-Robbins** Truly Free	70

ICE CREAM AND FROZEN BARS

1 bar or 1 piece unless noted

All flavors	
Crystal Light	14
Jell-O Gelatin Pops	35
Kool-Aid Cream Pops	50
Kool-Aid Kool Pops	40
Almond / **Eskimo**, Sugar Free	140
Amaretto-chocolate swirl / **Crystal Light** Cool n' Creamy	60

CALORIES

Bon Bons
    Chocolate ice cream with milk chocolate fl/coating /
        2.25 fl oz / **Nestlé**   190
    Vanilla ice cream with dk/chocolate fl/coating / 2.25
        fl oz / **Nestlé**   190
    Vanilla ice cream with m/chocolate fl/coating / 2.25
        fl oz / **Nestlé**   160
Butterfinger / 2.5 fl oz / **Nestlé**   180
Caramel cone / 1 cone / **Eskimo Pie** Sugar Free   260
Caramel almond / **Häagen-Dazs**   240
Cherry / **Dole** Fresh Lites   25
Chocolate
    Jell-O Pudding Pops   80
    Nestlé Crunch / 2 fl oz   150
    Nestlé Crunch / 3 fl oz   230
Chocolate caramel / **Baskin-Robbins** Light Sundae Bars   150
Chocolate chip
    Baskin-Robbins Chillyburgers   270
    Weight Watchers One-ders / 4 oz   120
    Dole Fresh Lites   60
Chocolate-dark chocolate / **Häagen-Dazs**   390
Chocolate dip / 1.7 oz / **Weight Watchers**   110
Chocolate fudge / **Crystal Light** Cool n' Creamy   50
Chocolate fudge / **Jell-O** Pudding Pops   80
Chocolate milk / **Jell-O** Pudding Pops   80
Chocolate mousse / 1.75 oz / **Weight Watchers**   35
Chocolate nuggets / 2.25 fl oz / **Nestlé** Crunch   180
Chocolate treat / 2.75 oz / **Weight Watchers**   100
Chocolate-vanilla / **Crystal Light** Cool n' Creamy   50
Chocolate-vanilla swirl / **Jell-O** Pudding Pops   80
Chocolate-peanut butter swirl / **Jell-O** Pudding Pops   80
Double chocolate swirl / **Jell-O** Pudding Pops   80
English toffee crunch / 1.7 oz / **Weight Watchers**   120
Eskimo Pie / 3 fl oz   180
Eskimo Pie w dark chocolate / 2.5 fl oz   140
Eskimo Pie w dark chocolate / 3.5 fl oz   210
Eskimo Pie w dark chocolate / 5 fl oz   290
Eskimo Pie w milk choc crispy / 2.5 fl oz   150
Eskimo Pie w milk choc crispy, sugar free / 2.5 fl oz   150
Fudge / 1.75 oz / **Weight Watchers**   60
Fudge bar pop / **Häagen-Dazs**   210

CALORIES

Fudge sundae / **Bakers** Fudgetastic	220
Fudge sundae crunchy / **Bakers** Fudgetastic	230
Grape / **Dole** Sun Tops	40
Grapefruit and cream bar / **Welch's** Juice Bar, No Sugar Added / 3 fl oz	45
Grapefruit juice bar / 1.75 oz / **Welch's** Juice Bars	45
Grapefruit juice bar / 3 fl oz / **Welch's** Juice Bars	80
Heavenly hash / 4 oz / **Weight Watchers** One-ders	120
Jamoca almond fudge / **Baskin-Robbins** Sundae Bars	300
Lemon / **Dole** Fresh Lites	25
Lemon / **Jell-O** Snowburst	45
Lemonade / **Dole** Sun Tops	40
Mint chocolate chip / **Baskin-Robbins** Chillyburgers	260
Oh Henry / 3 fl oz / **Nestlé**	320
Orange / **Dole** Sun Tops	40
Orange / **Jell-O** Snowburst	45
Orange cream pop / **Häagen-Dazs**	130
Orange-vanilla / **Crystal Light** Cool n' Creamy	30
Orange-vanilla treat / 1.75 oz / **Weight Watchers**	30
Peach / **Dole** Fruit n' Cream Bar	90
Peach passion fruit / **Dole** Fruit n' Juice Bar	70
Peanut butter / **Häagen-Dazs**	270
Pine-orange-banana / **Dole** Fruit n' Juice Bar	70
Pineapple / **Dole** Fruit n' Juice Bar	70
Pineapple-orange / **Dole** Fresh Lites	25
Pralines 'n cream / 4 oz / **Weight Watchers** One-ders	120
Pralines 'n cream / **Baskin-Robbins** Sundae Bars	310
Punch / **Dole** Sun Tops	40
Raspberry	
Dole Fresh Lites	25
Dole Fruit n' Cream Bar	90
Dole Fruit n' Juice Bar	60
Raspberry fruit and cream bar / 3 fl oz / **Welch's** Juice Bar, No Sugar Added	45
Raspberry fruit juice bar	
Welch's Juice Bar, No Sugar Added / 3 fl oz	25
Welch's Juice Bars / 1.75 fl oz	45
Welch's Juice Bars / 3 fl oz	80
Sandwich snacks / 1.5 oz / **Weight Watchers**	90
Strawberry	
Baskin-Robbins Tiny Toon Bars	210

CALORIES

Dole Fruit n' Cream Bar	90
Dole Fruit n' Juice Bar	70
Weight Watchers One-ders / 4 fl oz	110
Strawberry fruit and cream bar / 3 fl oz / **Welch's** Juice Bar, No Sugar Added	45
Strawberry fruit juice bar	
Welch's Juice Bar, No Sugar Added / 3 fl oz	25
Welch's Juice Bars / 1.75 fl oz	45
Welch's Juice Bars / 3 fl oz	80
Strawberry royal / **Baskin-Robbins** Sundae Bars	280
Strawberry very berry / **Baskin-Robbins** Chillyburgers	230
Sundae Cone / 4.2 fl oz / **Eskimo Pie**	230
Vanilla	
Baskin-Robbins Chillyburgers	240
Häagen-Dazs	220
Jell-O Pudding Pops	80
Nestlé Crunch / 3 fl oz	180
Vanilla-chocolate / **Baskin-Robbins** Light Sundae Bars	155
Vanilla-dark chocolate / **Häagen-Dazs**	390
Vanilla-milk chocolate / **Häagen-Dazs**	360
Vanilla-milk chocolate almond / **Häagen-Dazs**	370
Vanilla-milk chocolate brittle / **Häagen-Dazs**	370
Vanilla nuggets / 2.25 fl oz / **Nestlé** Crunch	190
Vanilla sandwich / 2.75 oz / **Weight Watchers**	150

ICE MILK

½ cup unless noted

Caramel nut / **Light n' Lively**	120
Chocolate	
Borden	100
Breyers Light	120
Weight Watchers Premium	110
Chocolate chip / **Light n' Lively**	120
Chocolate chip / **Weight Watchers**	120
Chocolate fudge twirl / **Breyers** Light	130
Chocolate swirl / **Weight Watchers** Premium	120
Coffee / **Light n' Lively**	100
Cookies n' cream / **Light n' Lively**	110
Heavenly hash / **Breyers** Light	150

CALORIES

Heavenly hash / **Light n' Lively**	120
Neapolitan / **Weight Watchers** Premium	110
Pecan pralines 'n creme / **Weight Watchers**	120
Praline almond / **Breyers** Light	130
Strawberry / **Borden**	90
Strawberry / **Breyers** Light	110
Toffee fudge parfait / **Breyers** Light	140
Vanilla	
Borden	90
Breyers Light	120
Weight Watchers Premium	100
Vanilla-chocolate-strawberry / **Breyers** Light	120
Vanilla-flavored / **Light n' Lively**	100
Vanilla-flavored, chocolate, strawberry / **Light n' Lively**	100
Vanilla-flavored fudge twirl / **Light n' Lively**	110
Vanilla-flavored w chocolate-covered almonds / **Light n' Lively**	120
Vanilla-flavored w red raspberry swirl / **Light n' Lively**	110
Vanilla-red raspberry / **Breyers** Light	130

SHERBET AND ICES

½ cup unless noted

Blueberry / **Häagen-Dazs** Sorbet and Cream	190
Blueberry-strawberry / **Breyers** Sorbet In Cream	150
Daiquiri ice / 1 scoop / **Baskin-Robbins**	140
Keylime / **Häagen-Dazs** Sorbet and Cream	190
Lemon / **Breyers** Sorbet In Cream	160
Lemon / **Häagen-Dazs**	140
Lime / **Sealtest**	130
Mandarin orange / **Dole** Sorbet	110
Orange	
Baskin-Robbins / 1 scoop	160
Borden	110
Häagen-Dazs / 4 fl oz	113
Häagen-Dazs Sorbet and Cream / 4 fl oz	190
Sealtest	130
Peach / **Dole** Sorbet	110
Pineapple / **Dole** Sorbet	110
Rainbow / 1 scoop / **Baskin-Robbins**	160

CALORIES

Rainbow / **Sealtest**	130
Raspberry	
Dole Sorbet	110
Frusen Glädjé Sorbet	140
Häagen-Dazs	93
Häagen-Dazs Sorbet and Cream	180
Red raspberry / **Sealtest**	130
Strawberry / **Dole** Sorbet	100

Italian Foods

CALORIES

See also **Dinners, Pizza and Spaghetti**

Angel hair pasta / frozen / 10 oz / **Weight Watchers** Entrees	210
Cannelloni	
Beef w mornay sauce / frozen / 9-⅝ oz / **Stouffer's** Lean Cuisine	210
Cheese / frozen / 9 oz / **Dining Light**	310
Cheese w tomato sauce / frozen / 9-⅛ oz / **Stouffer's** Lean Cuisine	270
Cheddar pasta and sauce, mix / ½ cup / **Hain**	310
Chicken	
Cacciatore / frozen / 10.95 oz / **Swanson** Homestyle	260
Cacciatore w vermicelli / frozen / 10-⅞ oz / **Stouffer's** Lean Cuisine	280
Fettucini / frozen / 9 oz / **Stouffer's** Lean Cuisine	280
Italiano / frozen / 9 oz / **Stouffer's** Lean Cuisine	290
Marsala w vegetables / frozen / 8-⅛ oz / **Stouffer's** Lean Cuisine	190
Parmesan / frozen / 10.80 oz / **Banquet**	300
Parmesan / frozen / 10-⅞ oz / **Stouffer's** Lean Cuisine	270
Parmigiana / frozen / 11-¾ oz / **Le Menu**	410
w vegetables and vermicelli / frozen / 11-¾ oz / **Stouffer's** Lean Cuisine	250

	CALORIES
Dill multi-bran pasta, creamy, mix / ½ cup / **Hain**	150
Fettucini	
Alfredo / frozen / 8 oz / **Healthy Choice**	240
Alfredo / frozen / 5 oz / **Stouffer's**	270
Alfredo / frozen / 9 oz / **Weight Watchers** Entrees	210
Alfredo and sauce, mix / ½ cup / **Hain**	350
Primavera / frozen / 1 pkg / **Green Giant** Garden Gourmet	230
Italian herb pasta and sauce, mix / ½ cup / **Hain**	180
Italian multi-bran pasta, mix / ½ cup / **Hain**	120
Lasagna	
Stouffer's / frozen / 10.5 oz	360
Weight Watchers Entrees / frozen w cheese / 11 oz	350
Stouffer's frozen fiesta / 10.25 oz	430
Weight Watchers Entrees / frozen garden / 11 oz	290
Banquet / frozen w meat sauce / 7 oz	270
Healthy Choice Light / frozen w meat sauce / 10 oz	260
Le Menu / frozen w meat sauce / 10 oz	290
Stouffer's Lean Cuisine / frozen w meat sauce / 10-¼ oz	260
Swanson Homestyle / frozen w meat sauce / 10-½ oz	400
Ultra Slim-Fast / frozen w meat sauce / 12 oz	330
Weight Watchers Entrees / frozen w meat sauce / 11 oz	320
Stouffer's Lean Cuisine / frozen tuna w spinach noodles and vegetables / 9-¾ oz	240
Le Menu Light / frozen w garden vegetables / 10-½ oz	260
Stouffer's / frozen vegetables / 10.5 oz	420
Ultra Slim-Fast / frozen vegetables / 12 oz	240
Healthy Choice / frozen zucchini / 11.50 oz	240
Stouffer's Lean Cuisine / frozen zucchini / 11 oz	260
Healthy Choice / microwave cup w meat sauce / 7.50 oz	220
Chef Boy-ar-dee / Microwave w garden vegetables / 7.5 oz	170
Linguini w clam sauce / frozen / 9-⅝ oz / **Stouffer's** Lean Cuisine	280
Linguini w shrimp / frozen / 9.50 oz / **Healthy Choice**	230

CALORIES

Manicotti
     Cheese / frozen / 9.25 oz / **Healthy Choice**   230
     Cheese / frozen / 9.25 oz / **Weight Watchers** Entrees   280
     w three cheeses / frozen / 11-¾ oz / **Le Menu**   390
Mostaccioli w meat sauce / frozen / 7 oz / **Banquet**   170
Parmesan pasta and sauce, mix / ½ cup / **Hain**   220
Pasta carbonara / frozen / 5 oz / **Stouffer's**   620
Pasta Dijon / frozen / 1 pkg / **Green Giant** Garden Gourmet   260
Pasta Florentine / frozen / 1 pkg / **Green Giant** Garden Gourmet   230
Pasta primavera / frozen / 5.3 oz / **Stouffer's**   270
Pasta primavera / frozen / 8.50 oz / **Weight Watchers** Entrees   260
Pasta rigati / frozen / 10.63 oz / **Weight Watchers** Entrees   300
Pepperoni French roll / frozen / 1 sandwich / **Quaker** Ovenstuffs   370
Primavera pasta and sauce, mix / ½ cup / **Hain**   240
Ravioli
     Cheese / frozen / 9 oz / **Healthy Choice**   240
     Cheese / frozen / 8-½ oz / **Stouffer's** Lean Cuisine   240
     Cheese / frozen / 12 oz / **Ultra Slim-Fast**   330
     Cheese / frozen / 9 oz / **Weight Watchers** Entrees   290
Raviolio's, beef in meat sauce / canned / 7-½ oz / **Franco-American**   250
Rigatoni in meat sauce / frozen / 9.50 oz / **Healthy Choice**   240
Rigatoni w meat sauce and cheese / frozen / 9-¾ oz / **Stouffer's** Lean Cuisine   250
Rotini cheddar / frozen / 1 pkg / **Green Giant** Garden Gourmet   230
Salsa multi-bran pasta, mix / ½ cup / **Hain**   130
Sausage French roll / frozen / 1 sandwich / **Quaker** Ovenstuffs   390
Shells, stuffed w three cheeses / frozen / 10 oz / **Le Menu** Light   280
Shells / frozen cheese w tomato sauce / 9.25 oz / **Stouffer's**   330
Shrimp Marinara / frozen / 12 oz / **Ultra Slim-Fast**   290

Spaghetti w meatballs / frozen / 13 oz / **Swanson** Home-style	490
Swiss pasta and sauce, mix / ½ cup / **Hain**	280
Tortellini	
Stouffer's / frozen beef w marinara sauce / 10 oz	360
Birds Eye For One / frozen cheese / 5.5 oz	210
Le Menu Light / frozen cheese / 10 oz	230
Weight Watchers Entrees / frozen cheese / 9 oz	310
Stouffer's / frozen cheese in Alfredo sauce / 9 oz	600
Le Menu Light / frozen cheese and meat sauce / 8 oz	250
Stouffer's / frozen cheese w tomato sauce / 9.6 oz	360
Tortellini Provencale / frozen / 1 pkg / **Green Giant** Garden Gourmet	260
Veal	
Marsala / frozen / 10 oz / **Le Menu** Light	230
Parmigiana / frozen / 11.25 oz / **Armour Classics**	400
Parmigiana / frozen / 11-½ oz / **Le Menu**	390
Parmigiana / frozen / 10 oz / **Swanson** Homestyle	330
Parmigiana / frozen / 18-¼ oz / **Swanson** Hungry Man	590
Patty parmigiana / frozen / 8.44 oz / **Weight Watchers** Entrees	190
Veal parmigiana and pasta / frozen / 9.25 oz / **Stouffer's**	350
Ziti in tomato sauce / frozen / 11 oz / **Healthy Choice**	350

Jams, Jellies, Preserves, Butters, Marmalade and Spreads

1 tsp unless noted

Butters
    Apple

	CALORIES
Bama	12
Empress	12
Lucky Leaf	14
Musselman's / 4 oz	14
Smucker's	12
Apple-spiced / **Empress**	12
Autumn harvest / **Smucker's**	12
Autumn harvest, pumpkin / **Smucker's**	12
Cider / **Smucker's**	12
Natural / **Smucker's**	12
Peach / **Smucker's**	15
Simply fruit / **Smucker's**	12

Jams
    All flavors

	CALORIES
Country Pure	35
Empress	17
Knott's Berry Farm	18
Kraft	17
Smucker's	18
Welch's	14
Grape / **Welch's**	17
Red plum / **Bama**	15

CALORIES

Jellies
    All flavors
        Bama   15
        Knott's Berry Farm   18
        Kraft   17
        Smucker's   18
    Grape / **Kraft** Reduced Calorie   6
    Grape / **Welch's**   17
Marmalade, orange / **Smucker's**   18
Marmalade, orange / **Welch's**   14
Preserves
    All flavors
        Empress   17
        Knott's Berry Farm   18
        Kraft   17
        Smucker's   18
    Peach / **Bama**   15
    Strawberry / **Bama**   15
    Strawberry / **Kraft** Reduced Calorie   6
Spreads
    All flavors / **Smucker's** Low Sugar   8
    Fruit
        Knott's Berry Farm Light   8
        Smucker's Light   7
        Smucker's Slenderella   7
    Grape / **Weight Watchers**   8
    Grape / **Welch's**   14
    Raspberry / **Weight Watchers**   8
    Raspberry-apple / **Welch's**   17
    Simply fruit / **Smucker's**   8
    Strawberry / **Weight Watchers**   8
    Strawberry / **Welch's**   17

Liqueurs and Brandies

BRANDIES

CALORIES

1 fl oz

Coffee / **Hiram Walker** Dubochett	88
Fruit-flavored / **Hiram Walker** Garnier	86
Ginger / **Hiram Walker** Garnier	74

LIQUEURS

1 fl oz

Anisette / **Hiram Walker**	111
B & B / **Hiram Walker**	94
Benedictine / **Hiram Walker**	112
Cherry Heering / **Hiram Walker**	80
Citrus Gin / **Hiram Walker** Old Mr. Boston	76
Citrus Vodka / **Hiram Walker** Old Mr. Boston	100
Coffee, Southern / **Hiram Walker**	85
Creme de Almonde / **Hiram Walker** Dubochett	101
Creme de Banana / **Hiram Walker** Garnier	96
Creme de Cacao / **Hiram Walker** Bols	101
Creme de Cassis / **Hiram Walker** Garnier	83
Creme de Menthe / **Hiram Walker** Garnier	101
Curacao / **Hiram Walker** Garnier	100
Drambuie / **Hiram Walker**	110
Kirsch / **Hiram Walker** Garnier	83

CALORIES

Kummel / **Hiram Walker** Garnier	75
Maraschino / **Hiram Walker** Garnier	94
Peppermint Schnapps / **Hiram Walker** Garnier	83
Pernod / **Hiram Walker**	79
Rock & Rye / **Hiram Walker** Old Mr. Boston	94
Sloe Gin / **Hiram Walker** Garnier	83
Southern Comfort / **Hiram Walker**	120
Tia Maria / **Hiram Walker**	92
Triple Sec / **Hiram Walker** Garnier	83

Macaroni

Plain, all types, cooked to firm "al dente" stage / 1 cup	190
Plain, all types, cooked to tender stage / 1 cup	155
Macaroni and beef / frozen / 5.75 oz / **Stouffer's**	170
Macaroni and beef in tomato sauce / frozen / 10 oz / **Stouffer's** Lean Cuisine Entree	240
Macaroni and cheese	
Franco-American / canned / 7-⅜ oz	170
Banquet Family Entrees / frozen / 7 oz	260
Green Giant One Servings / frozen / 5.7 oz	220
Healthy Choice / frozen / 9 oz	280
Stouffer's / frozen / 6 oz	250
Stouffer's / frozen / 5 oz	210
Stouffer's Lean Cuisine Entree / frozen / 9 oz	290
Swanson / frozen / 7 oz	200
Swanson Entree / frozen / 10 oz	390
Golden Grain Cheddar / mix, dry / 1.81 oz	190

Mayonnaise

CALORIES

1 tbsp

Bama	100
Bennett's	110
Hain Canola	100
Hain Canola, Reduced Calorie	60
Hain Cold Processed	110
Hain Eggless, No Salt	110
Hain Light, Low Sodium	60
Hain, No Salt	110
Hain Safflower	110
Hollywood Canola	100
Hollywood Safflower	100
Kraft Free	12
Kraft Light	50
Kraft Real	100
Nu Made	100
Nu Made Light	40
Weight Watchers	50
Weight Watchers, Cholesterol Free	50
Sandwich spread / **Kraft**	50

Meat

FRESH

CALORIES

3 oz unless noted

Beef
   Brisket

	CALORIES
Whole, braised, lean, trimmed to ¼-in fat	206
Whole, braised, lean and fat, trimmed to ¼-in fat	327
Flat half, braised, lean, trimmed to ¼-in fat	189
Flat half, braised, lean and fat, trimmed to ¼-in fat	309
Point half, braised, lean, trimmed to ¼-in fat	222
Point half, braised, lean and fat, trimmed to ¼-in fat	343

   Chuck

	CALORIES
Arm pot roast, braised, lean, trimmed to ¼-in fat	183
Arm pot roast, braised, lean and fat, trimmed to ¼-in fat	282
Blade roast, braised, lean, trimmed to ¼-in fat	213
Blade roast, braised, lean and fat, trimmed to ¼-in fat	293
Flank, broiled, lean, trimmed to 0-in fat	176
Flank, broiled, lean and fat, trimmed to 0-in fat	192

   Ground beef

	CALORIES
Baked, medium, 80% lean	224
Baked, medium, extra lean	200
Baked, well done, 80% lean	245
Baked, well done, extra lean	220
Broiled, medium, 80% lean	228
Broiled, medium, extra lean	204
Broiled, well done, 80% lean	235
Broiled, well done, extra lean	213
Pan fried, medium, 80% lean	231

CALORIES

Pan fried, medium, extra lean	203
Pan fried, well done, 80% lean	233
Pan fried, well done, extra lean	211
Rib	
Large end, roasted, lean, trimmed to ¼-in fat	201
Large end, roasted, lean and fat, trimmed to ¼-in fat	310
Small end, broiled, lean, trimmed to ¼-in fat	188
Small end, broiled, lean and fat, trimmed to ¼-in fat	285
Round	
Bottom round, braised, lean, trimmed to ¼-in fat	178
Bottom round, braised, lean and fat, trimmed to ¼-in fat	234
Eye of round, roasted, lean, trimmed to ¼-in fat	143
Eye of round, roasted, lean and fat, trimmed to ¼-in fat	195
Full cut, broiled, lean, trimmed to ¼-in fat	162
Full cut, broiled, lean and fat, trimmed to ¼-in fat	204
Tip round, roasted, lean, trimmed to ¼-in fat	157
Tip round, roasted, lean and fat, trimmed to ¼-in fat	199
Top round, broiled, lean, trimmed to ¼-in fat	153
Top round, broiled, lean and fat, trimmed to ¼-in fat	183
Shank, crosscuts, simmered, lean, trimmed to ¼-in fat	171
Shank, crosscuts, simmered, lean and fat, trimmed to ¼-in fat	224
Short loin	
Porterhouse steak, broiled, lean, trimmed to ¼-in fat	185
Porterhouse steak, broiled, lean and fat, trimmed to ¼-in fat	260
T-bone steak, broiled, lean, trimmed to ¼-in fat	182
T-bone steak, broiled, lean and fat, trimmed to ¼-in fat	253
Tenderloin, broiled, lean, trimmed to ¼-in fat	179
Tenderloin, broiled, lean and fat, trimmed to ¼-in fat	246

Top loin, broiled, lean, trimmed to ¼-in fat	176
Top loin, broiled, lean and fat, trimmed to ¼-in fat	244
Top sirloin, broiled, lean, trimmed to ¼-in fat	165
Top sirloin, broiled, lean and fat, trimmed to ¼-in fat	219
Short ribs, braised, lean, trimmed to ¼-in fat	251
Short ribs, braised, lean and fat, trimmed to ¼-in fat	400

Brains

Calf, braised	115
Calf, pan-fried	181
Lamb, braised	124
Lamb, pan-fried	232

Elk, roasted	124
Goat, roasted	122

Heart

Beef, lean, braised	150
Calf, braised	158
Lamb, braised	158

Kidney

Calf, braised	139
Lamb, braised	117

Lamb

Chops

Loin, broiled, lean and fat / 2.8 oz (3 chops per lb)	235
Loin, broiled, lean / 2.3 oz (3 chops per lb)	140
Loin, roasted, lean and fat	263
Loin, roasted, lean	171
Rib, broiled, lean and fat	307
Rib, broiled, lean	200
Rib, roasted, lean and fat	315
Rib, roasted, lean	130

Ground, broiled	240
Leg, roasted, lean and fat	205
Leg, roasted, lean / 2.6 oz	140
Shoulder, braised, lean and fat / 2.2 oz	220
Shoulder, braised, lean / 1.7 oz	135
Shoulder and leg cubed, broiled as kabobs, lean	158

Liver

Beef, fried	185
Calf, braised	140

CALORIES

Calf, fried	208
Lamb, braised	187
Lamb, fried	202
Moose, roasted	114
Pork	
Chop,	
Loin, broiled, lean and fat / 3.1 oz	275
Loin, broiled, lean / 2.5 oz	165
Loin, pan-fried, lean and fat / 3.1 oz	335
Loin, pan-fried, lean / 2.4 oz	180
Ham	
Light cure, roasted, lean and fat	205
Light cure, roasted, lean / 2.4 oz	105
Fresh, roasted, leg, lean and fat	250
Fresh, roasted, leg, lean / 2.5 oz	160
Rib, roasted, lean and fat	270
Rib, roasted, lean / 2.5 oz	175
Shoulder, braised, lean and fat	295
Shoulder, braised, lean / 2.4 oz	165
Rabbit, wild, stewed	147
Raccoon, roasted	217
Squirrel, roasted	116
Sweetbreads, calf, braised	148
Tongue	
Calf, braised	171
Lamb, braised	234
Veal	
Cutlet, braised or broiled, boneless, medium fat	185
Ground, broiled	146
Leg (top round), braised, lean and fat	180
Leg (top round), braised, lean	172
Leg (top round), pan-fried, breaded, lean and fat	194
Leg (top round), pan-fried, breaded, lean	175
Leg (top round), pan-fried, not breaded, lean and fat	179
Leg (top round), pan-fried, not breaded, lean	156
Leg (top round), roasted, lean	128
Loin	
Braised, lean and fat	242
Braised, lean	192
Roasted, lean and fat	184
Roasted, lean	149

CALORIES

Rib
    Braised, lean and fat   214
    Braised, lean   185
    - Roasted, lean and fat   230
    Roasted, lean   151

	CALORIES
Rib	
Braised, lean and fat	214
Braised, lean	185
Roasted, lean and fat	230
Roasted, lean	151
Shoulder, arm, braised, lean and fat	201
Shoulder, arm, braised, lean	171
Shoulder, arm, roasted, lean and fat	156
Shoulder, arm, roasted, lean	139
Shoulder, blade, braised, lean and fat	191
Shoulder, blade, braised, lean	168
Shoulder, blade, roasted, lean and fat	158
Shoulder, blade, roasted, lean	146
Shoulder and leg cubed, braised, lean	160
Sirloin, braised, lean and fat	214
Sirloin, braised, lean	173
Sirloin, roasted, lean and fat	171
Sirloin, roasted, lean	143
Venison, roasted	134

CANNED, CURED AND PROCESSED

CALORIES

1 slice unless noted

	CALORIES
Bacon, cooked	
Oscar Mayer	33
Oscar Mayer Center Cut	25
Oscar Mayer Lower Salt	33
Oscar Mayer Thick Sliced	58
Bits / ¼ oz / **Oscar Mayer**	20
Canadian / **Oscar Mayer**	28
Bar-B-Q loaf / **Oscar Mayer**	46
Beef, corned / **Oscar Mayer**	17
Beef, sliced thin, roast / **Oscar Mayer**	14
Beef, smoked / **Oscar Mayer**	14
Bologna	
Eckrich Lite	70
Oscar Mayer	90
Oscar Mayer Light	64
Beef / **Oscar Mayer**	89
Beef / **Oscar Mayer** Light	64

Beef, Lebanon / **Oscar Mayer**	46
Garlic beef / **Oscar Mayer**	90
w cheese / **Oscar Mayer**	74
Bratwurst links, smoked / 1 link / **Eckrich** Lite	190
Braunschweiger	
Oscar Mayer / 1 slice	96
Oscar Mayer / 1 oz	97
Oscar Mayer German / 1 oz	96
Frankfurters	
Eckrich Bunsize Lite / 1 frank	150
Eckrich Lite / 1 frank	120
Oscar Mayer Bun Length / 1 link	184
Oscar Mayer Light / 1 link	127
Oscar Mayer Little Wieners / 1 link	28
Oscar Mayer Wieners / 1 link	144
Bacon and cheddar cheese / **Oscar Mayer** / 1 link	137
Beef / **Oscar Mayer** / 1 link	143
Beef / **Oscar Mayer** Bun Length / 1 link	182
Beef / **Oscar Mayer** Light / 1 link	131
Beef w cheddar / **Oscar Mayer** / 1 link	136
Cheese / **Oscar Mayer** / 1 link	143
w noodles / canned / 1 cup / **Van Camp's**	245
Ham: 1 slice unless noted	
Oscar Mayer Breakfast	47
Oscar Mayer Honey	23
and cheese loaf / **Oscar Mayer**	66
Baked / **Oscar Mayer**	21
Boiled / **Oscar Mayer**	23
Canned / 1 oz / **Oscar Mayer** Jubilee	29
Chopped / **Oscar Mayer**	41
Chopped / **Oscar Mayer** Peppered	55
Cooked / **Eckrich** Lite / 1 oz	25
Cooked, smoked / **Oscar Mayer**	22
Pepper, black, cracked / **Oscar Mayer**	22
Slice / 1 oz / **Oscar Mayer** Jubilee	29
Slice / **Oscar Mayer** Lower Salt	23
Sliced thin / **Oscar Mayer**	13
Sliced thin / **Oscar Mayer** Honey	13
Smoked, boneless / 1 oz / **Oscar Mayer** Jubilee	43
Steaks / **Oscar Mayer** Jubilee	57
Head cheese / **Oscar Mayer**	54

Honey loaf / **Oscar Mayer**	34
Kielbasa / 1 oz / **Eckrich** Polska Lite	70
Liver cheese / **Oscar Mayer**	116
Luncheon meat / **Oscar Mayer**	94
Old-fashioned loaf / **Oscar Mayer**	62
Olive loaf / **Oscar Mayer**	63
Pastrami, sliced / **Oscar Mayer**	16
Peppered loaf / **Oscar Mayer**	39
Pickle and pimento loaf / **Oscar Mayer**	66
Picnic loaf / **Oscar Mayer**	61
Salami	
Beer / **Oscar Mayer**	50
Beer, beef / **Oscar Mayer**	63
Cotto / **Oscar Mayer**	52
Cotto, beef / **Oscar Mayer**	45
Genoa / **Oscar Mayer**	34
Hard / **Oscar Mayer**	33
Sausage	
New England / **Oscar Mayer**	29
Smoked / 1 oz / **Eckrich** Lite	70
Smoked / 1 link /**Eckrich** Lite	150
Sausage links / 1 link / **Oscar Mayer** Little Friers	82
Sausage links, smoked	
Eckrich Beef Lite / 1 link	200
Eckrich Cheddar Lite / 1 link	190
Eckrich Lite / 1 link	200
Eckrich Polish Lite / 1 link	180
Eckrich Smoky Links Lite / 2 links	120
Oscar Mayer, Beef Smokies / 1 link	124
Oscar Mayer Cheese Smokies / 1 link	126
Oscar Mayer Little Smokies / 1 link	27
Oscar Mayer Smokie Links / 1 link	126
Summer sausage / **Oscar Mayer**	69
Summer sausage, beef / **Oscar Mayer**	70
Vienna sausage, chicken / canned / 2 oz / **Libby's**	123

MEAT ENTRÉES, FROZEN

Beef	
and noodles w gravy / 7 oz / **Banquet**	180
Chipped / 4 oz / **Banquet** Cookin' Bag	100

CALORIES

Chipped, creamed / 11 oz / **Stouffer's**	230
Patties w mushroom gravy / 7 oz / **Banquet**	260
Patties w onion gravy / 7 oz / **Banquet**	260
Patty w mushroom gravy / 7 oz / **Banquet** Entree Express	350
Pepper steak / 11.25 oz / **Armour** Classics Lite	220
Sirloin tips / 7 oz / **Swanson** Homestyle	160
Sirloin tips and mushroom in wine sauce / 7.50 oz / **Weight Watchers**	220
Stroganoff / 11.25 oz / **Armour** Classics Lite	250
Stroganoff / 8.50 oz / **Weight Watchers**	290
Tips w vegetables / 12 oz / **Ultra Slim-Fast**	230
and bean enchaladas / 9-1/4 oz / **Stouffer's** Lean Cuisine	240
and noodles w vegetables / 8-3/8 oz / **Stouffer's**	230
cheddar deli melt / 1 sandwich / **Quaker** Ovenstuffs	390
Pepper steak / 9.50 oz / **Healthy Choice**	250
Pepper steak and rice / 12.00 oz / **Ultra Slim-Fast**	270
Sandwich, BBQ / 1 sandwich / **Tyson**	200
Sliced / 7 oz / **Banquet**	140
Sliced London broil in mushroom sauce / 7.37 oz / **Weight Watchers**	140
Sliced w gravy / 4 oz / **Banquet** Cookin' Bag	100
Stroganoff w noodles / 9.75 oz / **Stouffer's**	390
Teriyaki in sauce w rice and vegetables / 9.75 oz / **Stouffer's**	290
Beefsteak ranchero / 9-1/4 oz / **Stouffer's** Lean Cuisine	260
Green peppers stuffed w beef / 7.75 oz / **Stouffer's**	200
Green pepper steak w rice / 10.5 oz / **Stouffer's**	330
Homestyle barbecue / 10.25 oz / **Banquet** Healthy Balance	270
Meatballs, Swedish in gravy w noodles / 11 oz / **Stouffer's**	480
Meatballs, Swedish in gravy w pasta / 9-1/8 oz / **Stouffer's** Lean Cuisine	290
Meatloaf	
Armour Classics / 11.25 oz	360
Banquet Healthy Balance / 11 oz	270
Lipton Microeasy / 1/4 pkg	87
w tomato sauce / 7 oz / **Banquet** Entree Express	330
w tomato sauce / 10.50 oz / **Ultra Slim-Fast**	340

CALORIES

w whipped potatoes / 9.8 oz / **Stouffer's**	360
Salisbury parmigiana / 11.50 oz / **Armour** Classics	410
Salisbury steak	
Armour Classics / 11.25 oz	350
Armour Classics Lite / 11.5 oz	300
Banquet Cookin' Bag / 5 oz	190
Banquet Healthy Balance / 10.50 oz	260
Swanson Homestyle / 10 oz	320
and macaroni and cheese / 8-⅝ oz / **Stouffer's**	350
Romana / 8.75 oz / **Weight Watchers**	190
w gravy / 7 oz / **Banquet**	260
w gravy / 7 oz / **Banquet** Entree Express	300
w gravy and scalloped potatoes / 9-½ oz / **Stouffer's**	
Lean Cuisine	240
w mushroom gravy / 10.50 oz / **Ultra Slim-Fast**	290
Sandwich, burger pattie w cheese / 1 sandwich / **Morningstar Farms**	370
Sandwich, pattie w biscuit / 1 sandwich / **Morningstar Farms**	280
Scalloped potatoes and ham / 9 oz / **Swanson** Homestyle	300
Stew, beef / 7 oz / **Banquet**	140
Stew, beef / ¼ package / **Lipton** Microeasy	71
Stuffed cabbage w meat in tomato sauce / 10-¾ oz / **Stouffer's** Lean Cuisine	210
Swedish meatballs / 11.25 oz / **Armour** Classics	330
Swedish meatballs / 8 oz / **Le Menu** Lightstyle	260
Swedish meatballs / 8-½ oz / **Swanson** Homestyle	360
Veal parmigiana / 7 oz / **Banquet**	320
Veal parmigiana / 11.25 oz / **Armour** Classics	400

MEAT ENTRÉES CANNED

CALORIES

Beef, corned / 2.4 oz / **Libby's** 12-oz can	160
Beef, corned / 2.3 oz / **Libby's** 7-oz can	160
Bologna, chicken / 1 slice / **Tyson**	44
Frankfurters, cheese / each / **Weaver**	145
Frankfurters, chicken / each / **Weaver**	115
Hash, corned beef / 7-½ oz / **Libby's** 15-oz can	400
Hash, corned beef / 8 oz / **Libby's** 24-oz can	420
Potted meats / 1.83 oz / **Libby's**	110

CALORIES

Roast beef w gravy / 6 oz / **Libby's**	210
Stew, beef	
Healthy Choice / 7.5 oz	140
Healthy Choice Microwavable / 7.5 oz	140
Libby's / 7-½ oz	160
Libby's / 8 oz	170
Wolf / scant cup	179

Mexican Foods

CALORIES

See also **Dinners**

Beans, chili	
Gebhardt / canned / 1 cup	115
Green Giant 50% Less Salt / canned / ½ cup	100
Green Giant Spicy / canned / ½ cup	100
Hunt's / canned / 4 oz	100
Libby's / canned / 7-½ oz	270
Hot / canned / 7-¾ oz / **Campbell's**	180
Hot in chili gravy / canned / 7.5 oz / **Luck's**	200
Mexican style / canned / 1 cup / **Van Camp's**	210
Extra spicy / canned / ½ cup / **Green Giant**	100
Garbanzo / canned / ½ cup / **Old El Paso**	190
Mexe / canned / ½ cup / **Old El Paso**	163
Pinto / canned / ½ cup / **Old El Paso**	100
Refried	
Gebhardt / canned / 4 oz	100
Old El Paso / canned / ¼ cup	55
Rosarita / canned / 4 oz	100
w bacon / canned / 4 oz / **Rosarita**	110
w cheese / canned / 4 oz / **Rosarita**	110
w green chili / canned / ½ cup / **Little Pancho**	80
w green chilies / canned / ¼ cup / **Old El Paso**	49
w green chillies / canned / 4 oz / **Rosarita**	90
Jalapeno / canned / 4 oz / **Gebhardt**	115
w onions / canned / 4 oz / **Rosarita**	110

w sausage / canned / ¼ cup / **Old El Paso**	180
Spicy / canned / 4 oz / **Rosarita**	100
Vegetarian / canned / 4 oz / **Hain**	70
Vegetarian / canned / 4 oz / **Old El Paso**	70
Vegetarian / canned / 4 oz / **Rosarita**	100
Burritos / dinner kit / 1 / **Old El Paso**	299
Burritos, frozen	
Bean and cheese / 1 / **Old El Paso**	330
Beef / 3 oz / **Patio** Britos Nacho	220
Beef and bean / 3 oz / **Patio** Britos	210
Beef and bean	
Hot red chili / 5 oz / **Patio**	340
Medium / 5 oz / **Patio**	370
Mild green chili / 5 oz / **Patio**	330
Red hot and red chili / 5 oz / **Patio**	360
Cheese / 3.63 oz / **Patio** Britos	250
Chicken and cheese, spicy / 3 oz / **Patio** Britos	210
Hot beef and bean / 1 / **Old El Paso**	310
Mild beef and bean / 1 / **Old El Paso**	320
Chicken / 7.62 oz / **Weight Watchers**	310
Red beef and bean / 1 / **Old El Paso**	330
Burritos seasoning mix / ⅛ pkg / **Old El Paso**	17
Chili con carne, canned	
Gebhardt / 1 cup	530
Hain Spicy Tempeh / 7-½ oz	160
Hain Spicy Vegetarian / 7-½ oz	160
Hain Spicy Vegetarian, Reduced Salt / 7-½ oz	170
Just Rite / 4 oz	180
Libby's / 7.5 oz	390
Van Camp's / 1 cup	412
Wolf / 1 cup	387
Wolf Extra Spicy / scant cup	363
Chili con carne, frozen / 8-¼ oz / **Swanson** Entree	270
Chili con carne w beans, canned	
Dennison's Lite / 7.5 oz	180
Gebhardt / 1 cup	495
Gebhardt Hot / 1 cup	470
Just Rite / 4 oz	200
Just Rite Hot / 4 oz	195
Old El Paso / 1 cup	217
Van Camp's / 1 cup	352

Wolf / scant cup	345
Wolf Extra Spicy / scant cup	324
Chili con carne w beans / frozen / 8.75 oz / **Stouffer's**	260
Chili con carne w beans and chicken / canned / 7.5 oz /	
Dennison's Lite	190
Chili con carne w chicken / canned / 7-½ oz / **Hain**	130
Chili seasoning mix / ⅕ pkg / **Old El Paso**	21
Chili w turkey and beans	
Canned / 7.5 oz / **Healthy Choice**	200
Microwave cup / 7.5 oz / **Healthy Choice**	200
Spicy / canned / 7.5 oz / **Healthy Choice**	210
Spicy / microwave cup / 7.5 oz / **Healthy Choice**	210
Chili-Mac / canned / scant cup / **Wolf**	317
Chilies, chopped / canned / 2 tbsp / **Old El Paso**	8
Chilies, whole / canned / 1 chili / **Old El Paso**	8
Chimichangas, beef / frozen / 1 / **Old El Paso**	370
Chimichangas, chicken / frozen / 1 / **Old El Paso**	360
Chimichangas entree	
Bean and cheese / frozen / 1 / **Old El Paso**	380
Beef / frozen / 1 / **Old El Paso**	380
Beef and pork / frozen / 1 / **Old El Paso**	340
Chicken / frozen / 1 / **Old El Paso**	370
Dips, Mexican style	
Avocado / canned / 2 tbsp / **Kraft**	50
Bean, hot / canned / 4 tbsp / **Hain**	70
Bean, jalapeno / 1 tbsp / **Old El Paso**	14
Bean, jalapeno-flavored / canned / 2 tbsp / **Wise**	25
Bean, Mexican / canned / 4 tbsp / **Hain**	60
Bean w onion / canned / 4 tbsp / **Hain**	70
Jalapeno bean / canned / 1 oz / **Frito-Lay**	30
Jalapeno cheese / canned / 2 tbsp / **Kraft**	50
Jalapeno pepper / canned / 2 tbsp / **Kraft**	50
Nacho cheese / canned / 2 tbsp / **Kraft**	55
Picante / canned / 2 tbsp / **Wise**	12
Picante sauce / canned / 1 oz / **Frito-Lay**	10
Taco / canned / 2 tbsp / **Wise**	12
Taco and sauce / canned / ¼ cup / **Hain**	35
Enchiladas	
Gebhardt / canned / 2 pieces	310
Old El Paso / dinner kit / 1	145
Beef / frozen / 13.25 oz / **Patio**	520

CALORIES

Cheese / frozen / 12 oz / **Patio**	370
Chicken / frozen / 11 oz / **Banquet**	300
Enchiladas entrée, frozen	
Beef / 1 / **Old El Paso**	210
Beef ranchero / 9.12 oz / **Weight Watchers**	230
Beef w chili sauce / 7 oz / **Banquet**	270
Cheese / 1 / **Old El Paso**	250
Cheese / 10 -⅛ oz / **Stouffer's**	590
Chicken	
Healthy Choice / 9.5 oz	280
Old El Paso / 1	220
Stouffer's / 10 oz	490
Chicken ranchero / 8.87 oz / **Weight Watchers**	360
Chicken suiza / 9 oz / **Weight Watchers**	280
Chicken w sour cream sauce / 1 / **Old El Paso**	280
Enchiladas seasoning mix / ⅟₁₈ pkg / **Old El Paso**	6
Fajita marinade / 1 oz / **Old El Paso**	14
Fajitas	
Beef / frozen / 7 oz / **Healthy Choice**	210
Beef / frozen / 6.75 oz / **Weight Watchers**	250
Chicken / frozen / 7 oz / **Healthy Choice**	200
Chicken / frozen / 6.75 oz / **Weight Watchers**	230
Fiesta dinner / frozen / 12 oz / **Patio**	460
Guacamole seasoning mix / ⅟₇ pkg / **Old El Paso**	7
Jalapeno peppers	
Peeled / canned / 2 peppers / **Old El Paso**	na
Pickled / canned / 2 peppers / **Old El Paso**	na
Slices / canned / 2 tbsp / **Old El Paso**	na
Jalapeno relish / canned / 2 tbsp / **Old El Paso**	16
Menudo / canned / ½ can / **Old El Paso**	476
Mexican style dinner / frozen / 13.25 oz / **Patio**	540
Salsa	
Green chile / 1 tbsp / **Ortega**	6
Hot / 1 oz / **Frito-Lay** Chunky	12
Medium / 1 oz / **Frito-Lay** Chunky	12
Mild / 1 oz / **Frito-Lay** Chunky	12
Spanish rice / canned / 1 cup / **Van Camp's**	160
Taco shell	
Gebhardt / 1 shell	50
Old El Paso / 1 shell	55
Rosarita / 1 shell	50

CALORIES

Mini / 3 shells / **Old El Paso**	70
Super / 1 shell / **Old El Paso**	100
Tamales, canned	
Derby / 2 tamales	160
Gebhardt / 2 tamales	290
Gebhardt Jumbo / 2 tamales	400
Old El Paso / 2 tamales	190
Wolf / scant cup	328
w sauce / canned / 1 cup / **Van Camp's**	293
Tamales dinner / frozen / 13 oz / **Patio**	470
Tomatoes and green chilies / canned / ¼ cup / **Old El Paso**	14
Tomatoes and jalapenos / canned / ¼ cup / **Old El Paso**	11
Tortillas	
Corn, Enchilada style / 1 shell / **Tyson**	54
Flour / 1 shell / **Old El Paso**	150
Flour	
Burrito-style, heat-pressed / 1 shell / **Tyson**	173
Burrito-style, large / 1 shell / **Tyson**	182
Burrito-style, small / 1 shell / **Tyson**	106
Fajita-style / 1 shell / **Tyson**	84
Soft taco / 1 shell / **Tyson**	121
Tortillas grande / frozen / 9-⅝ oz / **Stouffer's**	530
Tostada shell: 1 shell	
Old El Paso	100
Pancho Villa	55
Rosarita	60
Old El Paso	55

Milk

1 cup (8 fl oz) unless noted

Non-brand names
Buttermilk	100
Whole, 3.3% fat	150
Lowfat, 2% fat	120
Lowfat, 1% fat	100
Nonfat, skim	85

Buttermilk
Lucerne	120
Lucerne Bulgarian	150
1.5% fat / **Borden**	120
1.5% fat / **Friendship**	120

Condensed, canned: ⅓ cup
Meadow Gold	320
sweetened / **Borden** Eagle Brand	320
sweetened / **Carnation**	320

Dry nonfat
Carnation Instant mix / 5 tbsp dry	80
Fearn / mix / 3 tbsp /	90
Weight Watchers Dairy Creamer / mix / 1 packet	10
Reconstituted, mix / **Lucerne**	80

Evaporated, canned
Carnation / ½ cup	170
Lucerne / 4 fl oz	170
Pet/Dairymate / ½ cup	170
Pet/Dairymate Filled / ½ cup	150
Pet/Dairymate Skim / ½ cup	100
Goatmilk / 4 oz undiluted / **Miracle**	160
Lowfat / ½ cup / **Carnation**	110
Skim / ½ cup / **Carnation** Lite	100

Low fat
Nestlé Quik, Banana	190

CALORIES

Nestlé Quik, Chocolate	200
Nestlé Quik, Strawberry	200
Nestlé Quik, Vanilla	200
Low fat, .5% fat / **Lucerne**	90
Low fat, 1% fat	
Borden	100
Lactaid Lactose Reduced	100
Lucerne	100
Low fat, 2% fat	
Borden	140
Borden Dutch Brand Chocolate	180
Dairy Ease Lactose Free	120
Hershey's Chocolate	190
Lucerne	120
Lucerne Two Ten	140
Viva w Extra Calcium	120
Skim	
Borden	90
Borden Nonfat	100
Weight Watchers	90
Whole	
Borden	150
Borden Hi Calcium	150
Lucerne	150
Meadow Gold, Chocolate	210
Whole, 3.5% fat / **Hershey's** Chocolate	210

FLAVORED MILK BEVERAGES

Banana flavor	
Nestlé Quik / mix / ¾ oz	90
Nestlé Quik / mix / 8 fl oz prepared w whole milk	230
Nestlé Quik / mix / 8 fl oz prepared w low fat milk	210
Nestlé Quik / mix / 8 fl oz prepared w skim milk	170
Chocolate	
Carnation Liquid Slender / canned / 10 fl oz	220
Sego Lite / canned / 10 oz	150
Sego Very / canned / 10 oz	225
Borden Frostee / dairy pack / 1 cup	200
Lucerne Lowfat / dairy pack / 8 fl oz	180
Nestlé Quik / dairy pack / 8 fl oz	230

CALORIES

Weight Watchers / mix / 1 env	60
Dutch / canned / 10 oz / **Sego** Lite	150
Low fat / dairy pack / **Hershey**	190
Malt / canned / 10 oz / **Sego** Very	225
Chocolate-flavor syrup	
Nestlé Quik / 1.22 oz	100
Nestlé Quik / 8 fl oz prepared w whole milk	240
Nestlé Quik / 8 fl oz prepared w low fat milk	220
Nestlé Quik / 8 fl oz prepared w skim milk	180
Chocolate fudge / canned / 10 fl oz / **Carnation** Liquid Slender	220
Chocolate malt / canned / 10 fl oz / **Carnation** Liquid Slender	220
Chocolate milk / ready to drink / 8 fl oz / **Nestlé** Quik	230
Chocolate milk / ready to drink / 8 fl oz / **Nestlé** Quik Lowfat Lite	130
Chocolate mixes	
Alba '77 / 1 env	70
Carnation Instant Breakfast / 1 env dry	130
Carnation Instant Breakfast, Diet / 1 env, dry	70
Hershey's / 3 tsp	90
Lucerne / 8 fl oz prepared	240
Lucerne Instant Breakfast / 1 env	130
Nestlé Quik / ¾ oz	90
Nestlé Quik / 8 fl oz prepared w whole milk	230
Nestlé Quik / 8 fl oz prepared w low fat milk	210
Nestlé Quik / 8 fl oz prepared w skim milk	170
Nestlé Quik, Sugar Free / 5.6 g	18
Nestlé Quik, Sugar Free / 8 fl oz prepared w 2% milk	140
Pillsbury Instant Breakfast / 1 env, prepared	250
Chocolate fudge / 1 env / **Weight Watchers**	70
Malt	
Carnation Instant Breakfast / 1 env, dry	130
Carnation Instant Breakfast, Diet / 1 env, dry	70
Pillsbury Instant Breakfast / 1 env, prepared	250
Chocolate mocha / dairy pack / 8 fl oz / **Nescafe** Mocha Cooler	150
Coffee mix / 1 env dry / **Carnation** Instant Breakfast	130
Coffee mix / 1 env / **Lucerne** Instant Breakfast	130
Eggnog / canned / 4 fl oz / **Borden**	160

CALORIES

Malt / mix, as packaged / 3 tsp / **Kraft** Instant Chocolate	90
Malt / mix, as packaged / 3 tsp / **Kraft** Instant Natural	90
Marshmallow-flavored / mix / 1 env / **Weight Watchers**	60
Milk chocolate / canned / 10 fl oz / **Carnation** Liquid Slender	220
Orange sherbet / mix / 1 env / **Weight Watchers**	70

Strawberry

Borden Frostee / canned / 1 cup	180
Sego Lite / canned / 10 oz	150
Sego Very / canned / 10 oz	225

Strawberry-flavor syrup

Nestlé Quik / 1.22 oz	100
Nestlé Quik / 8 fl oz prepared w whole milk	240
Nestlé Quik / 8 fl oz prepared w low fat milk	220
Nestlé Quik / 8 fl oz prepared w skim milk	180
Strawberry milk / ready to drink / 8 fl oz / **Nestlé** Quik	230

Strawberry mixes

Alba '77 / 1 env	70
Carnation Instant Breakfast / 1 env, dry	130
Carnation Instant Breakfast, Diet / 1 env, dry	70
Lucerne Instant Breakfast / 1 env	130
Nestlé Quik / ¾ oz	80
Nestlé Quik / 8 fl oz prepared w whole milk	220
Nestlé Quik / 8 fl oz prepared w low fat milk	200
Nestlé Quik / 8 fl oz prepared w skim milk	160
Pillsbury Instant Breakfast / 1 env, prepared	250

Vanilla

Carnation Liquid Slender / canned / 10 fl oz	220
Sego Lite / canned / 10 oz	150
Sego Very / canned / 10 oz	225
Vanilla, French / canned / 10 oz / **Sego** Lite	150

Vanilla mixes

Alba '77 / 1 env	70
Carnation Instant Breakfast / 1 env, dry	130
Carnation Instant Breakfast, Diet / 1 env, dry	70
Lucerne Instant Breakfast / 1 env	130
Pillsbury Instant Breakfast / 1 env, prepared	260

Muffins: English and Sweet

CALORIES

1 muffin unless noted

Apple cinnamon / mix, prepared / **Betty Crocker**	120
Apple cinnamon / mix, prepared, no cholesterol / **Betty Crocker**	110
Apple spice	
Health Valley	130
Healthy Choice / frozen	190
Weight Watchers / microwave / 2.5 oz	160
Applesauce / ⅙ mix, prepared **Gold Medal** Pouch Mixes	160
Banana / **Health Valley**	130
Banana / ⅙ mix prepared / **Gold Medal** Pouch Mixes	150
Banana nut	
Thomas' Toast-R-Cakes	110
Healthy Choice / frozen	180
Weight Watchers / microwave / 2.5 oz	170
Betty Crocker / mix, prepared	120
Betty Crocker / mix, prepared, no cholesterol	110
Banana nut, mini / **Tastykake**	60
Blueberry	
Thomas' Toast-R-Cakes	100
Healthy Choice / frozen	190
Pepperidge Farm / frozen	170
Weight Watchers / microwave / 2.5 oz	170
Betty Crocker / mix, prepared	120
Betty Crocker Light / mix, prepared	70
Betty Crocker Streusel / mix, prepared	210
Betty Crocker Twice the Blueberries / mix, prepared	120
Duncan Hines / mix, prepared	120

CALORIES

Duncan Hines / Bakery Style / mix, prepared	190
Gold Medal Pouch Mixes / ⅙ mix, prepared	170
Pillsbury / mix, prepared	100
Betty Crocker / mix, prepared, no cholesterol	110
Betty Crocker Light / mix, prepared, no cholesterol	70
Betty Crocker Twice the Blueberries / mix, prepared, no cholesterol	110
Pillsbury / mix, prepared w egg whites	100
Blueberry-apple / **Health Valley**	140
Blueberry, mini / **Tastykake**	50
Bran / ⅙ mix / **Fearn**	110
Caramel / ⅙ mix, prepared / **Gold Medal** Pouch Mixes	150
Carrot multi-bran / **Health Valley**	130
Carrot-raisin nut, mini / **Tastykake**	60
Cinnamon streusel / mix, prepared / **Betty Crocker**	200
Cinnamon swirl / mix, prepared / **Duncan Hines**	200
Corn	
Thomas' Toast-R-Cakes	120
Fearn / ⅙ mix	160
Arrowhead Mills Blue Corn / mix, prepared	11
Flako / mix, prepared	116
Gold Medal Pouch Mixes / ⅙ mix, prepared	180
English	
Millbrook	130
Pepperidge Farm	140
Pritikin	150
Roman Meal	150
Thomas'	120
Weber	130
Bran nut / **Thomas'**	140
Cinnamon-apple / **Pepperidge Farm**	140
Cinnamon chip / **Pepperidge Farm**	160
Cinnamon raisin / **Millbrook**	130
Cinnamon raisin / **Pepperidge Farm**	150
Honey wheat / **Thomas'**	120
Oat bran / **Millbrook**	140
Oat bran / **Thomas'**	120
Raisin / **Sunmaid**	160
Raisin / **Thomas'**	150
Sourdough	

CALORIES

Millbrook	130
Pepperidge Farm	135
Thomas'	130
Weber	130
Whole wheat / **Millbrook**	120
Grain cakes	
Corn / 1 cake / **Quaker**	35
Rye / 1 cake / **Quaker**	35
Wheat / 1 cake / **Quaker**	34
Honey bran / ⅙ mix, prepared / **Gold Medal** Pouch Mixes	170
Oat / ⅙ mix, prepared / **Gold Medal** Pouch Mixes	150
Oat / ⅙ mix, prepared, no cholesterol / **Gold Medal** Pouch Mixes	140
Oat bran / mix, prepared / **Betty Crocker**	190
Oat bran / mix, prepared, no cholesterol / **Betty Crocker**	180
Oat bran, almond date / **Health Valley**	140
Oat bran, apple spice / mix, prepared / **Arrowhead Mills**	120
Oat bran, blueberries / **Health Valley**	140
Oat bran, raisin / **Health Valley**	140
Oat bran, wheat free / mix, prepared / **Arrowhead Mills**	100
Oatbran w apple, cholesterol free / frozen / **Pepperidge Farm**	190
Raisin bran / **Thomas'** Toast-R-Cakes	100
Raisin bran / frozen / **Pepperidge Farm** Cholesterol Free	170
Raisin spice / **Health Valley**	130
Raspberry / **Health Valley**	130
Rice cakes	
Apple cinnamon / ½ oz / **Hollywood** Mini Cakes	50
Cheese / ½ oz / **Hollywood** Mini Cakes	60
Corn, lightly salted / 1 cake / **Quaker**	35
Honeynut / ½ oz / **Hollywood** Mini Cakes	60
Multigrain, lightly salted / 1 cake / **Quaker**	34
Plain, lightly salted / 1 cake / **Quaker**	35
Plain, salt free / 1 cake / **Quaker**	35
Sesame, lightly salted / 1 cake / **Quaker**	35
Sesame, salt free / 1 cake / **Quaker**	35
Wheat bran / mix, prepared / **Arrowhead Mills**	270

Nuts

UNSALTED AND UNFLAVORED

	CALORIES
Almonds	
Dried, in shell / 10 nuts	60
Dried, in shell / 1 cup	185
Dried, shelled, chopped / 1 tbsp	50
Dried, shelled, chopped / 1 cup	775
Dried, shelled, slivered / 1 cup	795
Dried, shelled, whole / 1 oz	165
Roasted, in oil / 1 cup	985
Beechnuts, in shell / 1 lb	1570
Beechnuts, shelled / 1 lb	2575
Brazil nuts, in shell / 1 cup	385
Brazil nuts, shelled / 1 oz	185
Brazil nuts, shelled / 1 cup	915
Butternuts, in shell / 1 lb	400
Butternuts, shelled / 1 lb	2850
Cashew nuts, roasted in oil / 1 cup	785
Cashew nuts, roasted in oil / 1 lb	2545
Chestnuts	
Fresh, in shell / 1 cup	190
Fresh, in shell / 1 lb	715
Fresh, shelled / 1 cup	310
Fresh, shelled / 1 lb	880
Roasted (European), shelled / 1 cup	350
Filberts, in shell / 1 lb	1325

	CALORIES
Filberts, shelled, chopped / 1 oz	180
Filberts, shelled, whole / 1 cup	855
Hickory nuts, shelled / 1 oz	200
Macadamia nuts, roasted in oil, shelled / 1 oz	205
Peanuts, roasted	
in shell / 10 jumbo nuts	105
in shell / 1 lb	1770
Spanish and Virginia / 1 lb	2655
Spanish and Virginia, chopped / 1 cup	840
Pecans	
Chopped or pieces / 1 tbsp	50
Chopped or pieces / 1 cup	810
Halves	
10 large (451–550 per lb)	60
10 jumbo (301–350 per lb)	95
10 mammoth (250 or fewer per lb)	125
1 cup	720
1 oz	190
Pine nuts, pignolias, shelled / 1 oz	155
Pine nuts, pinyon, shelled / 1 oz	160
Pistachio nuts, in shell / 1 lb	1345
Pistachio nuts, dried, shelled / 1 oz	165
Walnuts	
Black, chopped / 1 oz	170
English or Persian, pieces or chips / 1 oz	180

ROASTED AND FLAVORED

	CALORIES
1 oz unless noted (1 oz equals about ⅕ cup)	
Almonds	
Blue Diamond Smokehouse	150
Dole	170
Fisher	170
Barbecue / **Blue Diamond**	160
Chili w lemon / **Blue Diamond**	160
Chopped, natural / **Blue Diamond**	150
Dry roasted, unsalted / **Blue Diamond**	150
Honey roasted / **Blue Diamond**	140
Honey roasted / **Planters**	170

CALORIES

Lightly salted / **Blue Diamond**	150
Sliced, natural / **Blue Diamond**	150
Slivered / **Safeway** Party Pride	170
Slivered, blanched / **Blue Diamond**	150
Sour cream and onion / **Blue Diamond**	150
Toasted, unsalted / **Blue Diamond**	150
Whole, blanched / **Blue Diamond**	150
Whole, natural / **Blue Diamond**	150
Cashew halves, oil roasted / **Planters**	170
Cashew halves, unsalted, oil roasted / **Planters**	170
Cashews	
Frito-Lay	170
Safeway Party Pride	170
Dry roasted, lightly salted / **Planters**	160
Dry roasted / **Safeway** Party Pride	170
Honey roasted / **Planters**	170
Oil roasted, lightly salted / **Planters**	160
Whole, salted / **Guy's**	170
Cashews, fancy, oil roasted / **Planters**	170
Cashews, fancy, unsalted / **Planters**	170
Corn nuts / 1.38 oz / **Frito-Lay** Toasted Corn Nuggets	170
Macadamias, lightly salted / **Blue Diamond**	190
Mix, peanut, cashew, honey roasted / **Planters**	170
Mixed	
Fisher	170
Guy's	180
Cashews, almonds, peanuts / **Planters** Vacuum Bag	170
Cashews, almonds, pecans / **Planters** Vacuum Bag	180
Cashews, pecans, peanuts / **Planters** Vacuum Bag	180
Dry roasted / **Planters**	160
Dry roasted / **Safeway** Party Pride	170
Honey roasted / **Planters**	170
Oil roasted / **Planters**	180
Oil roasted, deluxe / **Planters**	180
Oil roasted, lightly salted / **Planters**	180
Oil roasted, unsalted / **Planters**	180
Sesame nut / **Planters**	160
w peanuts / **Safeway** Party Pride	180
w o peanuts / **Safeway** Party Pride	180
Nut toppings / **Fisher**	160

CALORIES

Peanuts	
Planters Fresh Roast Vacuum Bag	170
Planters Lightly Salted	170
Planters Salted	170
Safeway Party Pride	170
Weight Watchers / 1 pouch	100
Cocktail / **Planters**	170
Cocktail, salted / **Frito-Lay**	170
Cocktail, unsalted / **Planters**	170
Dry roasted / 1-⅛ oz / **Frito-Lay**	190
Dry roasted / **Guy's**	170
Dry roasted / **Planters**	160
Dry roasted / **Planters** Lightly Salted Vacuum Bag	170
Dry roasted, honey roasted / **Planters**	160
Dry roasted, lightly salted / **Planters**	170
Dry roasted, unsalted / **Planters**	170
Honey roasted / **Planters**	170
Oil roasted / **Planters** Unsalted, Vacuum Bag	170
Redskin / **Planters**	170
Roasted in shell / **Fisher**	160
Roasted in shell, salted / **Planters**	170
Roasted in shell, unsalted / **Planters**	170
Spanish / **Guy's**	170
Spanish / **Safeway** Party Pride	180
Spanish, oil roasted / **Planters**	170
Spanish, raw / **Fisher**	160
Spanish, roasted / **Fisher**	170
Sweet 'n Crunchy / **Planters**	140
Pecan halves / **Safeway** Party Pride	200
Pecans / **Fisher**	190
Pecans, honey roasted / **Planters**	200
Pignoli, imported / 1 tbsp / **Progresso**	60
Pistachios, natural / **Blue Diamond**	140
Pistachios, red / **Blue Diamond**	140
Pistachios, natural, dry roasted / **Planters**	170
Pistachios, red, dry roasted / **Planters**	170
Pistachios, shelled / **Dole**	160
Sunflower kernels, dry roasted / **Safeway** Party Pride	190
Sunflower nuts, dry roasted	
Planters	160
Fisher	170
Sunflower nuts, oil roasted / **Fisher**	170

CALORIES

Sunflower nuts, oil roasted / **Planters**	170
Sunflower seeds / **Frito-Lay**	160
Tasty mix / **Guy's**	130
Walnuts, black / **Fisher**	170
Walnuts, raw / **Fisher**	180

Oils

1 tbsp unless noted

Corn	125
Olive	125
Peanut	125
Safflower	125
Soybean	125
Soybean-cottonseed blend	125
Sunflower	125

Brand names

All Blend / **Hain**	120
Almond / **Hain**	120
Apricot kernel / **Hain**	120
Avocado / **Hain**	120
Canola	
Hain Organic	120
Hollywood	120
Weight Watchers Cooking Spray / 1 sec	2
Wesson	120
Coconut / **Hain**	120
Cooking spray / 1 sec / **Weight Watchers**	2
Corn	
Crisco	120
Hain	120
Nu Made	120

	CALORIES
Pam Cooking Spray / 1 sec	2
Wesson	120
Cottonseed / **Nu Made**	120
Garlic and oil / **Hain**	120
Olive	
Hain	120
Pam Cooking Spray / 1 sec	2
Wesson	120
Olive, extra virgin / **Progresso**	125
Olive, imported / **Progresso**	125
Peanut	
Hain	120
Hollywood	120
Planters	120
Popcorn / **Planters**	120
Rice bran / **Hain**	120
Rice bran / **Hollywood**	120
Safflower	
Hain Hi Oleic	120
Hain Organic	120
Hollywood	120
Salad / **Nu Made**	120
Sesame / **Hain**	120
Soy / **Hain**	120
Soy / **Hollywood**	120
Sunflower	
Hain	120
Hollywood	120
Nu Made	120
Wesson	120
Vegetable	
Crisco	120
Nu Made	120
Puritan	120
Wesson	120
Wesson Cooking Spray Lite / 1 sec	<1
Walnut / **Hain**	120

Olives

CALORIES

10 olives

Green
    Small   33
    Medium   38
    Extra large   50
Ripe, black
    Ascolano
      Extra large   61
      Giant   89
      Jumbo   105
    Manzanillo
      Small   38
      Medium   44
      Large   51
      Extra large   61
    Mission
      Small   50
      Medium   63
      Large   75
      Extra large   87
    Sevillano
      Giant   64
      Jumbo   76
      Collosal   95
      Supercollosal   114
    Greek style / medium   65
    Greek style / extra large   89

Pancakes, Waffles and Similar Breakfast Foods

See also Eggs

Breakfast, frozen entree

Belgian waffles / 1.5 oz / **Weight Watchers** Microwave   120

Belgian waffles and sausage / 2.85 oz / **Swanson**
Great Starts   280

Belgian waffles and strawberries and sausage / 3-½ oz
/ **Swanson** Great Starts   210

Blueberry pancakes / 3.47 oz / **Kid Cuisine**   210

Buttermilk pancakes / 4.17 oz / **Kid Cuisine**   180

Buttermilk pancakes / 2.5 oz / **Weight Watchers**
Microwave   140

Egg patties w cheese / 4.8 oz / **Kid Cuisine**   190

English muffin sandwich / 4.25 oz / **Healthy Choice**   200

English muffin sandwich / 4 oz / **Weight Watchers**
Microwave   230

French toast

   Kid Cuisine / 4.11 oz   260

   and sausages / 5.3 oz / **Aunt Jemima** Home-
style   360

   mini w sausage / 2-½ oz / **Swanson** Great
Starts   190

   oatmeal w lite links / 4.65 oz / **Swanson** Great
Starts   310

   sticks and syrup / 5.2 oz / **Aunt Jemima** Home-
style   400

	CALORIES
w cinnamon / 3 oz / **Weight Watchers** Microwave	160
w links / 4.50 oz / **Weight Watchers** Microwave	270
w sausage / 5-½ oz / **Swanson** Great Starts	380
Ham w cheese on bagel / 3 oz / **Swanson** Great Starts	240
Omelet, western style on English muffin / 4.75 oz / **Healthy Choice**	200
Pancakes	
Lite and lite syrup / 6 oz / **Aunt Jemima** Homestyle	260
Lite and two lite links / 6 oz / **Aunt Jemima** Homestyle	310
Rolled, w apples / 3.85 oz / **Kid Cuisine**	210
Silver dollar w sausage / 3-¾ oz / **Swanson** Great Starts	310
w blueberry topping / 4.75 oz / **Weight Watchers** Microwave	200
w links / 4 oz / **Weight Watchers** Microwave	220
w strawberry topping / 4.75 oz / **Weight Watchers** Microwave	200
w bacon / 4-½ oz / **Swanson** Great Starts	400
w sausages / 6 oz / **Aunt Jemima** Homestyle	420
w sausages / 6 oz / **Swanson** Great Starts	460
Whole wheat w lite links / 5-½ oz / **Swanson** Great Starts	350
Sandwich / 4.90 oz / **Kid Cuisine**	330
Sausage biscuit / 3 oz / **Weight Watchers** Microwave	220
Sausage on a biscuit / 4.70 oz / **Swanson** Great Starts	410
Scrambled eggs / 4.10 oz / **Kid Cuisine**	280
Scrambled eggs and sausage w hash browns / 5.7 oz / **Aunt Jemima** Homestyle	290
Scrambled eggs, cheddar cheese and fried potatoes / 5.9 oz / **Aunt Jemima** Homestyle	250
Scrambled eggs w sausage and pancakes / 5.2 oz / **Aunt Jemima** Homestyle	270
Turkey sausage omelet on English muffin / 4.75 oz / **Healthy Choice**	210

CALORIES

Waffle w bacon / 2.20 oz / **Swanson** Great Starts	230
French toast	
Cinnamon swirl / frozen / 3 oz / **Aunt Jemima**	171
Original / frozen / 3 oz / **Aunt Jemima**	166
Regular / frozen / 2 slices / **Downyflake**	270
Pancakes	
Batter, frozen / 3.6 oz / **Aunt Jemima** Original	183
Batter, frozen, blueberry / 3.6 oz / **Aunt Jemima**	204
Batter, frozen, buttermilk / 3.6 oz / **Aunt Jemima**	180
Microwave / 3.48 oz / **Aunt Jemima** Original	211
Microwave / 3 cakes / **Pillsbury** Hungry Jack Original	240
Microwave, blueberry / 3.48 oz / **Aunt Jemima**	220
Microwave, blueberry / 3 cakes / **Pillsbury** Hungry Jack	230
Microwave, buttermilk	
Aunt Jemima / 3.48 oz	210
Aunt Jemima Lite / 3.48 oz	140
Pillsbury Hungry Jack / 3 cakes	260
Microwave, harvest wheat / 3 cakes / **Pillsbury** Hungry Jack	230
Microwave, oat bran / 3 cakes / **Pillsbury** Hungry Jack	230
Mix, dry / .5 cup / **Arrowhead Mills**	260
Mix, dry / 1 serv / **Aunt Jemima** Original	116
Mix, dry / 1 serv / **Aunt Jemima** Original Complete	253
Mix, dry / ½ cup / **Fearn**	190
Mix, dry, buckwheat / 1 serv / **Aunt Jemima**	143
Mix, dry, buckwheat / ½ cup / **Fearn**	235
Mix, dry, buttermilk	
Aunt Jemima / 1 serv	122
Aunt Jemima Complete / 1 serv	231
Aunt Jemima Lite Complete / 1 serv	130
Mix, dry, seven grain buttermilk / ½ cup / **Fearn**	200
Mix, dry, seven grain buttermilk / ½ cup / **Fearn** Low Sodium	200
Mix, dry, stoneground wholewheat / ½ cup / **Fearn**	220
Mix, dry, wheat and soya / ½ cup / **Fearn**	235
Mix, dry, wheat and soya / ½ cup / **Fearn** Low Sodium	230
Mix, dry, whole wheat / 1 serv / **Aunt Jemima**	120

CALORIES

Mix, prepared / 3 cakes, 4-in diam / **Pillsbury** Hungry Jack Extra Lights ... 190

Mix, prepared / 3 cakes, 4-in diam / **Pillsbury** Hungry Jack Extra Lights Complete ... 180

Mix, prepared, buttermilk / 3 cakes, 4-in diam / **Pillsbury** Hungry Jack ... 210

Mix, prepared, blueberry / 3 cakes, 4-in diam / **Pillsbury** Hungry Jack ... 320

Mix, prepared, buttermilk / 3 cakes, 4-in diam / **Betty Crocker** ... 280

Mix, prepared, buttermilk 3 cakes, 4-in diam / **Betty Crocker** Complete ... 210

Mix, prepared, buttermilk / ⅛ mix / **Gold Medal** Pouch Mixes ... 110

Mix, prepared, buttermilk / 3 cakes, 4-in diam / **Pillsbury** Hungry Jack Complete ... 180

Mix, prepared, buttermilk w egg whites / 3 cakes, 4-in diam / **Pillsbury** Hungry Jack ... 200

Mix, prepared, packets / 3 cakes, 4-in diam / **Pillsbury** Hungry Jack ... 180

Mix, prepared, w egg whites, 3 cakes, 4-in diam / **Pillsbury** Hungry Jack Extra Lights ... 170

Pancake-waffle mix

Mix, dry / .5 cup / **Arrowhead Mills** Multigrain ... 350

Mix, dry, blue corn / .5 cup / **Arrowhead Mills** ... 330

Mix, dry, buckwheat / .5 cup / **Arrowhead Mills** ... 270

Mix, dry, oat bran / .5 cup / **Arrowhead Mills** ... 200

Mix, prepared / 3 cakes, 4-in diam / **Bisquick** Shake 'n Pour ... 240

Waffles, frozen: 1 waffle unless noted

Aunt Jemima Original / 2.5 oz ... 173

Eggo Nutri-Grain / ... 120

Kid Cuisine / 3.6 oz ... 160

Nutri-Grain ... 130

Roman Meal / 2 waffles ... 280

CALORIES

Apple cinnamon / 2.5 oz / **Aunt Jemima**	176
Apple cinnamon / **Eggo**	130
Blueberry	
Aunt Jemima / 2.5 oz	175
Downyflake / 2 waffles	180
Eggo	130
Buttermilk / 2.5 oz / **Aunt Jemima**	179
Buttermilk / **Eggo**	120
Buttermilk, jumbo / 2 waffles / **Downyflake**	190
Homestyle / **Eggo**	120
Hot and buttery / 2 waffles / **Downyflake**	180
Mini's / **Eggo**	90
Multi-bran / **Eggo** Nutri-Grain	110
Multi-grain / 2 waffles / **Downyflake**	250
Nut and honey / **Eggo**	130
Oat bran	
Common Sense	110
2 waffles / **Downyflake**	260
Eggo	110
w fruit and nut / **Common Sense**	120
w fruit and nut / **Eggo**	120
Raisin and bran / **Eggo**	120
Raisin and bran / **Nutri-Grain**	130
Regular / 2 waffles / **Downyflake**	120
Regular, jumbo / 2 waffles / **Downyflake**	170
Special K / **Eggo**	80
Strawberry / **Eggo**	130
Wholegrain / 2.5 oz / **Aunt Jemima**	154

Pastry

FROZEN

	CALORIES
Apple crisp / 4-¾ oz / **Pepperidge Farm**	250
Apple dumplings / 3 oz / **Pepperidge Farm**	260
Apple fruit squares / 1 piece / **Pepperidge Farm**	220
Broccoli w cheese / 1 pastry / **Pepperidge Farm**	230
Cobbler: ⅙ pie	
Apple / **Pet-Ritz**	290
Blackberry / **Pet-Ritz**	250
Blueberry / **Pet-Ritz**	370
Cherry / **Pet-Ritz**	280
Peach / **Pet-Ritz**	260
Strawberry / **Pet-Ritz**	290
Turnover: 1 turnover	
Apple / **Pepperidge Farm**	300
Blueberry / **Pepperidge Farm**	310
Cherry / **Pepperidge Farm**	310
Peach / **Pepperidge Farm**	310
Raspberry / **Pepperidge Farm**	310

TOASTER PASTRY

Pop Tarts: 1 portion	
Blueberry / **Kellogg's**	210
Blueberry, frosted / **Kellogg's**	210
Brown sugar cinnamon / **Kellogg's**	210
Brown sugar cinnamon, frosted / **Kellogg's**	210
Cherry / **Kellogg's**	210
Cherry, frosted / **Kellogg's**	200
Chocolate fudge, frosted / **Kellogg's**	200
Chocolate vanilla creme, frosted / **Kellogg's**	200

CALORIES

Dutch apple, frosted / **Kellogg's**	210
Grape, frosted / **Kellogg's**	200
Raspberry, frosted / **Kellogg's**	200
Strawberry / **Kellogg's**	210
Strawberry, frosted / **Kellogg's**	200
Toaster Strudel: 1 portion	
Apple / **Pillsbury**	200
Blueberry / **Pillsbury**	190
Cinnamon / **Pillsbury**	200
Strawberry / **Pillsbury**	190
Toaster tart: 1 tart	
Apple cinnamon / **Pepperidge Farm**	170
Cheese / **Pepperidge Farm**	190
Strawberry / **Pepperidge Farm**	190
Toastettes, all varieties / 1 tart / **Nabisco**	190

Pickles and Relishes

CALORIES

Artichoke hearts, drained / ½ cup / **Progresso**	16
Artichoke hearts, marinated / ½ cup / **Progresso**	190
Artichoke hearts, undrained / ½ cup / **Progresso**	20
Capers, imported / 1 tbsp / **Progresso**	0
Cauliflower, sweet / 1 oz / **Vlasic**	35
Eggplant, Caponata / ¼ cup / **Progresso**	70
Garden Mix, hot and spicy / 1 oz / **Vlasic**	4
Mushrooms, marinated / ¼ cup / **Progresso**	160
Olive appetizer / ½ cup / **Progresso**	180
Olive salad / ½ cup / **Progresso**	130
Onions, cocktail, lightly salted / 1 oz / **Vlasic**	4
Pepperoncini / 1 oz / **Vlasic** Mild Greek	4
Peppers	
Hot / 1 oz / **Vlasic** Banana Rings	4
Hot cherry / ½ cup / **Progresso**	190

Hot cherry / 1 oz / **Vlasic**	10
Hot cherry, pickled / ½ cup / **Progresso**	130
Jalapeno, Mexican hot / 1 oz / **Vlasic**	8
Mexican, tiny, hot / 1 oz / **Vlasic**	6
Mild, cherry / 1 oz / **Vlasic**	8
Piccalilli / ½ cup / **Progresso**	190
Roasted / ½ cup / **Progresso**	20
Sweet, fried / ½ jar / **Progresso**	37
Tuscan / ½ cup / **Progresso**	20

Pickles: 1 oz
  Bread and butter

Chips / **Vlasic**	30
Chips / **Vlasic** Deli	25
Chunks / **Vlasic**	25
Stixs / **Vlasic**	18

  Dill

Chips / **Vlasic** Hamburger, Half The Salt	2
Chunks / **Vlasic** Kosher Snack	4
Chunks / **Vlasic** Original Polish	4
Chunks / **Vlasic** Original Zesty Snack	4
Gerkins / **Vlasic** Kosher	4
Halves / **Vlasic** Deli	4
Slices / **Heinz** Hamburger	4
Spears / **Vlasic** Original Zesty	4
Spears / **Vlasic** Kosher	4
Spears / **Vlasic** Kosher, Half The Salt	4
Spears / **Vlasic** No Garlic	4
Whole / **Heinz** Kosher, Baby	4
Whole / **Vlasic** Kosher, Baby	4
Whole / **Vlasic** Kosher Crunchy	4
Whole / **Vlasic** Kosher Crunchy, Half The Salt	4
Whole / **Vlasic** Original	2
Whole / **Vlasic** Original Zesty Crunchy	4

  Sweet

Chips / **Vlasic** Butter, Half The Salt	30
Whole / **Heinz** Gerkins	25–30
Whole / **Heinz** Mixed	25–30

Relishes: 1 oz

Dill / **Vlasic**	2
Hamburger / **Vlasic**	40
Hot dog / **Vlasic**	40

	CALORIES
Hot piccalilli / **Vlasic**	35
India / **Vlasic**	30
Piccalilli / **Heinz**	30
Sweet / **Heinz**	35
Sweet / **Vlasic**	30

Pies

FROZEN

	CALORIES
Apple	
Banquet Familey Size / 3.33 oz	250
McMillin / 4 oz	430
Pet-Ritz / ⅙ pie	330
Weight Watchers / 3.50 oz	200
Mrs. Smith's 8 in / ⅛ pie	220
Mrs. Smith's 10 in / ⅛ pie	390
Apple, natural juice / 9 in / **Mrs. Smith's** / ⅛ pie	370
Apple cobbler / ⅙ pie / **Pet-Ritz**	290
Apple-cranberry / 8 in / ⅛ pie / **Mrs. Smith's**	230
Banana cream	
Banquet / 2.33 oz	180
Pet-Ritz / ⅙ pie	170
Mrs. Smith's 8 in / ⅛ pie	140
Berry / 4 oz / **McMillin**	430
Berry / 8 in / ⅛ pie / **Mrs. Smith's**	230
Blackberry / 3.33 oz / **Banquet** Family Size	270
Blackberry / 8 in / ⅛ pie / **Mrs. Smith's**	230
Blackberry cobbler / ⅙ pie / **Pet-Ritz**	250
Blueberry	
Banquet Familey Size / 3.33 oz	270
Pet-Ritz / ⅙ pie	370
Mrs. Smith's 8 in / ⅛ pie	210
Blueberry / **Mrs. Smith's** 9 in / natural juice / ⅛ pie	350
Blueberry cobbler / ⅙ pie / **Pet-Ritz**	370

CALORIES

Boston cream / 3 oz / **Weight Watchers**	160
Boston cream / 8 in / ⅛ pie / **Mrs. Smith's**	180
Cherry	
Banquet Family Size / 3.33 oz	250
McMillin / 4 oz	430
Pet-Ritz / ⅙ pie	300
Mrs. Smith's 10 in / ⅛ pie	390
Mrs. Smith's 8 in / ⅛ pie	220
Mrs. Smith's 9 in / natural juice / ⅛ pie	350
Cherry cobbler / ⅙ pie / **Pet-Ritz**	280
Chocolate cream / 2.33 oz / **Banquet**	190
Chocolate cream / ⅙ pie / **Pet-Ritz**	190
Chocolate cream / 8 in / ⅛ pie / **Mrs. Smith's**	150
Chocolate meringue / 8 in / ⅛ pie / **Mrs. Smith's**	260
Chocolate mocha / 2.75 oz / **Weight Watchers**	160
Chocolate pudding / 4 oz / **McMillin**	420
Coconut cream / 2.33 oz / **Banquet**	190
Coconut cream / ⅙ pie / **Pet-Ritz**	190
Coconut cream / 8 in / ⅛ pie / **Mrs. Smith's**	150
Coconut custard / 10 in / ⅛ pie / **Mrs. Smith's**	280
Coconut custard / 8 in / ⅛ pie / **Mrs. Smith's**	180
Coconut pudding / 4 oz / **McMillin**	450
Dutch apple / 10 in / ⅛ pie / **Mrs. Smith's**	430
Dutch apple / 8 in / ⅛ pie / **Mrs. Smith's**	250
Dutch apple / 9 in / natural juice / ⅛ pie / **Mrs. Smith's**	380
Egg custard / ⅙ pie / **Pet-Ritz**	200
French silk cream / 8 in / ⅛ pie / **Mrs. Smith's**	280
Hearty pumpkin / 8 in / ⅛ pie / **Mrs. Smith's**	190
Lemon / 4 oz / **McMillin**	450
Lemon cream / 2.33 oz / **Banquet**	170
Lemon cream / ⅙ pie / **Pet-Ritz**	190
Lemon cream / 8 in / ⅛ pie / **Mrs. Smith's**	140
Lemon meringue / 8 in / ⅛ pie / **Mrs. Smith's**	210
Mince / ⅙ pie / **Pet-Ritz**	280
Mince / 10 in / ⅛ pie / **Mrs. Smith's**	430
Mince / 8 in / ⅛ pie / **Mrs. Smith's**	220
Mincemeat / 3.33 oz / **Banquet** Family Size	260
Neapolitan cream/ ⅙ pie / **Pet-Ritz**	180
Peach	
Banquet Family Size / 3.33 oz	245
McMillin / 4 oz	430

CALORIES

Pet-Ritz / ⅙ pie	320
Mrs. Smith's 10 in / ⅛ pie	360
Mrs. Smith's 8 in / ⅛ pie	200
Mrs. Smith's 9 in / natural juice / ⅛ pie	330
Peach cobbler / ⅙ pie / **Pet-Ritz**	260
Pecan / 10 in / ⅛ pie / **Mrs. Smith's**	490
Pecan / 8 in / ⅛ pie / **Mrs. Smith's**	330
Pumpkin / 3.33 oz / **Banquet** Family Size	200
Pumpkin custard / ⅙ pie / **Pet-Ritz**	250
Pumpkin custard / 10 in / ⅛ pie / **Mrs. Smith's**	300
Pumpkin custard / 8 in / ⅛ pie / **Mrs. Smith's**	180
Red raspberry / 8 in / ⅛ pie / **Mrs. Smith's**	220
Strawberry / 4 oz / **McMillin**	400
Strawberry cobbler / ⅙ pie / **Pet-Ritz**	290
Strawberry cream / 2.33 oz / **Banquet**	170
Strawberry cream / ⅙ pie / **Pet-Ritz**	170
Strawberry-rhubarb / 8 in / ⅛ pie / **Mrs. Smith's**	230
Sweet potato / ⅙ pie / **Pet-Ritz**	150

PIE FILLING, CANNED

4 oz unless noted

Apple	
Comstock / ½ cup	120
Lucky Leaf	110
Lucky Leaf Deluxe	110
Lucky Leaf Plus	120
Musselman's	110
Musselman's Deluxe	110
Musselman's Plus	120
Turnover filling, diced / **Lucky Leaf**	110
Turnover filling, diced / **Musselman's**	110
Apricot / **Lucky Leaf**	140
Apricot / **Mussleman's**	140
Banana / ½ cup / **Comstock**	110
Black raspberry / **Lucky Leaf**	180
Black raspberry / **Musselman's**	180
Blackberry	
Lucky Leaf	110
Lucky Leaf Plus	120

CALORIES

Musselman's	110
Musselman's Plus	120
Blueberry	
Lucky Leaf	110
Lucky Leaf Plus	150
Musselman's	110
Mussleman's Plus	150
Comstock / ½ cup	110
Boysenberry / **Lucky Leaf**	110
Boysenberry / **Musselman's**	110
Cherry	
Comstock / ½ cup	110
Lucky Leaf	110
Lucky Leaf Plus	110
Musselman's	110
Musselman's Plus	110
Cherry Lite / ½ cup / **Comstock**	80
Chocolate / ½ cup / **Comstock**	130
Coconut / ½ cup / **Comstock**	120
Lemon	
Comstock / ½ cup	140
Lucky Leaf	150
Musselman's	150
Lemon, French / **Lucky Leaf**	160
Lemon, French / **Musselman's**	160
Mincemeat	
Lucky Leaf	180
Musselman's	180
None Such / ⅓ cup	200
None Such w Brandy and Rum / ⅓ cup	220
Mincemeat, condensed / ¼ pkg / **None Such**	220
Peach	
Lucky Leaf	140
Lucky Leaf Plus	110
Musselman's	140
Musselman's Plus	110
Pineapple / **Lucky Leaf**	100
Pineapple / **Musselman's**	100
Pumpkin	
Libby's Plain / 1 cup	210
Libby's Solid Pack / 1 cup	80

CALORIES

Lucky Leaf	160
Musselman's	160
Raisin / **Lucky Leaf**	120
Raisin / **Musselman's**	120
Red Raspberry / **Lucky Leaf**	180
Red Raspberry / **Musselman's**	180
Strawberry	
Lucky Leaf	110
Lucky Leaf Plus	140
Musselman's	110
Mussleman's Plus	140
Strawberry-rhubarb / **Lucky Leaf**	110
Strawberry-rhubarb / **Musselman's**	110
Vanilla creme / **Lucky Leaf**	140
Vanilla creme / **Musselman's**	140

PIE MIXES

⅛ pie unless noted

Banana cream / mix, prepared w whole milk / ⅙ pie / **Jell-O**	100
Banana cream / mix, prepared w whole milk / **Jell-O** No Bake Desserts	240
Boston cream / mix, prepared / **Betty Crocker** Classic	270
Cheesecake / mix, prepared w whole milk / **Jell-O** No Bake Desserts	280
Cheesecake, lemon / mix, prepared w whole milk / **Jell-O** No Bake Desserts	270
Cheesecake, NY Style / mix, prepared w whole milk / **Jell-O** No Bake Desserts	280
Chocolate mousse / mix / **Royal** No Bake	130
Chocolate mousse / mix, prepared w whole milk / **Jell-O** No Bake Desserts	260
Coconut cream / mix, prepared w whole milk / ⅙ pie / **Jell-O**	110
Coconut cream / mix, prepared w whole milk / **Jell-O** No Bake Desserts	260
Key lime / dry mix / ½ cup / **Royal**	50
Lemon / dry mix / ½ cup / **Royal**	50
Lemon / mix, prepared as directed / ⅙ pie / **Jell-O**	170

CALORIES

Lemon meringue / mix / **Royal** No Bake	210
Pumpkin / mix, prepared w whole milk / **Jell-O** No Bake Desserts	250

PIE CRUSTS AND PASTRY SHELLS

Mini puff / frozen / 1 shell / **Pepperidge Farm**	50
Pie crust	
Mix / 1/16 pkg / **Betty Crocker**	120
Mix / 1 serv / **Flako**	247
Mix / 1/8 pkg / **Pillsbury**	200
Refrigerated / 1/8 pkg / **Pillsbury** All Ready	240
Sticks / 1/8 stick / **Betty Crocker**	120
Pie shell / 9 in / frozen / 1/6 shell / **Oronoque**	120
Pic shell / 9 in / frozen / 1/6 shell / **Pet-Ritz**	120
Pie shell / 9 in, deep dish / frozen / 1/6 shell / **Oronoque**	130
Pie shell / 9 in, deep dish / frozen / 1/6 shell / **Pet-Ritz**	130
Pie shell / 9.5 in / frozen / 1/6 shell / **Pet-Ritz**	170
Pie shell, graham cracker / frozen / 1/6 shell / **Pet-Ritz**	110
Pie shell, vegetable shortening / frozen / 1/6 shell / **Pet-Ritz**	110
Pie shell, vegetable shortening, deep dish / frozen / 1/6 shell / **Pet-Ritz**	140
Puff / frozen / 1 shell / **Pepperidge Farm**	210
Puff dough, sheets / frozen / 1/4 sheet / **Pepperidge Farm**	260
Tart shell / 3 in / frozen / **Pet-Ritz**	150

READY TO SERVE PIES AND PASTRIES

1 piece unless noted

Apple / 1/8 pie / **Mrs. Smith's**	210
Apple, French pie / **Tastykake**	350
Apple pastry / **Stella D'Oro** Dietetic	80
Apple pastry, pocket / **Tastykake**	320
Apple pie / **Tastykake**	300
Banana cream pie / **Tastykake**	380
Blueberry / 1/8 pie / **Mrs. Smith's**	220
Blueberry pie / **Tastykake**	310
Cheese pastry, pocket / **Tastykake**	330
Cherry / 1/8 pie / **Mrs. Smith's**	220

Cherry pastry, pocket / **Tastykake**	330
Cherry pie / **Tastykake**	300
Coconut cream pie / **Tastykake**	380
Lemon pie / **Tastykake**	320
Lemon-lime pie / **Tastykake**	320
Peach / ⅛ pie / **Mrs. Smith's**	210
Peach-apricot pastry / **Stella D'Oro** Dietetic	90
Peach pie / **Tastykake**	300
Pineapple cheese pie / **Tastykake**	340
Prune pastry / **Stella D'Oro** Dietetic	90
Pumpkin pie / **Tastykake**	320
Strawberry pie / **Tastykake**	340
Tasty klair pie / **Tastykake**	400

Pizza

CALORIES

Canadian bacon

Frozen / ½ pizza / **Jeno's**	240
Frozen / 1 piece / **Stouffer's** French Bread	360
Frozen / ½ pizza / **Totino's**	330

Cheese

Frozen / 1 pizza / **Celeste** For One	500
Frozen / ¼ pizza / **Celeste** Large	315
Frozen / 5.60 oz / **Healthy Choice** French Bread	300
Frozen / ½ pizza / **Jeno's**	240
Frozen / 3 oz / **Jeno's** Pizza Rolls	200
Frozen / 6.85 oz / **Kid Cuisine**	380
Frozen / 9.70 oz / **Kid Cuisine** Mega Meal	430
Frozen / ⅕ pizza / **Pappalo's** Pan Pizza, Three Cheese	310
Frozen / 1 pizza / **Pepperidge Farm**	430
Frozen / 5.7 oz / **Pillsbury** French Bread, Microwave	350
Frozen / ½ pizza / **Pillsbury** Microwave	250
Frozen / 4.25 oz / **Stouffer's**	320

	CALORIES
Frozen / 1 piece / **Stouffer's** Double Cheese French Bread	410
Frozen / 4.75 oz / **Stouffer's** Extra Cheese	370
Frozen / 1 piece / **Stouffer's** French Bread	340
Frozen / 5-⅛ oz / **Stouffer's** Lean Cuisine French Bread	300
Frozen / 6-⅛ oz / **Stouffer's** Lean Cuisine French Bread, Deluxe	320
Frozen / 5-½ oz / **Stouffer's** Lean Cuisine French Bread, Extra Cheese	330
Frozen / ½ pizza / **Totino's**	290
Frozen / ⅓ pizza / **Totino's** Family Size	320
Frozen / 1 pizza / **Totino's** Microwave	250
Frozen / ⅙ pizza / **Totino's** Pan	290
Frozen / 5.86 oz / **Weight Watchers**	300
Combination	
Frozen / 1 pizza / **Celeste** For One Deluxe	580
Frozen / 1 pizza / **Celeste** For One, Four Cheese Original	540
Frozen / 1 pizza / **Celeste** For One, Four Cheese Zesty	550
Frozen / 1 pizza / **Celeste** For One, Suprema	680
Frozen / ¼ pizza / **Celeste** Large Deluxe	380
Frozen / ¼ pizza / **Celeste** Large Suprema	380
Frozen / 6.25 oz / **Healthy Choice** French Bread, Deluxe	330
Frozen / ½ pizza / **Jeno's**	280
Frozen / 1 pocket / **Jeno's** Pizza Pockets, Supreme	370
Frozen / 3 oz / **Jeno's** Pizza Rolls	220
Frozen / ½ pizza / **Pappalo's** 9-in Crust, Supreme	400
Frozen / ½ pizza / **Pappalo's** 9-in Crust, Three Cheese	350
Frozen / ¼ pizza / **Pappalo's** 12-in Crust, Supreme	350
Frozen / ¼ pizza / **Pappalo's** 12-in Crust, Three Cheese	310
Frozen / ⅕ pizza / **Pappalo's** Pan Pizza, Supreme	340
Frozen / 1 pizza / **Pepperidge Farm** Deluxe	440
Frozen / 6.5 oz / **Pillsbury** French Bread, Microwave	420
Frozen / ½ pizza / **Pillsbury** Microwave	310
Frozen / ½ pizza / **Pillsbury** Microwave Supreme	310

CALORIES

Frozen / 5 oz / **Stouffer's** Deluxe	370
Frozen / 1 piece / **Stouffer's** Deluxe French Bread	430
Frozen / 1 piece / **Stouffer's** Hamburger French Bread	410
Frozen / 1 piece / **Stouffer's** Pepperoni, Mushroom French Bread	430
Frozen / 1 piece / **Stouffer's** Pepperoni and Sausage	380
Frozen / 1 piece / **Stouffer's** Sausage, Pepperoni French Bread	450
Frozen / ½ pizza / **Totino's**	370
Frozen / ⅓ pizza / **Totino's**, Family Size	400
Frozen / 1 pizza / **Totino's** Microwave	290
Frozen / 7.15 oz / **Weight Watchers** Deluxe	330
Frozen / 6.12 oz / **Weight Watchers** French Bread Deluxe	330

Hamburger

Frozen / ½ pizza / **Jeno's**	280
Frozen / 3 oz / **Jeno's** Pizza Rolls	220
Frozen / ½ pizza / **Totino's**	350

Pepperoni

Frozen / 1 pizza / **Celeste** For One	545
Frozen / ¼ pizza / **Celeste**, Large	370
Frozen / 6.25 oz / **Healthy Choice** French Bread	320
Frozen / ½ pizza / **Jeno's**	280
Frozen / 1 pocket / **Jeno's** Pizza Pockets	370
Frozen / 3 oz / **Jeno's** Pizza Rolls	220
Frozen / ½ pizza / **Pappalo's** 9-in Crust	390
Frozen / ¼ pizza / **Pappalo's** 12-in Crust	350
Frozen / ⅕ pizza / **Pappalo's** Pan Pizza	350
Frozen / 1 pizza / **Pepperidge Farm**	420
Frozen / 6 oz / **Pillsbury** French Bread, Microwave	410
Frozen / ½ pizza / **Pillsbury** Microwave	300
Frozen / 1 piece / **Stouffer's**	350
Frozen / 1 piece / **Stouffer's** French Bread	410
Frozen / 5-¼ oz / **Stouffer's** Lean Cuisine French Bread	330
Frozen / ½ pizza / **Totino's**	380
Frozen / ⅓ pizza / **Totino's** Family Size	410
Frozen / 1 pizza / **Totino's** Microwave	270
Frozen / ⅙ pizza / **Totino's** Pan	330
Frozen / 6.09 oz / **Weight Watchers**	320

CALORIES

	CALORIES
Frozen / 5.25 oz / **Weight Watchers** French Bread Sausage	320
Frozen / 1 pizza / **Celeste** For One	570
Frozen / ¼ pizza / **Celeste** Large	375
Frozen / 6.45 oz / **Healthy Choice** French Bread, Turkey	320
Frozen / ½ pizza / **Jeno's**	280
Frozen / 1 pocket / **Jeno's** Pizza Pockets	360
Frozen / 1 pocket / **Jeno's** Pizza Pockets and Pepperoni	360
Frozen / 3 oz / **Jeno's** Pizza Rolls	210
Frozen / ½ pizza / **Pappalo's** 9-in Crust	380
Frozen / ½ pizza / **Pappalo's** 9-in Crust w Pepperoni	390
Frozen / ¼ pizza / **Pappalo's** 12-in Crust	350
Frozen / ¼ pizza / **Pappalo's** 12-in Crust w Pepperoni	360
Frozen / ⅕ pizza / **Pappalo's** Pan Pizza	350
Frozen / ⅕ pizza / **Pappalo's** Pan Pizza	360
Frozen / 6.3 oz / **Pillsbury** French Bread, Microwave	400
Frozen / ½ pizza / **Pillsbury** Microwave	290
Frozen / 1 piece / **Stouffer's**	360
Frozen / 1 piece / **Stouffer's** French Bread	420
Frozen / 6 oz / **Stouffer's** Lean Cuisine French Bread	330
Frozen / ½ pizza / **Totino's**	370
Frozen / ⅓ pizza / **Totino's** Family Size	410
Frozen / 1 pizza / **Totino's** Microwave	280
Frozen / ⅙ pizza / **Totino's** Pan	320
Frozen / ⅙ pizza / **Totino's** Pan w Pepperoni	330
Frozen / 6.26 oz / **Weight Watchers**	320
Vegetable / Frozen / 1 pizza / **Celeste** For One	490
Vegetable, deluxe / frozen / 1 piece / **Stouffer's** French Bread	420
Pizza crust mix / ⅙ mix / **Gold Medal** Pouch Mixes	110

Popcorn

CALORIES

3 cups popped unless noted

Plain
Jiffy Pop	80
Jolly Time, White	60
Jolly Time, Yellow	60
Weight Watchers, Lightly Salted / .66 oz	80

Microwave
Weight Watchers / 1 oz	100

Butter flavored
Chesters	120
Country Light / 4 cups	120
Jolly Time	90
Merry Poppin' / 4 cups	190
Merry Poppin' Light / 4 cups	120
Orville Redenbacher Gourmet	100
Orville Redenbacher Gourmet, Frozen	100
Orville Redenbacher Gourmet, Salt Free	100
Planters	140
Pop Secret	100
Pop Secret Light	70
Pop Secret Light Singles / 6 cups	140
Pop Secret Pop Quiz	100
Pop Secret, Salt Free	100
Pop Secret Singles / 6 cups	200
TV Time Micro Gourmet / 4 cups	230

Butter flavored, light / **Jolly Time**	60
Butter flavored, light / **Orville Redenbacher** Gourmet	70
Butter toffee-flavored / 2.5 cups / **Orville Redenbacher** Gourmet	210
Caramel-flavored / 2.5 cups / **Orville Redenbacher** Gourmet	240

CALORIES

Cheddar cheese-flavored / **Orville Redenbacher** Gourmet	130
Cheese-flavored / **Chesters**	110
Cheese-flavored / **Jolly Time**	180
Natural / **Orville Redenbacher** Gourmet	100
Natural / **Orville Redenbacher** Gourmet, Salt Free	100
Natural-flavored	
Chesters	110
Country Light / 4 cups	120
Jolly Time	130
Merry Poppin' / 4 cups	190
Merry Poppin' Light / 4 cups	120
Orville Redenbacher Gourmet, Frozen	100
Planters	140
Pop Secret	100
Pop Secret Light	70
Pop Secret Light Singles / 6 cups	150
Pop Secret Pop Quiz	100
TV Time Micro Gourmet	230
Natural-flavored, light / **Jolly Time**	70
Natural-flavored, light / **Orville Redenbacher** Gourmet	70
Sour cream 'n onion-flavored / **Orville Redenbacher** Gourmet	160

Ready to eat: ½ oz unless noted

Baby / **Wise**	70
Butter light / **Smartfood**	70
Cheddar cheese / **Chesters**	80
Cheddar cheese / **Smartfood**	80
Cheddar cheese-flavor / **Chee•tos**	80
Cheddar cheese, white / .66 oz / **Weight Watchers**	100
Cheese flavor / **Wise**	70
Cracker Jack / **Cracker Jack**	120

Pot Pies

CALORIES

Frozen: 1 whole pie

Beef
Banquet / 7 oz	510
Morton / 7 oz	430
Stouffer's / 10 oz	500
Swanson / 7 oz	370
Swanson Hungry Man / 16 oz	610

Chicken
Banquet / 7 oz	550
Morton / 7 oz	420
Stouffer's / 10 oz	530
Swanson / 7 oz	380
Swanson Homestyle Entree / 8 oz	410
Swanson Hungry Man / 16 oz	630
Tyson / 9 oz	390
w white meat / 9 oz / **Tyson**	400

Turkey
Banquet / 7 oz	510
Morton / 7 oz	420
Stouffer's / 10 oz	540
Swanson / 7 oz	380
Swanson Hungry Man / 16 oz	650
Tyson / 9 oz	370

Poultry and Poultry Entrées

FRESH

CALORIES

3½ oz unless noted

Chicken, fryer or broiler, batter-fried: ½ chicken	1350
Chicken, fryer or broiler	
Breast, meat and skin, raw: ½ breast (5 oz)	250
Breast, meat and skin, fried: ½ breast	220
Drumstick, meat and skin, raw: 1 drumstick (2½ oz)	117
Drumstick, meat and skin, fried: 1 drumstick	120
Thigh, meat and skin, raw: 1 thigh (3.3 oz)	200
Thigh, meat and skin, batter-fried: 1 thigh	238
Wing, meat and skin, raw: 1 wing (¾ oz)	109
Wing, meat and skin, batter-fried: 1 wing	159
Wing, meat and skin, roasted: 1 wing	100
Chicken, roasting, meat and skin: ½ chicken (1 lb)	1070
Chicken, roasting	
Dark meat wo skin, roasted	178
Light meat wo skin, roasted	153
Dark meat wo skin: 1 cup (5 oz)	250
Light meat wo skin: 1 cup (5 oz)	215
Chicken, stewed wo skin	177
Chicken, stewed w skin	219
Cornish game hen, roasted w skin	239
Cornish game hen, roasted wo skin	190
Duck, w skin, roasted	337
Duck, wo skin, roasted	201
Goose, roasted, domesticated, wo skin	233

CALORIES

Goose, roasted, domesticated, w skin	441
Goose, roasted, wild	309
Pheasant, cooked	208
Pheasant, cooked: ½ breast	278
Pheasant, cooked, leg	138
Quail, cooked: 1 average-size	364
Squab, cooked: 1 average-size	293
Turkey, dark meat, w skin, roasted	221
Turkey, dark meat, wo skin, roasted	187
Turkey, white meat, w skin, roasted	197
Turkey, white meat, wo skin, roasted	157
Heart, chicken, cooked: 1 oz	42
Heart, turkey, cooked: 1 oz	60
Liver, chicken, cooked: 1 oz	47
Liver, goose, raw: 1 oz	50
Liver, turkey, cooked: 1 oz	50

CANNED, FROZEN AND PROCESSED

CALORIES

Chicken

À l'orange / frozen / 9 oz / **Healthy Choice**	240
À l'orange w almond rice / frozen / 8 oz / **Stouffer's** Lean Cuisine	280
À la King / canned / 5-¼ oz / **Swanson**	190
Frozen / 11.25 oz / **Armour** Classics Lite	290
Frozen / 8-¼ oz / **Le Menu** Light	240
Frozen / 9 oz / **Weight Watchers**	240
À la King w rice / frozen / 9.5 oz / **Stouffer's**	290
Baked breast w vegetables / frozen / 7-⅜ oz / **Stouffer's**	190
Barbecue style / microwaveable / ¼ pkg / **Lipton** Microeasy	108
Breast strips, grilled / frozen / 2.75 oz / **Tyson**	100
Breast strips, Oriental / frozen / 2.75 oz / **Tyson**	110
Breast tenders, hot and spicy / frozen / 2.75 oz / **Tyson**	110
Breast tenders, mesquite / frozen / 2.75 oz / **Tyson**	110
Burgundy / frozen / 10 oz / **Armour** Classics Lite	210
Chow mein w rice / frozen / 9 oz / **Stouffer's** Lean Cuisine	240

Chunks and slices

Boneless / frozen / 17-¾ oz / **Swanson** Hungry Man	700
Breast / oven-roasted, thin sliced / 1 slice / **Louis Rich**	12
Breast chunks / frozen / 3 oz / **Tyson**	240
Chunk / frozen 2.6 oz / **Tyson**	220
Chunk / frozen / 2.6 oz / **Tyson** Chick'n Cheddar	220
Chunk, white / canned / 2-½ oz / **Swanson**	100
Chunk, white and dark / canned / 2-½ oz / **Swanson**	100
Chunks / canned / 2-½ oz / **Swanson** Mixin	130
Diced / frozen / 3 oz / **Tyson**	130
Patties / frozen / 2.6 oz / **Tyson**	220
Slices, breast, hickory smoked / 1 slice / **Louis Rich**	30
Slices, breast, oven roasted / 1 slice / **Oscar Mayer**	29
Slices, breast, smoked / 1 slice / **Oscar Mayer**	25
Slices, breast, smoked hickory / 1 slice / **Tyson**	25
Slices, breast, honey flavored / 1 slice / **Tyson**	25
Slices, breast, mesquite / 1 slice / **Tyson**	25
Slices, breast, oven roasted / 1 slice / **Tyson**	25
Slices, roll / 1 slice / **Tyson**	26
Slices, smoked / 1 oz / **Eckrich** Lite	30
Slices, thin, breast / 1 slice / **Oscar Mayer**	13
Slices, white, oven roasted / 1 slice / **Louis Rich**	35
Cordon bleu / frozen / 8 oz / **Weight Watchers**	220
Country style / microwaveable / ¼ pkg / **Lipton** Microeasy	78
Creamed / frozen / 6.5 oz / **Stouffer's**	300
Croquettes w gravy / frozen / 2 pieces / **Weaver**	280
Dijon / frozen / 8 oz / **Le Menu Light**	240
Divan / frozen / 8.5 oz / **Stouffer's**	320
Divan / frozen / 11 oz / **Weight Watchers**	280
and dumplings entree / frozen / 7 oz / **Banquet**	280
Empress / frozen / 8-¼ oz / **Le Menu Light**	210
Enchiladas / frozen / 8 oz / **Le Menu Light**	280

CALORIES

Enchiladas / frozen / 9-⅞ oz / **Stouffer's** Lean Cuisine	290
Escalloped and noodles / frozen / 10 oz / **Stouffer's**	420
Fettucini	
Frozen / 1 pkg / **Armour** Classics	260
Frozen / 8.5 oz / **Healthy Choice**	240
Frozen / 9 oz / **Stouffer's** Lean Cuisine	280
Frozen / 12 oz / **Ultra Slim-Fast**	380
Frozen / 8.25 oz / **Weight Watchers**	280
Fiesta / frozen / 8-½ oz / **Stouffer's** Lean Cuisine	240
Fillets / frozen / 4.5 oz / **Weaver**	270
Fillets, tenders / frozen / 2.25 oz / **Banquet** Healthy Balance	120
Fillets, BBQ / frozen / 3 oz / **Tyson**	110
Fillets, breast / frozen / 3 oz / **Tyson**	190
Fillets, grilled / frozen / 2.75 oz / **Tyson**	100
Fillets, lemon pepper / frozen / 2.75 oz / **Tyson**	100
Fillets, marinated, barbecue / frozen / 3.75 oz / **Tyson**	120
Fillets, marinated, butter garlic / frozen / 3.75 oz / **Tyson**	120
Fillets, marinated, Italian / frozen / 3.75 oz / **Tyson**	120
Fillets, marinated, lemon pepper / frozen / 3.75 oz / **Tyson**	130
Fillets, marinated, Teriyaki / frozen / 3.75 oz / **Tyson**	130
Fried, frozen	
Swanson, Homestyle / 7+ oz	390
Assorted pieces / 6.4 oz / **Banquet** Hot 'n Spicy	330
Assorted pieces / 5.6 oz / **Banquet** Original	290
Assorted pieces / 5.6 oz / **Banquet** Southern	290
Assorted pieces / 3.6 oz / **Weaver**	290
Assorted, Southern / 6.5 oz / **Weight Watchers**	320
Breast and whipped potatoes / 7-⅛ oz / **Stouffer's**	350
Breast, fillet strips / 3.3 oz / **Weaver**	200
Breast, fillets / 3 oz / **Tyson**	220
Breast portions / 5.75 oz / **Banquet**	220
Breast tenders / 2.25 oz / **Banquet**	160
Breast tenders / 2.25 oz / **Banquet** Boneless Chicken	150

CALORIES

Breast tenders / 3 oz / **Tyson**	225
Breasts / 4-½ oz / **Swanson**	360
Breasts / 4.4 oz / **Weaver**	310
Breasts, Dutch frye / 4.5 oz / **Weaver**	350
Breasts, skinless / 2.9 oz / **Weaver**	170
Chunks / 3 oz / **Country Skillet**	260
Chunks / 2.6 oz / **Tyson** Chick'n Chunks	220
Chunks, Southern / 3 oz / **Country Skillet**	270
Dark meat / 14-¼ oz / **Swanson** Hungry Man	860
Drum snackers / 2.5 oz / **Banquet** Boneless Chicken	210
Drums / 3 oz / **Weaver**	210
Drums and thighs / 3 oz / **Weaver**	210
Drums and thighs, Dutch frye / 3.5 oz / **Weaver**	290
Drums, herb and spice / 3 oz / **Weaver**	200
Nibbles / 3-¼ oz / **Swanson**	300
Nibbles / 4-¼ oz / **Swanson** Homestyle	340
Nuggets	
Banquet / 2.5 oz	200
Country Skillet / 3 oz	250
Swanson / 3 oz	230
Weaver / 2.6 oz	190
Weight Watchers / 5.9 oz	270
Banquet Healthy Balance / 2.25 oz	120
Nuggets, hot & spicy / 2.5 oz / **Banquet**	240
Nuggets w cheddar / 2.5 oz / **Banquet**	240
Parts / 3-¼ oz / **Swanson**	270
Patties	
Banquet / 2.5 oz	190
Banquet / 2.5 oz	200
Banquet Healthy Balance / 2.25 oz	120
Country Skillet / 3 oz	230
Tyson Thick & Crispy / 2.6 oz	220
Weaver/ 3 oz	205
Patties, Southern / 3 oz / **Country Skillet**	240
Patties, Southern style / 2.6 oz / **Tyson**	220
Rondelet / 3 oz / **Weaver**	190
Rondelet, Italian / 2.6 oz / **Weaver**	190
Rondelet w cheese / 2.6 oz / **Weaver**	190

CALORIES

Sticks / 2.5 oz / **Banquet**	210
Tenders / 3. oz / **Weaver**	170
Tenders, honey batter / 3 oz / **Weaver**	220
Thighs and drumsticks / 6.25 oz / **Banquet**	250
Thighs and drumsticks / 3-¼ oz / **Swanson**	290
White meat / 14-¼ oz / **Swanson** Hungry Man	870
Wings / 3.6 oz / **Weaver**	280
Wings / 2.7 oz / **Weaver** Zesty	170
Wings, barbecue / 6–7 wings / **Tyson**	218
Wings, Dutch frye / 4 oz / **Weaver**	400
Wings, hot and spicy / 6–7 wings / **Tyson**	218
Wings, teriyaki / 6–7 wings / **Tyson**	218
Glazed / frozen/ 8.5 oz / **Healthy Choice**	220
Glazed w vegetable rice / frozen / 8-½ oz / **Stouffer's** Lean Cuisine	260
Herb roasted / frozen / 7-¾ oz / **Le Menu** Light	260
Hot 'n spicy / frozen / 3.75 oz / **Banquet** Snack 'n Chicken	140
Imperial / frozen / 9.25 oz / **Weight Watchers**	240
in barbecue sauce / frozen / 8-¾ oz / **Stouffer's** Lean Cuisine	260
Italiano / frozen / 9 oz / **Stouffer's** Lean Cuisine	290
Kiev / frozen / 7 oz / **Weight Watchers**	230
Mandarin / frozen / 11 oz / **Healthy Choice**	260
Marsala / frozen / 10.5 oz / **Armour** Classics Lite	250
Mesquite	
Frozen / 1 pkg / **Armour** Classics	370
Frozen / 10.5 oz / **Banquet** Healthy Balance	310
Frozen / 12 oz / **Ultra Slim-Fast**	360
and noodles	
Frozen / 1 pkg / **Armour** Classics	230
Frozen / 8.5 oz / **Banquet**	240
Frozen / 10 oz / **Stouffer's**	290
Frozen / 9 oz / **Weight Watchers**	240
Oriental / frozen / 10 oz / **Armour** Classics Lite	180
Oriental w vegetables and vermicelli / frozen / 9 oz / **Stouffer's** Lean Cuisine	280
Parmigiana / frozen / 11.5 oz / **Armour** Classics	370
Parmigiana and pasta / frozen / 9.8 oz / **Stouffer's**	360
Roasted, wings / frozen / 6–7 wings / **Tyson**	218
Sandwich, BBQ / frozen / 4 oz / **Tyson** Microwave	230

Sandwich, breast / frozen / 4.25 oz / **Tyson** Microwave	328
Sandwich, breast, grilled / frozen / 3.5 oz / **Tyson**	150
Sandwich, grilled / frozen / 3.5 oz / **Tyson**	200
Stew / canned / 7-⅝ oz / **Swanson**	160
Sweet and sour	
Frozen / 11 oz / **Armour** Classics Lite	240
Frozen / 10.25 oz / **Banquet** Healthy Balance	270
Frozen / 12 oz / **Ultra Slim-Fast**	330
Tenderloins in herb cream sauce / frozen / 9-½ oz / **Stouffer's** Lean Cuisine	240
Tenderloins in peanut sauce / frozen / 9 oz / **Stouffer's** Lean Cuisine	290
and vegetables / frozen / 11.5 oz / **Healthy Choice**	210
and vegetables / frozen / 12 oz / **Ultra Slim-Fast**	290
Vegetables and primavera / frozen / 4 oz / **Banquet** Cookin' Bag	100
Vegetables and primavera entree / frozen / 7 oz / **Banquet**	140
w dumplings / canned / 7-½ oz / **Swanson**	220
w dumplings / frozen / 7 oz / **Banquet** Family Entrees	280
w mushroom sauce, roasted / frozen / 12 oz / **Ultra Slim-Fast**	280
w wine and mushroom sauce / frozen / 10.75 oz / **Armour** Classics	280
Turnover, entree / frozen / 1 sandwich / **Quaker** Ovenstuffs	350
Turkey, slices and pieces	
Frozen / 8 oz / **Le Menu** Light	200
Frozen / 17 oz / **Swanson** Hungry Man	550
and gravy, entree / frozen / 7 oz / **Banquet**	220
and gravy w dressing / frozen / 11.25 oz / **Banquet** Healthy Balance	270
and mushrooms in gravy, entree / frozen / 8.5 oz / **Healthy Choice**	200
Baked potato, homestyle / frozen / 12 oz / **Weight Watchers**	300
Breast	
Tyson 1 slice	20
Barbecued / 1 oz / **Louis Rich**, Skinless	29

CALORIES

Fresh cooked / 1 oz / **Louis Rich**	47
Fresh cooked / 1 oz / **Louis Rich** Hen	50
Hickory smoked / 1 oz / **Louis Rich**, Skinless	28
Honey roasted / 1 slice / **Louis Rich**	32
Honey roasted / 1 oz / **Louis Rich**, Skinless	31
Oven roasted / 1 oz / **Eckrich** Lite	30
Oven roasted / 1 slice / **Louis Rich**	31
Oven roasted / 1 slice / **Louis Rich**, Deluxe	30
Oven roasted / 1 oz / **Louis Rich**, Skinless	26
Oven roasted / 1 slice / **Louis Rich**, Thin Sliced	12
Oven roasted / 1 slice / **Oscar Mayer**	23
Roast, fresh-cooked / 1 oz / **Louis Rich**	42
Smoked / 1 oz / **Eckrich** Lite	30
Smoked / 1 oz / **Louis Rich**	33
Smoked / 1 slice / **Louis Rich**	21
Smoked / 1 slice / **Louis Rich**, Thin Sliced	11
Sliced thin / 1 slice / **Oscar Mayer**	12
Slices, fresh-cooked / 1 oz / **Louis Rich**	39
Steak, cooked / 1 oz / **Louis Rich**	39
Tenderloin, cooked / 1 oz / **Louis Rich**	39
Smoked / 1 slice / **Oscar Mayer**	20
Breast, stuffed / frozen / 8.5 oz / **Weight Watchers**	260
Chunk, white / canned / 2-½ oz / **Swanson**	80
Drumsticks, fresh-cooked / 1 oz / **Louis Rich**	56
Glazed / frozen / 8-¼ oz / **Le Menu** Light	260
Ground	
Fresh-cooked / 1 oz / **Louis Rich**	60
Fresh-cooked / 1 oz / **Louis Rich** Lean	52
Fresh-cooked / 1 oz / **Louis Rich** Lean w Natural flv	50
Homestyle w vegetables and pasta / frozen / 9-⅜ oz / **Stouffer's** Lean Cuisine	230
Medallions in herb sauce, entree / frozen / 12 oz / **Ultra Slim-Fast**	280
Nuggets, breaded / cooked / 1 nugget / **Louis Rich**	62
Patties, breaded / cooked / 1 pattie / **Louis Rich**	209
Slices	
Smoked / 1 slice / **Louis Rich**	32
in mushroom sauce / frozen / 8 oz / **Stouffer's** Lean Cuisine	220
w dressing / frozen / 7-⅞ oz / **Stouffer's** Lean Cuisine	200

Slices and gravy / frozen / 5 oz / **Banquet** Cookin' Bag	100
Slices w gravy, entree / frozen / 7 oz / **Banquet**	120
Sticks, breaded / cooked / 1 stick / **Louis Rich**	81
Thigh / fresh-cooked / 1 oz / **Louis Rich**	64
w dressing, entree / frozen / 10.5 oz / **Ultra Slim-Fast**	340
w dressing and potatoes / frozen / 9 oz / **Swanson** Homestyle	290
w dressing and gravy / frozen / 11.5 oz / **Armour** Classics	320
w stuffing / frozen / 7.8 oz / **Stouffer's**	300
Wing drumettes / fresh-cooked / 1 oz / **Louis Rich**	51
Wing portion / fresh-cooked / 1 oz / **Louis Rich**	54
Wings / fresh-cooked / 1 oz / **Louis Rich**	54

Turkey

and ham deli melt, entree / frozen / 1 sandwich / **Quaker** Ovenstuffs	360
Casserole w gravy and dressing / frozen / 9.75 oz / **Stouffer's**	360
Chili / frozen / 4 oz / **Banquet** Cookin' Bag	80
Dijon / frozen / 9-½ oz / **Stouffer's** Lean Cuisine	230
Bacon / cooked / 1 slice / **Louis Rich**	32
Bologna / 1 slice / **Louis Rich**	61
Bologna, mild / 1 slice / **Louis Rich**	59
Breakfast sausage links / cooked / 1 link / **Louis Rich**	46
Breakfast sausage / cooked / 1 oz / **Louis Rich**	56
Cotto salami / 1 slice / **Louis Rich**	53

Franks

Louis Rich / 1 link	101
Bun length / 1 link / **Louis Rich**	128
Cheese / 1 link / **Louis Rich**	109

Ham

Louis Rich / 1 oz	33
Louis Rich Round / 1 slice	34
Louis Rich Square / 1 slice	24
Louis Rich Thin Sliced / 1 slice	12
Tyson / 1 slice	23
Chopped / 1 slice / **Louis Rich**	46
Honey-cured / 1 slice / **Louis Rich**	25

CALORIES

Luncheon loaf / 1 slice / **Louis Rich**	45
Pastrami	
Louis Rich / 1 slice	32
Louis Rich Square / 1 slice	24
Louis Rich Thin Sliced / 1 slice	11
Polska kielbasa / 1 oz / **Louis Rich**	40
Salami / 1 slice / **Louis Rich**	54
Sausage / smoked / 1 oz / **Louis Rich**	43
Sausage w cheese / smoked / 1 oz / **Louis Rich**	47
Summer sausage / 1 slice / **Louis Rich**	55
Tetrazzini / frozen / 10 oz / **Stouffer's**	380
Turnover, entree / frozen / 1 sandwich / **Quaker** Ovenstuffs	350

Pretzels

CALORIES

1 oz

Bachman Butter Twist	110
Bachman Nutzels	110
Bachman Rods	110
Bachman Stix	110
Bachman Thin 'n Light	110
Bachman Twist	110
Mister Salty Sticks	110
Quinlan/Borden Beer Pretzels	110
Quinlan/Borden Hard Sourdough Pretzels	100
Quinlan/Borden Logs	110
Quinlan/Borden Nuggets	110
Quinlan/Borden Sticks	110
Quinlan/Borden Thin Pretzels	100
Rold Gold Bavarian	120
Rold Gold Rods	110
Rold Gold Sticks	110
Rold Gold Tiny Twists	110
Rold Gold Twists	110

CALORIES

Rold Gold, Unsalted	110
Seyfert's Pretzel Rods	110

Puddings

CALORIES

½ cup unless noted

Banana	
Canned, ready to serve / 5 oz / **Del Monte** Pudding Cup	180
Canned, ready to serve / 4 oz / **Lucky Leaf**	150
Canned, ready to serve / 4 oz / **Musselman's**	150
Mix, prepared w 2% milk / **Jell-O** Sugar Free, Instant	80
Banana cream	
Mix, prepared w whole milk / **Jell-O** Instant	160
Mix, prepared w whole milk / **Jell-O** Microwave	150
Butter pecan / mix, prepared w whole milk / **Jell-O** Instant	170
Butterscotch	
Canned, ready to serve / 5 oz / **Del Monte** Pudding Cup	180
Canned, ready to serve / 4 oz / **Hunt's** Snack Pack	150
Canned, ready to serve / 4 oz cup / **Jell-O** Pudding Snacks	180
Canned, ready to serve / 4 oz / **Lucky Leaf**	170
Canned, ready to serve / 4 oz / **Musselman's**	170
Mix / **Weight Watchers**	50
Mix, prepared w 2% milk / **Jell-O** Sugar Free, Instant	90
Mix, prepared w skim milk / **D-Zerta**	70
Mix, prepared w skim milk / **Weight Watchers**	90
Mix, prepared w whole milk / **Jell-O**	90
Mix, prepared w whole milk / **Jell-O** Instant	160
Mix, prepared w whole milk / **Jell-O** Microwave	170
Caramello / canned, ready to serve / 4 oz / **Hershey's**	180

	CALORIES
Cherry vanilla / mix / **Royal** Instant	90
Chocolate	
Canned, ready to serve / 5 oz / **Del Monte** Pudding Cup	190
Canned, ready to serve / 4 oz / **Hershey's**	180
Canned, ready to serve / 4 oz / **Hunt's** Snack Pack	150
Canned, ready to serve / 4 oz / **Hunt's** Snack Pack, Lite	100
Canned, ready to serve / **Jell-O** Light Snacks	100
Canned, ready to serve / 4 oz cup / **Jell-O** Pudding Snacks	180
Canned, ready to serve / 4 oz cup / **Jell-O** Pudding Snacks	170
Canned, ready to serve / 5.5 oz cup / **Jell-O** Pudding Snacks	230
Canned, ready to serve / 4 oz / **Lucky Leaf**	180
Canned, ready to serve / 4 oz / **Musselman's**	180
Mix / **Weight Watchers**	50
Mix, prepared w 2% milk / **Jell-O** Sugar Free	90
Mix, prepared w 2% milk / **Jell-O** Sugar Free, Instant	90
Mix, prepared w skim milk / **D-Zerta**	60
Mix, prepared w skim milk / **Weight Watchers**	90
Mix, prepared w whole milk / **Jell-O**	160
Mix, prepared w whole milk / **Jell-O** Instant	180
Mix, prepared w whole milk / **Jell-O** Microwave	170
Chocolate and almond / canned, ready to serve / 4 oz / **Hershey's**	180
Chocolate and vanilla / canned, ready to serve / 4 oz / **Hershey's**	180
Chocolate caramel swirl / canned, ready to serve / 4 oz cup / **Jell-O** Pudding Snacks	170
Chocolate fudge	
Canned, ready to serve / 5 oz / **Del Monte** Pudding Cup	190
Canned, ready to serve / 4 oz cup / **Jell-O** Light Snacks	100
Canned, ready to serve / 4 oz cup / **Jell-O** Pudding Snacks	170
Canned, ready to serve / 4 oz / **Lucky Leaf**	180
Canned, ready to serve / 4 oz / **Musselman's**	180

CALORIES

Mix, prepared w 2% milk / **Jell-O** Sugar Free, Instant	100
Mix, prepared w whole milk / **Jell-O**	160
Mix, prepared w whole milk / **Jell-O** Instant	180
Chocolate fudge-milk chocolate swirl / canned, ready to serve / 4 oz cup / **Jell-O** Pudding Snacks	170
Milk chocolate	
Canned, ready to serve / 4 oz cup / **Jell-O** Pudding Snacks	170
Mix, prepared w whole milk / **Jell-O**	160
Mix, prepared w whole milk / **Jell-O** Instant	180
Mix, prepared w whole milk / **Jell-O** Microwave	160
Milk chocolate-chocolate fudge swirl / canned, ready to serve / 4 oz cup / **Jell-O** Pudding Snacks	170
Chocolate-vanilla combo / canned, ready to serve / 4 oz cup / **Jell-O** Light Snacks	100
Chocolate-vanilla swirl / canned, ready to serve / 4 oz cup / **Jell-O** Pudding Snacks	170
Chocolate-vanilla swirl / canned, ready to serve / 5.5 oz cup / **Jell-O** Pudding Snacks	240
Coconut cream / mix, prepared w whole milk / **Jell-O** Instant	180
Egg custard / mix, prepared w whole milk / **Jell-O**	160
Flan / mix, prepared w whole milk / **Jell-O**	150
Lemon	
Canned, ready to serve / 4 oz / **Lucky Leaf**	130
Canned, ready to serve / 4 oz / **Musselman's**	130
Mix, prepared w whole milk / **Jell-O** Instant	170
Mousse	
Cheesecake / mix / **Weight Watchers**	50
Cheesecake / mix, prepared w skim milk / **Weight Watchers**	60
Chocolate	
Mix, prepared w whole milk / **Jell-O**	150
Mix, prepared w skim milk / **Weight Watchers**	60
Chocolate fudge / mix, prepared w whole milk / **Jell-O**	140
Raspberry / mix, prepared w skim milk / **Weight Watchers**	60
White chocolate-almond / mix, prepared w skim milk / **Weight Watchers**	60

Pistachio

    Mix, prepared w 2% milk / **Jell-O** Sugar Free,
      Instant   90

    Mix, prepared w whole milk / **Jell-O** Instant   170

Rice / canned, ready to serve / 4 oz / **Lucky Leaf**   120

Rice / canned, ready to serve / 4 oz / **Musselman's**   120

Rice / mix, prepared w whole milk / **Jell-O**   170

Special dark / canned, ready to serve / 4 oz / **Hershey's**   170

Tapioca

    Canned, ready to serve / 5 oz / **Del Monte** Pudding
      Cup   180

    Canned, ready to serve / 4 oz / **Hunt's** Snack Pack   150

    Canned, ready to serve / 4 oz cup / **Jell-O** Pudding
      Snacks   170

    Canned, ready to serve / 4 oz / **Lucky Leaf**   140

    Canned, ready to serve / 4 oz / **Musselman's**   140

Tapioca, vanilla / mix, prepared w whole milk / **Jell-O**   160

Vanilla

    Canned, ready to serve / 5 oz / **Del Monte** Pudding
      Cup   180

    Canned, ready to serve / 4 oz / **Hunt's** Snack Pack   160

    Canned, ready to serve / 4 oz cup / **Jell-O** Light
      Snacks   100

    Canned, ready to serve / 4 oz cup / **Jell-O** Pudding
      Snacks   180

    Canned, ready to serve / 5.5 oz cup / **Jell-O** Pudding
      Snacks   250

    Canned, ready to serve / 4 oz / **Lucky Leaf**   170

    Canned, ready to serve / 4 oz / **Musselman's**   170

    Mix / **Weight Watchers**   50

    Mix, prepared w 2% milk / **Jell-O** Sugar Free   80

    Mix, prepared w 2% milk / **Jell-O** Sugar Free,
      Instant   90

    Mix, prepared w skim milk / **D-Zerta**   70

    Mix, prepared w skim milk / **Weight Watchers**   90

    Mix, prepared w whole milk / **Jell-O**   160

    Mix, prepared w whole milk / **Jell-O** Instant   170

    Mix, prepared w whole milk / **Jell-O** Microwave   160

Vanilla-chocolate swirl / canned, ready to serve / 4 oz cup /
Jell-O Pudding Snacks   180

CALORIES

Vanilla, French / mix, prepared w whole milk / **Jell-O**   170
Vanilla, French / mix, prepared w whole mix / **Jell-O**
Instant   160
Vanilla swirl / canned, ready to serve / 4 oz cup / **Jell-O**
Pudding Snacks   180
York peppermint pattie / canned, ready to serve / 4 oz /
Hershey's   180

Rice and Rice Dishes

RICE, PLAIN

	CALORIES
Brown, long grain, parboiled / ⅔ cup cooked	200
White, instant / 1 cup cooked	180
White, long grain / ⅔ cup cooked	225
White, parboiled / 1 cup cooked	185

RICE DISHES, FROZEN

½ cup unless noted

Asparagus pilaf / 1 pkg / **Green Giant** Garden Gourmet	190
Country style / 3.3 oz / **Birds Eye** International	90
French style / 3.3 oz / **Birds Eye** International	110
Pilaf / **Green Giant** Originals	110
Rice 'n broccoli / **Green Giant** Originals	120
Rice and broccoli in cheese sauce / 5.5 oz / **Green Giant** One Servings	160
Rice Florentine / **Green Giant** Originals	140
Rice medley / **Green Giant** Originals	100
Spanish rice / 3.3 oz / **Birds Eye** International	110
White 'n wild rice / **Green Giant** Originals	130

CANNED OR MIXES

½ cup unless noted

Almond chicken w wild rice / mix, prepared / **Rice-A-Roni** Classics	140

CALORIES

Asparagus w Hollandaise sauce / mix, prepared / **Lipton**	123.3
Beef / mix, prepared / **Rice-A-Roni**	140
Beef / mix, prepared / **Rice-A-Roni** Classics	150
Beef and mushroom / mix, prepared / **Rice-A-Roni**	150
Beef flavor / mix, prepared / **Lipton** Rice and Sauce	119
Beef-flavored / mix, prepared w butter / **Minute** Family Size, Microwave	160
Beef-flavored / mix, prepared w butter / **Minute** Single Size, Microwave	150
Broccoli au gratin / mix, prepared / **Rice-A-Roni** Classics	180
Cajun / mix, prepared / **Lipton** Rice and Sauce	123.2
Cauliflower au gratin / mix, prepared / **Rice-A-Roni** Classics	170
Cheddar / mix, prepared / **Rice-A-Roni** Classics	180
Cheddar broccoli / mix, prepared / **Lipton** Rice and Sauce	124.6
Cheddar cheese w broccoli / mix, prepared w butter / **Minute** Family Size, Microwave	160
Cheddar cheese w broccoli / mix, prepared w butter / **Minute** Single Serve, Microwave	160
Chicken / mix, prepared / **Rice-A-Roni**	150
Chicken / mix, prepared / **Rice-A-Roni** Classics	140
Chicken and broccoli / mix, prepared / **Rice-A-Roni**	150
Chicken and broccoli Dijon / mix, prepared / **Rice-A-Roni** Classics	160
Chicken and mushroom / mix, prepared / **Rice-A-Roni**	180
Chicken and vegetables / mix, prepared / **Rice-A-Roni**	140
Chicken-broccoli / mix, prepared / **Lipton** Rice and Sauce	128.7
Chicken flavor / mix, prepared / **Lipton** Rice and Sauce	124.3
Chicken-flavored / mix, prepared w butter / **Minute** Family Size, Microwave	160
Chicken-flavored / mix, prepared w butter / **Minute** Single Serve, Microwave	150
Chicken Florentine / mix, prepared / **Rice-A-Roni** Classics	130
Creamy chicken / mix, prepared / **Lipton** Rice and Sauce	141.5
Drumstick / mix, prepared w butter / **Minute**	150
Fried, beef flavor / mix, prepared / **Lipton** Golden Saute	124.1
Fried, Oriental / mix, prepared / **Lipton** Golden Saute	127.3
Fried rice / mix, prepared / **Rice-A-Roni**	110
Fried rice / mix, prepared w oil / **Minute**	160

CALORIES

Garden pilaf / mix, prepared / **Rice-A-Roni** Classics	140
Green bean almondine / mix, prepared / **Rice-A-Roni** Classics	210
Herb & butter / mix, prepared / **Rice-A-Roni**	130
Herbs and butter / mix, prepared / **Lipton** Rice and Sauce	122.6
Long grain / mix, prepared / ⅔ cup / **Minute**	120
Long grain and wild / mix, prepared w butter / **Minute**	150
Long grain and wild rice	
Mix, prepared / **Lipton** Rice and Sauce, Mushrooms and Herbs	124.7
Mix, prepared / **Lipton** Rice and Sauce, Original	121.3
Mix, prepared / **Rice-A-Roni**	130
Long grain and wild rice, chicken w almonds / mix, prepared / **Rice-A-Roni**	140
Long grain and wild rice pilaf / mix, prepared / **Rice-A-Roni**	130
Mexican / box / **Old El Paso**	140
Mexican fiesta / mix, prepared / **Rice-A-Roni** Classics	170
Minute / mix, prepared / ⅔ cup / **Minute**	120
Minute / mix, prepared / **Minute** Boil In Bag	90
Mushroom / mix, prepared / **Lipton** Rice and Sauce	122.6
Oriental stir fry / mix, prepared / **Rice-A-Roni** Classics	150
Parmesan and herbs / mix, prepared / **Rice-A-Roni** Classics	170
Pilaf / mix, prepared / **Lipton** Rice and Sauce	121.8
Pilaf / mix, prepared / **Rice-A-Roni**	150
Pilaf, French style / mix, prepared w butter / **Minute** Family Size Microwave	130
Pilaf, French style / mix, prepared w butter / **Minute** Single Serve, Microwave	120
Rib roast / mix, prepared w butter / **Minute**	150
Risotto / mix, prepared / **Rice-A-Roni**	200
Spanish	
Can / **Old El Paso**	70
Mix, prepared / **Lipton** Rice and Sauce	117.7
Mix, prepared / **Rice-A-Roni**	150
Spanish rice and sauce / mix, as packaged / **Lipton** Skillet Style	103.7
Stroganoff / mix, prepared / **Rice-A-Roni**	200

CALORIES

Vegetables and cheese / mix, prepared / **Rice-A-Roni**
   Classics   170
Yellow rice / mix, prepared / **Rice-A-Roni**   140

Rolls, Buns and Bagels

BAGELS

CALORIES

1 bagel

Cinnamon raisin / **Thomas'**	160
Egg / **Thomas'**	150
Onion / **Thomas'**	150
Frozen	
Blueberry / **Lender's**	190
Cinnamon raisin / **Lender's**	190
Cinnamon raisin / **Lender's** Big Crusty	230
Egg / **Lender's**	150
Egg / **Lender's** Big Crusty	210
Onion / **Lender's**	150
Onion / **Lender's** Big Crusty	210
Original Soft / **Lender's**	200
Plain / **Lender's**	150
Plain / **Lender's** Big Crusty	210

BUNS FOR SANDWICHES

1 bun

Less Wheat Bun	90
Mrs. Wright's Soft Sandwich	110
Weber's Egg Bun / 1 oz	70
Weber's Egg Bun / 1.5 oz	120

Weber's Egg Bun / 2 oz	160
Weber's Egg Bun / 2.5 oz	200
Weber's Egg Bun / 3 oz	240
Weber's Egg Bun / 3.5 oz	280
Hamburger	
Butternut / 1 oz	80
Butternut / 1.5 oz	120
Butternut / 2 oz	150
Butternut / 2.5 oz	190
Butternut / 3 oz	240
Butternut / 3.5 oz	270
Cotton/Holsum	90
Cotton/Holsum / 1.5 oz	110
Cotton/Holsum / 1.75 oz	130
Cotton/Holsum / 2.5 oz	190
Cotton/Holsum / 2.75 oz	210
Cotton/Holsum / 3 oz	230
Cotton/Holsum / 3.5 oz	270
Eddy's / 1 oz	80
Eddy's / 1.5 oz	120
Eddy's / 2 oz	150
Eddy's / 2.5 oz	190
Eddy's / 3 oz	240
Eddy's / 3.5 oz	270
Holsum / 1 oz	80
Holsum / 1.5 oz	120
Holsum / 2 oz	150
Holsum / 2.5 oz	190
Holsum / 3 oz	240
Holsum / 3.5 oz	270
Merita / 1.25 oz	90
Merita / 1.5 oz	110
Merita / 1.75 oz	130
Merita / 2 oz	150
Merita / 2.25 oz	170
Merita / 2.5 oz	190
Millbrook / 1 oz	80
Millbrook / 1.5 oz	120
Millbrook / 2 oz	150
Millbrook / 2.5 oz	190
Millbrook / 3 oz	240

CALORIES

Millbrook / 3.5 oz	270
Mrs. Karl's / 1 oz	80
Mrs. Karl's / 1.5 oz	120
Mrs. Karl's / 2 oz	150
Mrs. Karl's / 2.5 oz	190
Mrs. Karl's / 3 oz	240
Mrs. Karl's / 3.5 oz	270
Roman Meal	120
Sweetheart / 1 oz	80
Sweetheart / 1.5 oz	120
Sweetheart / 2 oz	150
Sweetheart / 2.5 oz	190
Sweetheart / 3 oz	240
Sweetheart / 3.5 oz	270
Weber / 1 oz	80
Weber / 1.5 oz	120
Weber / 2 oz	150
Weber / 2.5 oz	190
Weber / 3 oz	240
Weber / 3.5 oz	270
Hoagie / **Pepperidge Farm**	210
Hot dog	
Butternut / 1 oz	80
Butternut / 1.5 oz	120
Cotton/Holsum	90
Cotton/Holsum / 1.5 oz	110
Cotton/Holsum / 1.75 oz	130
Eddy's / 1 oz	80
Eddy's / 1.5 oz	120
Holsum / 1 oz	80
Holsum / 1.5 oz	120
Merita / 1.25 oz	90
Merita / 1.5 oz	110
Merita / 1.75 oz	130
Millbrook / 1 oz	80
Millbrook / 1.5 oz	120
Mrs. Karl's / 1 oz	80
Mrs. Karl's / 1.5 oz	120
Pepperidge Farm	140
Roman Meal	110
Sweetheart / 1 oz	80

Sweetheart / 1.5 oz	120
Weber / 1 oz	80
Weber / 1.5 oz	120
Hot Dog, Dijon / **Pepperidge Farm**	160
Hot dog w sesame seeds / **Mrs. Wright's**	120
Onion w poppy seeds / **Pepperidge Farm**	150
Potato / **Pepperidge Farm**	160
Salad / **Pepperidge Farm**	110
Submarine roll / **Mrs. Wright's**	310
w sesame seeds / **Mrs. Wright's**	210
w sesame seeds / **Pepperidge Farm**	140
Croissant / **Pepperidge Farm**	170

DINNER ROLLS

1 bun

Soft

Butternut / 1 oz	90
Butternut / 1.5 oz	130
Butternut / 2 oz	170
Butternut / 2.5 oz	210
Butternut / 3 oz	250
Butternut / 3.5 oz	290
Butternut Brown 'n Serve / 1 oz	90
Butternut Brown 'n Serve / 1.5 oz	130
Butternut Brown 'n Serve / 2 oz	170
Butternut Steak Roll / 1 oz	80
Butternut Steak Roll / 1.5 oz	120
Butternut Steak Roll / 2 oz	150
Butternut Steak Roll / 2.5 oz	190
Butternut Steak Roll / 3 oz	230
Butternut Steak Roll / 3.5 oz	270
Eddy's Brown 'n Serve / 1 oz	90
Eddy's Brown 'n Serve / 1.5 oz	130
Eddy's Brown 'n Serve / 2 oz	170
Eddy's Hawkins Dinner Roll / 1 oz	70
Eddy's Hawkins Dinner Roll / 1.5 oz	110
Eddy's Hawkins Dinner Roll / 2 oz	150
Holsum / 1 oz	90
Holsum / 1.5 oz	130

CALORIES

Holsum / 2 oz	170
Holsum / 2.5 oz.	210
Holsum / 3 oz	250
Holsum / 3.5 oz	290
Holsum Brown 'n Serve / 1 oz	90
Holsum Brown 'n Serve / 1.5 oz	130
Holsum Brown 'n Serve / 2 oz	170
Merita Brown 'n Serve / .8 oz	60
Merita Brown 'n Serve / 1 oz	80
Millbrook Brown 'n Serve / 1 oz	90
Millbrook Brown 'n Serve / 1.5 oz	130
Millbrook Brown 'n Serve / 2 oz	170
Mrs. Karl's / 1 oz	90
Mrs. Karl's / 1.5 oz	130
Mrs. Karl's / 2 oz	170
Mrs. Karl's / 2.5 oz	210
Mrs. Karl's / 3 oz	250
Mrs. Karl's / 3.5 oz	290
Mrs. Karls Brown 'n Serve / 1 oz	90
Mrs. Karl's / Brown 'n Serve / 1.5 oz	130
Mrs. Karl's Brown 'n Serve / 2 oz	170
Mrs. Wright's / 4 rolls	190
Mrs. Wright's Buttermilk Biscuits / 2 rolls	100
Mrs. Wright's Cloverleaf Brown 'n Serve / 2 rolls	180
Mrs. Wright's Farmstyle	100
Mrs. Wright's Farmstyle, Sesame	100
Mrs. Wright's Sesame Brown 'n Serve	80
Mrs. Wright's Tea Rolls	70
Mrs. Wright's Twin Brown 'n Serve / 2 rolls	170
Mrs. Wright's Wheatberry	150
Pepperidge Farm Club, Enriched Brown & Serve	100
Pepperidge Farm Butter Crescent	110
Pepperidge Farm Country Classic	50
Pepperidge Farm Finger, Poppyseed	50
Pepperidge Farm French, Enriched Brown & Serve	120
Pepperidge Farm Golden Twist	110
Pepperidge Farm Hearth, Enriched Brown & Serve	50
Pepperidge Farm Hearty Potato Classic	90
Pepperidge Farm Old-Fashioned	50

CALORIES

Pepperidge Farm Parker House	60
Pepperidge Farm Party	30
Pepperidge Farm Soft, Family	100
Roman Meal / 2 rolls	155
Sweetheart Brown 'n Serve / 1 oz	90
Sweetheart Brown 'n Serve / 1.5 oz	130
Sweetheart Brown 'n Serve / 2 oz	170
Weber / 1 oz	90
Weber / 1.5 oz	130
Weber / 2 oz	170
Weber / 2.5 oz	210
Weber / 3 oz	250
Weber / 3.5 oz	290
Weber Brown 'n Serve / 1 oz	90
Weber Brown 'n Serve / 1.5 oz	130
Weber Brown 'n Serve / 2 oz	170

Hard Rolls
   French

Mrs. Wright's / 2 oz	160
Sweetheart / 2 oz	150
Sweetheart / 2.5 oz	180
Sweetheart / 3 oz	220
French sesame / **Mrs. Wright's** / 2 oz	145
French Style / **Pepperidge Farm**	100
Italian / **Mrs. Wright's**	150

   Kaiser

Dutch Hearth / 1.5 oz	110
Dutch Hearth / 2 oz	150
Dutch Hearth / 2.5 oz	180
Dutch Hearth / 3 oz	230
Millbrook / 1.5 oz	110
Millbrook / 2 oz	150
Millbrook / 2.5 oz	180
Millbrook / 3 oz	230
Mrs. Wright's	150
Sweetheart / 1.5 oz	110
Sweetheart / 2 oz	150
Sweetheart / 2.5 oz	180
Sweetheart / 3 oz	230
Kaiser, poppy / **Mrs. Wright's**	150
Kaiser, sesame / **Mrs. Wright's**	150

CALORIES

Potato / **Mrs. Wright's** Old-Fashioned	100
Sourdough, French Style / **Pepperidge Farm**	100
Steak, seeded / **Mrs. Wright's**	220

REFRIGERATOR ROLLS

1 roll

Pillsbury Butterflake	140
Pillsbury Crescent	100

SWEET ROLLS

1 piece unless noted:

Apple / **Dolly Madison**	210
Apple / microwave / 2.25 oz / **Weight Watchers**	160
Apple-cinnamon / 2 oz / **Aunt Fanny's**	178
Bear claw / **Dolly Madison**	290
Caramel nut / 2 oz / **Aunt Fanny's**	180
Caramel nut, rectangular / 2 oz / **Aunt Fanny's**	180
Caramel w nuts / refrigerated / **Pillsbury**	160
Cheese / microwave / 2.25 oz / **Weight Watchers**	180
Cherry / **Dolly Madison**	210
Cinnamon	
Aunt Fanny's / 2 oz	181
Aunt Fanny's / 3.75 oz	340
Aunt Fanny's / rectangular / 2 oz	181
Dolly Madison	210
Pepperidge Farm / frozen / 2-¼ oz	280
Cinnamon-raisin / rectangular / **Aunt Fanny's** / 2 oz	181
Cinnamon w icing / refrigerated / **Pillsbury**	110
Danish Apple / **Dolly Madison**	420
Danish Apple / frozen / **Pepperidge Farm**	220
Danish Cheese / frozen / **Pepperidge Farm**	240
Danish Cherry / **Dolly Madison**	410
Danish, cinnamon-raisin / **Dolly Madison**	410
Danish, cinnamon-raisin / frozen / **Pepperidge Farm**	250
Danish, cinnamon-raisin w icing / refrigerated / **Pillsbury**	150
Danish, creme cheese / **Dolly Madison**	380
Danish, orange w icing / refrigerated / **Pillsbury**	150

CALORIES

Danish, raspberry / frozen / **Pepperidge Farm**	220
Honey bun / 3 oz / **Aunt Fanny's**	346
Honey bun / **Dolly Madison**	450
Honey bun, golden / **Butternut**	120
Honey bun, glazed / **Tastykake**	360
Honey bun, iced / **Tastykake**	350
Pecan, rectangular / 2 oz / **Aunt Fanny's**	184
Pecan rollers / **Dolly Madison**	120
Pecan twirls / **Tastykake**	110
Strawberry / rectangular / 2 oz / **Aunt Fanny's**	165
Strawberry / microwave / 2.25 oz / **Weight Watchers**	170
Tasty twist / **Tastykake**	18

TURNOVERS

1 turnover

Apple / refrigerated / **Pillsbury**	170
Cherry / refrigerated / **Pillsbury**	170

Salad Dressings

1 tbsp unless noted

	CALORIES
Bottled	
Bama	50
Miracle Whip	70
Miracle Whip Free	20
Miracle Whip Light	45
Bacon / bottled / **Kraft** Creamy, Reduced Calorie	30
Bacon and tomato / bottled / **Kraft**	70
Bacon and tomato / bottled / **Kraft**, Reduced Calorie	30
Bleu cheese, bottled	
Hidden Valley Ranch	80
Hidden Valley Ranch Take Heart	12
Healthy Sensation	19
Henri's Light	35
Kraft Chunky	60
Kraft Chunky, Reduced Calorie	30
Kraft Roka	60
Kraft Roka, Reduced Calorie	16
Nu Made	60
Wish-Bone Chunky	73
Blue cheese, mix, prepared	
Good Seasons	70
Hain, No Oil	14
Buttermilk, bottled	
Hain Old Fashioned	70
Kraft Creamy, Reduced Calorie	30

239

CALORIES

Kraft Seven Seas Ranch, Light, Reduced Calories	50
Nu Made Creamy	50
Buttermilk, mix, prepared	
Good Seasons	60
Hain, No Oil	11
Buttermilk, creamy / bottled / **Kraft**	80
Buttermilk recipe / bottled / **Kraft** Seven Seas	80
Caesar, bottled	
Hain Creamy	60
Hain Creamy, Low Salt	60
Hollywood	70
Weight Watchers	4
Weight Watchers Single Serve	6
Caesar, mix, prepared	
Hain, No Oil	6
Suddenly Salad / ⅙ serv	170
Caesar, golden / bottled / **Kraft**	70
Caesar w olive oil / bottled / **Wish-Bone** Lite	28
Catalina / bottled / **Kraft** Free	16
Catalina / bottled / **Kraft**, Reduced Calorie	18
Cheese, garlic / mix, prepared / **Good Seasons**	70
Cheese, Italian / mix, prepared / **Good Seasons**	70
Cheese, Italian / mix, prepared / **Good Seasons** Lite	25
Citrus / bottled / **Hain** Tangy	50
Classic, herb / mix, prepared / **Good Seasons**	70
Classic, pasta / mix, prepared / **Suddenly Salad** / ⅙ serv	160
Coleslaw dressing / bottled / **Kraft**	70
Coleslaw dressing / bottled / **Miracle Whip**	70
Creamy dressing / bottled / **Kraft** Rancher's Choice	90
Creamy dressing / bottled / **Kraft** Rancher's Choice, Reduced Calorie	30
Creamy macaroni / mix, prepared / **Suddenly Salad** / ⅙ serv	200
Cucumber, creamy bottled	
Henri's Light	35
Kraft	70
Kraft, Reduced Calorie	25
Nu Made	70
Weight Watchers	18
Cucumber, dill / bottled / **Hain**	80
Dijon vinaigrette / bottled / **Hain**	50

CALORIES

Dijon vinaigrette / bottled / **Wish-Bone** Classic	557
Dijon vinaigrette / bottled / **Wish-Bone** Classic Lite	30
French, bottled	
Hain Creamy	60
Healthy Sensation	21
Henri's Bacon 'n Tomato	70
Henri's Frontier	70
Henri's Hearty	70
Henri's Hearty Light	35
Henri's Light	40
Henri's Original	60
Hidden Valley Ranch Take Heart	20
Kraft	60
Kraft Catalina	60
Kraft Free	20
Kraft Miracle	70
Kraft Reduced Calorie	20
Kraft Seven Seas, Creamy	60
Kraft Seven Seas, Light, Reduced Calories	35
Nu Made	60
Weight Watchers	10
Wish Bone, Red	64
Wish-Bone, Deluxe	57
Wish-Bone, Fat Free	6
Wish-Bone Lite	22
Wish-Bone Lite, Sweet 'n Spicy	17
Wish-Bone Sweet 'n Spicy	61
French mustard / bottled / **Hain** Spicy	50
French, Red / bottled / **Wish-Bone** Lite	17
French / mix, prepared / **Hain**, No Oil	12
Garden tomato vinaigrette / bottled / **Hain**	60
Garlic and cheese / mix, prepared / **Hain**, No Oil	6
Garlic and sour cream / bottled / **Hain**	70
Garlic, creamy / bottled / **Kraft**	50
Garlic, herbs / mix, prepared / **Good Seasons**	70
Green goddess / bottled / **Nu Made**	60
Herb / mix, prepared / **Hain**, No Oil	2
Herb / bottled / **Hain**, No Salt	90
Herb and spice / bottled / **Kraft** Seven Seas, Viva	60
Herbs and spices / bottled / **Kraft** Seven Seas, Light, Reduced Calories	30

CALORIES

Honey and sesame / bottled / **Hain**	60
Honey Dijon, bottled	
Healthy Sensation	26
Hidden Valley Ranch	80
Hidden Valley Ranch Take Heart	20
Italian, bottled	
Hain	80
Hain Creamy	80
Hain Creamy, No Salt	80
Hain, No Salt	60
Healthy Sensation	7
Henri's Creamy Garlic	50
Henri's Creamy Light	30
Henri's Herb	50
Henri's Traditional	50
Hollywood, Creamy	90
Kraft Creamy, Reduced Calorie	25
Kraft Free	6
Kraft House	60
Kraft House, Reduced Calorie	30
Kraft Oil Free, Reduced Calorie	4
Kraft Presto	70
Kraft Seven Seas, Creamy	70
Kraft Seven Seas, Creamy Light, Reduced Calories	45
Kraft Seven Seas, Free Viva	4
Kraft Seven Seas, Viva	50
Kraft Seven Seas, Viva Light, Reduced Calories	30
Kraft Zesty	50
Kraft Zesty, Reduced Calorie	20
Nu Made, Creamy	60
Nu Made, Tangy	80
Weight Watchers	6
Weight Watchers Single Serve	9
Wish-Bone	45
Wish-Bone Classic Olive Oil	33
Wish-Bone Creamy Lite	26
Wish-Bone Creamy	26
Wish-Bone Lite	6
Wish-Bone Robusto	446

Italian, mix, prepared
Good Seasons	70
Good Seasons, Lite	25
Good Seasons, Mild	70
Good Seasons, No Oil	6
Good Seasons, Zesty	70
Good Seasons, Zesty Lite	25
Hain, No Oil	2
Italian cheese vinaigrette / bottled / **Hain**	55

Italian, creamy, bottled
Kraft w Real Sour Cream	50
Weight Watchers	12
Wish-Bone	54
Italian olive oil / bottled / **Wish-Bone** Classic Lite	20
Italian pasta / mix, prepared / **Suddenly Salad** / ⅙ serv	160
Italian w cheese / bottled / **Wish-Bone**	86
Lemon and herbs / mix, prepared / **Good Seasons**	70
Oil and vinegar / bottled / **Kraft**	70
Olive oil / bottled / **Wish-Bone** Lite, Vinaigrette	16
Olive oil / bottled / **Wish-Bone** Vinaigrette	30
Pasta primavera / mix, prepared / **Suddenly Salad** / ⅙ serv	190
Peppercorn / bottled / **Weight Watchers**	8
Poppyseed, ranchers / bottled / **Hain**	60

Ranch, bottled
Healthy Sensation	15
Henri's	70
Henri's Light	40
Kraft Free	16
Kraft Seven Seas	16
Kraft Seven Seas, Light, Reduced Calories	50
Kraft Seven Seas, Viva	80
Nu Made	80
Weight Watchers Single Serve	35
Wish-Bone / ½ fl oz	76
Wish-Bone Lite	42

Ranch, mix, prepared
Good Seasons	60
Good Seasons Lite	30
Ranch and bacon / mix, prepared / **Suddenly Salad** / ⅙ serv	210

CALORIES

Ranch, creamy / bottled / **Weight Watchers**	25
Ranch, original / bottled / **Hidden Valley** Ranch	80
Ranch, original / bottled / **Hidden Valley** Ranch Take Heart	20
Ranch, parmesan / bottled / **Henri's**	70
Ranch, parmesan / bottled / **Henri's** Light	35
Ranch w bacon / bottled / **Hidden Valley** Ranch	80
Ranch w bacon / bottled / **Hidden Valley** Ranch Take Heart	20
Red wine olive oil / bottled / **Wish-Bone** Vinaigrette	34
Red wine olive oil / bottled / **Wish-Bone** Lite Vinaigrette	20
Red wine vinegar / bottled / **Kraft** Seven Seas	6
Red wine vinegar / bottled / **Kraft** Seven Seas, Viva, Reduced Calories	45
Red wine vinegar and oil / bottled / **Kraft** Seven Seas, Viva	70
Red wine vinegar and oil / bottled / **Kraft**	60
Russian, bottled	
Kraft Reduced Calorie	30
Wish-Bone	54
Wish-Bone Lite	21
Russian, creamy / bottled / **Kraft**	60
Russian w pure honey / bottled / **Kraft**	60
Sour / bottled / **Friendship** Non Butterfat / 1 fl oz	36
Swiss cheese vinaigrette / bottled / **Hain**	60
Tas-Tee / bottled / **Henri's**	60
Tas-Tee / bottled / **Henri's** Light	30
Thousand Island, bottled	
Hain	50
Healthy Sensation	20
Henri's	50
Henri's Light	30
Hidden Valley Ranch	80
Hidden Valley Ranch Take Heart	20
Kraft	60
Kraft Free	20
Kraft Reduced Calorie	20
Kraft Seven Seas, Creamy	50
Kraft Seven Seas, Light, Reduced Calories	30
Nu Made	60
Wish-Bone	62

CALORIES

Wish-Bone Lite	22
Thousand Island / mix, prepared / **Hain**, No Oil	12
Thousand Island and bacon / bottled / **Kraft**	60
Tomato vinaigrette / bottled / **Weight Watchers**	8
Tortellini Italiano / mix, prepared / **Suddenly Salad** / ⅕ serv	160

Sauces

CALORIES

A la King / 1 cup / **Durkee**	133
Alfredo, mix, prepared: 1 tbsp unless noted	
McCormick/Schilling Pasta Prima / ½ cup	253
Barbecue, bottled or canned: 1 tbsp unless noted	
Heinz Cajun	15
Heinz Chunky	15
Heinz Hawaiian	19
Heinz Hickory Smoke	19
Heinz Old-Fashioned	18
Heinz Original	15
Heinz Regular	18
Hunt's Country	20
Hunt's Hickory	20
Hunt's Homestyle	20
Hunt's Kansas City	20
Hunt's New Orleans	20
Hunt's Original	20
Hunt's Southern	20
Hunt's Texas	25
Hunt's Western	20
Kraft / 2 tbsp	45
Kraft Thick 'n Spicy Chunky / 2 tbsp	60
Kraft Thick 'n Spicy w Honey / 2 tbsp	60
Garlic / 2 tbsp / **Kraft**	40
Hickory smoke / 2 tbsp / **Kraft**	45
Hickory smoke / 2 tbsp / **Kraft** Thick 'n Spicy	50

CALORIES

Hickory smoke, onion bits / 2 tbsp / **Kraft**	50
Honey / 1 tbsp / **Hain**	14
Hot / 1 tbsp / **Heinz** Texas Style	15
Hot / 2 tbsp / **Kraft**	45
Hot, hickory smoke / 2 tbsp / **Kraft**	45
Italian seasonings / 2 tbsp / **Kraft**	50
Kansas style / 2 tbsp / **Kraft**	50
Kansas style / 2 tbsp / **Kraft** Thick 'n Spicy	60
Mesquite smoke / 2 tbsp / **Kraft**	45
Mesquite smoke / 2 tbsp / **Kraft** Thick 'n Spicy	50
Mushroom / 1 tbsp / **Heinz**	14
Onion / 1 tbsp / **Heinz**	15
Onion bits / 2 tbsp / **Kraft**	50
Original / 2 tbsp / **Kraft** Thick 'n Spicy	50
Beef stew / mix, prepared / ¼ pkg / **McCormick/Schilling**	33
Beef stroganoff / mix, prepared / ¼ pkg / **McCormick/Schilling**	32
Bernaise / mix, prepared / ¼ cup / **McCormick/Schilling**	129
Bread, molasses / ½ tsp / **La Choy**	7
Cheese	
Mix, prepared w milk / 1 cup / **Durkee**	316
Mix, prepared / ⅓ cup / **French's**	110
Mix, prepared / ¼ pkg / **McCormick/Schilling**	35
Cheddar / canned / 4 oz / **Lucky Leaf**	220
Cheddar / canned / 4 oz / **Musselman's**	220
Cheddar, aged / canned / 4 oz / **Lucky Leaf**	240
Cheddar, aged / canned / 4 oz / **Musselman's**	240
Nacho / canned / 4 oz / **Lucky Leaf**	220
Nacho / canned / 4 oz / **Musselman's**	220
Chili	
Hunt's Manwich / 5.3 oz	110
Canned / ¼ cup / **Del Monte**	70
Mix, prepared / ¼ pkg / **McCormick/Schilling**	27
Hot dog / canned / ⅙ cup / **Wolf**	44
Mild, green / 2 tbsp / **El Molino**	10
Red / ½ cup / **Las Palmas**	25
Hot dog / 2 tbsp / **Gebhardt**	30
Chili salsa, green, thick and chunky / canned / 2 tbsp / **Old El Paso**	3
Clam, red / jar / ½ cup / **Progresso**	70
Clam, white / jar / ½ cup / **Progresso**	110

Cocktail / bottle / 1 tbsp / **Kraft** Sauceworks	14
Dill, creamy / mix / 1 pkg / **Durkee** Roastin' Bag	153
Enchilada	
Gebhardt / 3 tbsp	25
Green / canned / 2 tbsp / **Old El Paso**	11
Hot / canned / 2 tbsp / **El Molino**	16
Hot / canned / ½ cup / **Las Palmas**	25
Hot / canned / ¼ cup / **Old El Paso**	30
Mild / canned / 2.5 oz / **Rosarita**	25
Mild / canned / ¼ cup / **Old El Paso**	25
Garlic, creamy / mix, prepared / ½ cup / **McCormick/ Schilling** Pasta Prima	277
Green peppercorn / mix, prepared / ¼ cup / **McCormick/ Schilling**	86
Herb and garlic / mix, prepared / ½ cup / **McCormick/ Schilling** Pasta Prima	326
Hollandaise, mix, prepared	
Durkee / ¾ cup	173
French's / 3 tbsp	30
McCormick/Schilling / ¼ cup	137
McCormick/Schilling ¼ pkg	51
Hot / ½ tsp / **Gebhardt**	<1
Hot dog / 2 oz / **Just Rite**	60
Hunter / mix, prepared / ¼ cup / **McCormick/Schilling**	104
Lemon butter / mix, w roasting bag / 1 pkg / **Durkee** Roastin' Bag	75
Marinara / mix, prepared / ½ cup / **McCormick/Schilling** Pasta Prima	329
Meat marinade / mix, prepared / ½ cup / **Durkee**	47
Mexican / 2.5 oz / **Hunt's** Manwich, Mexican	35
Nacho cheese / mix, prepared / ¼ pkg / **McCormick/Schilling**	42
Newburg w sherry / ⅓ cup / **Snow's**	120
Pasta / jar / ½ cup / **McCormick/Schilling** Sutter Home	100
Pasta salad / mix, prepared / ½ cup / **McCormick/Schilling** Pasta Prima	390
Pesto / mix, prepared / ½ cup / **McCormick/Schilling** Pasta Prima	193
Picante	
Hot chunky / 3 tbsp / **Rosarita**	18
Medium chunky / 3 tbsp / **Rosarita**	16
Mild chunky / 3 tbsp / **Rosarita**	25

CALORIES

Picante salsa, mild, med or hot / canned / 2 tbsp / **Old El Paso**	10
Picante sauce, mild, med or hot, chunky / canned / 2 tbsp / **Old El Paso**	7
Primavera / mix, prepared / ½ cup / **McCormick/Schilling** Pasta Prima	244
Primavera, creamy / jar / ½ cup / **Progresso**	190
Rock lobster / jar / ½ cup / **Progresso**	120
Salsa	
Hot / bottled / ¼ cup / **Hain**	22
Hot, chunky / 3 tbsp / **Rosarita**	25
Medium, chunky / 3 tbsp / **Rosarita**	25
Mild / bottled / ¼ cup / **Hain**	20
Mild, chunky / 3 tbsp / **Rosarita**	25
Mild, med or hot, thick and chunky / canned / 2 tbsp / **Old El Paso**	6
Taco, medium, chunky / 3 tbsp / **Rosarita**	25
Taco, mild, chunky / 3 tbsp / **Rosarita**	25
Salsa verde, thick and chunky / canned / 2 tbsp / **Old El Paso**	10
Sauce / 1 tbsp / **Durkee** Famous Sauce	70
Seafood / jar / ½ cup / **Progresso**	190
Seafood, creamy / mix, prepared / ½ cup / **McCormick/ Schilling** Pasta Prima	209
Seafood cocktail / canned / ¼ cup / **Del Monte**	70
Sicilian / jar / ½ cup / **Progresso**	30
Sloppy Joe	
Hunt's Manwich / 2.5 oz	40
Hunt's Manwich, Extra Thick / 2.5 oz	60
Mix, prepared / ¼ pkg / **McCormick/Schilling**	26
Sour cream / mix, prepared / ¼ pkg / **McCormick/Schilling**	44
Spaghetti	
Canned / 4 oz / **Hunt's** Chunky	50
Canned / 4 oz / **Hunt's** Homestyle	60
Canned / 4 oz / **Hunt's** Traditional	70
Jar / 4 oz / **Buitoni** Marinara	70
Jar / 4 oz / **Buitoni** Meatless	60
Jar / 4 oz / **Prego**	130
Jar / 4 oz / **Prego**, No Salt	110

CALORIES

Jar / ½ cup / **Progresso**	110
Mix, prepared / 2-½ cups / **Durkee**	224
Mix, prepared / ¼ pkg / **McCormick/Schilling**	32
Garden combination / jar / 4 oz / **Prego** Extra Chunky	80
Marinara / jar / 4 oz / **Prego**	100
Marinara / jar / ½ cup / **Progresso**	90
Meat-flavored	
Jar / 4 oz / **Buitoni**	85
Jar / 4 oz / **Prego**	140
Jar / ½ cup / **Progresso**	110
Jar / ⅓ cup / **Weight Watchers**	50
Mushroom-flavored / jar / ⅓ cup / **Weight Watchers**	40
Red clam / jar / 5 fl oz / **Buitoni**	190
w meat / canned / 4 oz / **Hunt's**	70
w meat / canned / 4 oz / **Hunt's** Homestyle	60
w mushrooms / mix, prepared / ½ cup / **French's**	100
w mushroom and extra spice / jar / 4 oz / **Prego** Extra Chunky	100
w mushroom and green pepper / jar / 4 oz / **Prego** Extra Chunky	100
w mushroom and onion / jar / 4 oz / **Prego** Extra Chunky	100
w mushroom and tomato / jar / 4 oz / **Prego** Extra Chunky	110
w mushrooms	
Canned / 4 oz / **Hunt's**	70
Canned / 4 oz / **Hunt's** Homestyle	50
Jar / 4 oz / **Buitoni**	60
Jar / 4 oz / **Prego**	130
Jar / ½ cup / **Progresso**	110
w onion and garlic / jar / 4 oz / **Prego**	110
w sausage and green pepper / jar / 4 oz / **Prego** Extra Chunky	160
w three cheese / jar / 4 oz / **Prego**	100
w tomato and basil / jar / 4 oz / **Prego**	100
w tomato and onion / jar / 4 oz / **Prego** Extra Chunky	110
White clam / jar / 5 fl oz / **Buitoni**	200
Sparerib / mix, w roasting bag / 1 pkg / **Durkee** Roastin' Bag	162

Stroganoff / mix, prepared / ⅓ pkg / **Durkee**	110
Swedish meatballs / mix, prepared / ¼ pkg / **McCormick/ Schilling**	57
Sweet and sour / 1 tbsp / **La Choy**	25
Sweet and sour / bottled / 1 tbsp / **Kraft** Sauceworks	25
Sweet and sour, duck / 1 tbsp / **La Choy**	25
Taco	
Canned / 2 tbsp / **Old El Paso**	15
Mix, prepared / ¼ pkg / **McCormick/Schilling**	31
Mild / 2 tbsp / **El Molino**	10
Mild and hot / canned / 1 tbsp / **Ortega**	8
Mild, med or hot / jar / 2 tbsp / **Old El Paso**	10
Teriyaki, ½ tsp	
La Choy	5
La Choy Basting	2
La Choy Lite	5
Tomato-basil / mix, prepared / ½ cup / **McCormick/Schilling** Pasta Prima	175
Tomato sauce, canned	
Contadina / ½ cup	30
Contadina, Italian Style / ½ cup	30
Del Monte / 1 cup	70
Del Monte, No Salt / 1 cup	70
Health Valley / 8 oz	70
Hunt's / 4 oz	30
Hunt's Herb / 4 oz	70
Hunt's Italian / 4 oz	60
Hunt's Special / 4 oz	35
w bits / 4 oz / **Hunt's**	30
w garlic / 4 oz / **Hunt's**	70
w garlic / 4 oz / **Hunt's**, No Salt Added	35
w mushrooms / 4 oz / **Hunt's**	25
w onions / 1 cup / **Del Monte**	100
w onions / 4 oz / **Hunt's**	40
Welsh rarebit / ½ cup / **Snow's**	170
White / mix, prepared w milk / 1 cup / **Durkee**	317
White / mix, prepared / ¼ cup / **McCormick/Schilling**	59

Seasonings

SEASONINGS

½ tsp unless noted

	CALORIES
Accent flavor enhancer / **Accent**	5
All purpose / **McCormick/Schilling** Parsley Patch	3
All purpose, sesame / **McCormick/Schilling** Parsley Patch	8
Bacon, imitation	
Bac'Os / 2 tsp	25
Durkee Bacon Bits / 1 tbsp	50
Durkee Bacon Chips / 1 tbsp	44
Libby's / 1 tbsp	25
McCormick/Schilling / 1 tbsp	26
Barbecue, powder / ¼ tsp / **McCormick/Schilling**	1
Beef flavor base / 1 tsp / **McCormick/Schilling**	5
Butter flavor, original / **McCormick/Schilling** Best O'Butter	4
Cheddar cheese flavor / **McCormick/Schilling** Best O'Butter	6
Chicken and fish seasoning, powder / 1 tsp **McCormick/Schilling** Grillmates	8
Chicken flavor base / 1 tsp / **McCormick/Schilling**	13
Chicken, fried, powder / ¼ tsp / **McCormick/Schilling**	1
Chili powder / 1 tsp / **Gebhardt**	15
Garlic / **McCormick/Schilling** Parsley Patch, Saltless	5
Garlic bread sprinkle, powder / ¼ tsp / **McCormick/Schilling**	5
Garlic, crushed, powder / 1 tsp / **McCormick/Schilling** Gilroy	8
Garlic flavor, powder / **McCormick/Schilling** Best O'Butter	4
Garlic, minced, powder / 1 tsp / **McCormick/Schilling** Gilroy	23

CALORIES

Garlic pepper, powder / 1 tsp / **McCormick/Schilling**	8
Garlic powder, powder / 1 tsp / **McCormick/Schilling**	12
Italian, powder / ¼ tsp / **McCormick/Schilling**	1
It's a dilly / **McCormick/Schilling** Parsley Patch	4
Lemon and herb, powder / ¼ tsp / **McCormick/Schilling**	1
Lemon and pepper, powder / ¼ tsp / **McCormick/Schilling**	2
Lemon pepper / **McCormick/Schilling** Parsley Patch	5
Meat marinade / ⅛ pkg / **French's**	10
Old bay seasoning / 1 tsp / **McCormick/Schilling** Old Bay	<1
Pepper, seasoned / 1 tsp / **French's**	8
Pepper, seasoned, powder / ¼ tsp / **McCormick/Schilling**	1
Pizza seasoning / 1 tsp / **French's**	8
Popcorn / **McCormick/Schilling** Parsley Patch	5
Salad supreme	
Powder / ¼ tsp / **McCormick/Schilling**	3
Garlic powder / 1 tsp / **McCormick/Schilling**	5
Seasoned powder / ¼ tsp / **McCormick/Schilling**	1
and spice, powder / ¼ tsp / **McCormick/Schilling**	1
Seafood, powder / ¼ tsp / **McCormick/Schilling** Ches. Bay	2
Season, All, powder / ¼ tsp / **McCormick/Schilling**	1
Season, All, powder / ¼ tsp / **McCormick/Schilling** Light	<1
Season, All, garlic, powder / ¼ tsp / **McCormick/Schilling**	2
Season, All, spice, powder / ¼ tsp / **McCormick/Schilling**	2
Soup greens / 2-½ oz jar / **Durkee**	216
Sour cream flavor / **McCormick/Schilling** Best O'Butter	4
Steak, broiled, powder / ¼ tsp / **McCormick/Schilling**	1
Steak seasoning, powder / 1 tsp / **McCormick/Schilling** Grillmates	7
Stir fry, powder / 1 tsp / **McCormick/Schilling** Gilroy	6

SEASONING MIXES

1 pkg unless noted

Beef stew
Mix, dry / **Durkee**	99

CALORIES

Mix, prepared / 1 cup / **Durkee**	379
French's / ⅙ pkg	25
Mix / **McCormick/Schilling** Bag'n Season	87

Chicken

Mix / **McCormick/Schilling** Bag'n Season	122
Mix, prepared / ¼ pouch / **Shake 'n Bake** Seasoning	80
Barbecue / mix, prepared / ¼ pouch / **Shake 'n Bake** Seasoning	90
Cacciatore / mix, dry / **McCormick/Schilling**	132
Country / mix / **McCormick/Schilling** Bag'n Season	134
Creamy curry / mix, dry / **McCormick/Schilling**	152
Creole / mix, dry / **McCormick/Schilling**	104
Dijon / mix, dry / **McCormick/Schilling**	151
Extra crispy / mix, prepared / **Shake 'n Bake** Oven Fry	110
Homestyle / mix, prepared / **Shake 'n Bake** Oven Fry	80
Italian / mix, dry / **McCormick/Schilling**	120
Mesquite / mix, dry / **McCormick/Schilling**	132
Parmesan / mix, dry / **McCormick/Schilling**	244
Southwest style / mix, dry / **McCormick/Schilling**	106
Stir fry / mix, dry / **McCormick/Schilling**	124
Sweet and sour / mix, dry / **McCormick/Schilling**	204
Teriyaki / mix, dry / **McCormick/Schilling**	172

Chili

Gebhardt / 1 tsp	10
Mix, dry / ¼ pkg / **McCormick/Schilling**	4
Texas / mix, dry / **Durkee**	151
Texas / mix, prepared / 1 cup / **Durkee**	772
con carne / mix, dry / **Durkee**	148
con carne / mix, prepared / 1 cup / **Durkee**	465
Chili-O / ⅙ pkg / **French's**	25
Chili-O w onions / ⅙ pkg / **French's**	35
Chop suey / mix, dry / **Durkee**	128
Chop suey / mix, prepared / ½ cup / **Durkee**	159
Country, mild / mix, prepared / ¼ pouch / **Shake 'n Bake** Seasoning	80
Crab cake, classic / pkg unprepared / **McCormick/Schilling** Old Bay	133
Fajitas / mix, dry / ¼ pkg / **McCormick/Schilling**	28

CALORIES

Fish / mix, prepared / ¼ pouch / **Shake 'n Bake** Seasoning	70
Fried rice / mix, dry / 1 oz / **Durkee**	62
Fried rice / mix, prepared / 1 cup / **Durkee**	215
Ground beef / mix, dry / **Durkee**	91
Ground beef / mix, prepared / 1 cup / **Durkee**	519
Ground beef w onions / mix, dry / **Durkee**	102
Ground beef w onions / mix, prepared / 1 cup / **Durkee**	659
Hamburger	
Mix, dry / **Durkee**	110
Mix, prepared / 1 cup / **Durkee**	663
Mix, dry / .25 oz / **Hunt's** Manwich	20
Italian herb / mix, prepared / ¼ pouch / **Shake 'n Bake** Seasoning	80
Italian herb, fish / mix / **McCormick/Schilling** Bag'n Season	94
Lemon butter for fish / mix w roasting bag / **Durkee** Roastin' Bag	75
Lemon and dill, fish / mix / **McCormick/Schilling** Bag'n Season	161
Meatball / mix, prepared / 1 cup / **Durkee**	619
Meatloaf / mix, dry / ⅛ pkg / **French's**	20
Meatloaf / mix / **McCormick/Schilling** Bag'n Season	11
Menudo / 1 tsp / **Gebhardt**	5
Nacho cheese / mix, dry / ¼ pkg / **McCormick/Schilling**	42
Oriental style / mix / **McCormick/Schilling** Bag'n Season	152
Pork / mix, prepared / ⅛ pouch / **Shake 'n Bake** Seasoning	40
Pork barbecue / mix, prepared / ⅛ pouch / **Shake 'n Bake** Seasoning	40
Pork chops / mix / **McCormick/Schilling** Bag'n Season	102
Pork, extra crispy / mix, prepared / **Shake 'n Bake** Oven Fry	120
Pot roast / mix **McCormick/Schilling** Bag'n Season	55
Roast turkey / mix / **McCormick/Schilling** Bag'n Season	146
Salmon, classic / pkg unprepared / **McCormick/Schilling** Old Bay	159
Sloppy Joe	
Mix, dry / **Durkee**	118
Mix, prepared / ½ cup / **Durkee**	291

CALORIES

Mix, dry / ⅛ pkg / **French's**	16
Italian mix, dry / **Durkee**	99
Italian mix, prepared / ½ cup / **Durkee**	298
Spaghetti / mix, dry / ¼ pkg / **McCormick/Schilling**	6
Spaghetti / mix, dry / ¼ pkg / **McCormick/Schilling** Thick and Zesty	34
Spare ribs / mix / **McCormick/Schilling** Bag'n Season	185
Swiss steak / mix / **McCormick/Schilling** Bag'n Season	81
Taco	
Mix, dry / **Durkee**	67
Mix, prepared / 1 cup / **Durkee**	619
Mix, dry / ⅙ pkg / **French's**	20
Mix, dry / ¼ pkg / **McCormick/Schilling**	26
Mix / for 1 shell / **Ortega**	90
Tortilla mix, corn / ⅓ cup uncooked / **Albers** Ricamasa	140
Tuna, classic / pkg unprepared / **McCormick/Schilling** Old Bay	117

Shortening

CALORIES

Solid	
Lard	
1 cup	1850
1 tbsp	115
Shortening, vegetable: 1 tbsp	
Crisco	110
Crisco, Butter Flavor	110
Nu Made	110
Wesson	110

Soft Drinks

	CALORIES
6 fl oz unless noted	
Birch beer	
Canada Dry	80
Shasta Diet	0
Bitter lemon	
Canada Dry	80
Schweppes	80
Black cherry	
Canada Dry	100
Cragmont	91
Cragmont Diet	0
Shasta	80
Shasta Diet	0
Cactus cooler / **Canada Dry**	80
Cherry	
Canada Dry	80
Canada Dry PM	80
Coca-Cola	76
Coca-Cola Diet	1
Crush	100
Sundrop	90
Cherry Cola	
Cragmont	79
Cragmont Diet	0
Shasta	74
Shasta Diet	0
Cherry-lemon-lime / **Cragmont**	82
Cherry-lemon-lime / **Cragmont** Diet	0
Cherry-lime / **Shasta** Spree	88
Chocolate / **Shasta** Diet	0
Citrus mist / **Shasta**	96
Club soda	

CALORIES

Cragmont	0
Canada Dry	0
Schweppes	0
Schweppes Sodium Free	0
Shasta	0

Cola

Canada Dry Diet	2
Canada Dry Jamaica	80
Canada Dry PM	80
Coca-Cola	77
Coca-Cola Classic	72
Coca-Cola Classic, Caffeine Free	72
Coca-Cola, Caffeine Free	77
Coke, Diet	1
Coke, Diet, Caffeine Free	1
Cragmont	82
Cragmont Diet	0
Pepsi, Caffeine Free / 8 fl oz	105
Pepsi, Diet / 8 fl oz	1
Pepsi, Diet, Caffeine Free / 8 fl oz	1
Pepsi-Cola / 8 fl oz	104.8
Shasta	80
Shasta, Caffeine Free	80
Shasta, Caffeine Free, Diet	0
Shasta, Diet	0
Shasta, Low Sodium / 8 fl oz	108
Shasta, Low Sodium, Diet	0
Shasta Spree / 12 fl oz	88
Tab	<1
Tab, Caffeine Free	<1
Country Time lemonade	72

Cream

A&W	84
A&W, Diet	1
Cragmont	84
Cragmont Diet	0
Hires	90
Hires, Diet	2
Shasta	82
Shasta, Diet	0
Dr. Diablo / **Shasta**	78

	CALORIES
Fresca	2
Ginger ale	
Canada Dry	70
Canada Dry, Cherry	80
Canada Dry, Cherry, Diet	2
Canada Dry, Diet	2
Canada Dry, Golden	70
Canada Dry, Lemon	70
Canada Dry, Lemon, Diet	4
Cragmont	63
Cragmont, Diet	0
Fanta	63
Health Valley	76
Schweppes	70
Schweppes, Diet	2
Schweppes, Diet, Raspberry	2
Schweppes, Raspberry	80
Shasta	66
Shasta, Diet	0
Shasta, Low Sodium / 8 fl oz	89
Shasta, Low Sodium, Diet	0
Shasta Spree	66
Ginger beer / **Schweppes**	70
Grape	
Canada Dry	100
Canada Dry PM	80
Cragmont	96
Cragmont, Sparkling	96
Crush	100
Fanta	86
Schweppes	100
Shasta	88
Shasta, Diet	0
Grapefruit	
Cragmont	84
Cragmont, Diet	0
Schweppes	80
Shasta, Diet	<2
Shasta Spree	88
Half & Half / **Canada Dry**	80
Hi Spot / **Canada Dry**	80

	CALORIES
Hi Spot / **Canada Dry** PM	90
Island lime / **Canada Dry**	100
Kiwi-strawberry / **Shasta**	88
Lemon lime	
Cragmont	74
Cragmont, Diet	0
Schweppes	70
Shasta / 12 fl oz	148
Shasta, Diet	0
Shasta, Low Sodium / 8 fl oz	100
Shasta, Low Sodium, Diet	0
Shasta Spree	86
Lemon, sour / **Schweppes**	80
Lemon-tangerine / **Shasta** Spree	94
Lemonade / **Canada Dry** Tahitian Treat PM	90
Lemonade / **Cragmont**	70
Mandarin-lime / **Shasta** Spree	88
Mello Yello	87
Mello Yello, diet	3
Mountain Dew / 8 fl oz	118
Mountain Dew, diet / 8 fl oz	2
Mr. Pibb	71
Orange	
Canada Dry	90
Canada Dry, Diet	0
Canada Dry PM	90
Cragmont	89
Cragmont, Diet	0
Crush	100
Crush, Diet	12
Fanta	88
Minute Maid	87
Minute Maid, Diet	3
Shasta	92
Shasta, Diet	0
Peach / **Canada Dry**	90
Peach / **Shasta**	176
Pineapple	
Canada Dry	80
Crush	100
Shasta	106

	CALORIES
Pineapple-orange / **Shasta**	94
Pineapple-orange / **Shasta** Diet	0
Raspberry creme / **Shasta**	90
Red cream / **Cragmont**	84
Red Pop / **Shasta** / 12 fl oz	80
Red Pop / **Shasta**, Diet / 12 fl oz	0
Root beer	
A&W	84
A&W, Diet	1
Canada Dry Barrelhead	80
Canada Dry Barrelhead, Diet	2
Canada Dry Barrelhead PM	80
Cragmont	84
Cragmont, Diet	0
Fanta	78
Health Valley Old-Fashioned	60
Health Valley Sarsaparilla	73
Hires	90
Hires, Diet	2
Ramblin'	88
Ramblin', Diet	1
Shasta	80
Shasta, Diet	0
Shasta Spree	86
Seltzer / **Manischewitz** / 8 fl oz	0
Seltzer water, all flavors	
Canada Dry	0
Schweppes	0
Skipper / **Cragmont**, Diet	0
Slice / 8 fl oz	102
Slice, diet / 8 fl oz	18
Slice, orange / 8 fl oz	129
Slice, orange, diet / 8 fl oz	13
Sparkling water, all flavors	
Canada Dry	0
Schweppes	0
Shasta	0
Sparkling water, plain / **Shasta**	0
Sprite	71
Sprite, diet	2
Squirt	78

CALORIES

Squirt, diet	1
Strawberry	
Canada Dry, California	80
Canada Dry, California PM	90
Cragmont	88
Crush	90
Shasta	76
Shasta, Diet	0
Strawberry-peach / **Shasta**	86
Strawberry-peach / **Shasta**, Diet	0
Sundrop	100
Sundrop, diet	2
Sweet and sour / **Canada Dry**	110
Tahitian treat / **Canada Dry**	100
Tahitian treat / **Canada Dry** PM, Non Carb	90
Tonic	
Canada Dry	60
Canada Dry, Diet	0
Canada Dry, Diet w Twist	4
Canada Dry PM	70
Canada Dry w Twist	70
Cragmont	70
Cragmont, Diet	0
Schweppes	70
Schweppes, Diet	0
Shasta	64
Tropical blend / **Shasta** Spree	80
Vanilla cream / **Canada Dry**	80
Vanilla cream / **Crush**	90
Vernors	72
Vernors, diet / 1 fl oz	1
Vichy water / **Canada Dry**	0
Vichy water / **Schweppes**	0
Wild berry / **Health Valley**	71
Wink / **Canada Dry**	90
Wink / **Canada Dry** PM	90
Wink II / **Canada Dry**	90
Wink II / **Canada Dry**, Diet	2

Soups

CALORIES

Prepared according to label directions unless noted

	CALORIES
Asparagus, cream of / canned / 8 fl oz / **Campbell's**	80
Asparagus, cream of / frozen / 6 fl oz / **Kettle Ready**	62
Bean, canned	
Campbell's Homestyle / 8 fl oz	130
and ham / 10-¾ fl oz / **Campbell's** Home Cookin'	210
and ham / 9-½ fl oz / **Campbell's** Home Cookin'	180
and ham / 7.50 oz / **Healthy Choice**	220
Black / 7-½ oz / **Health Valley** No Salt	150
Black w vegetable / 7-½ oz / **Health Valley**	70
w bacon / 8 fl oz / **Campbell's**	140
w bacon / 8 fl oz / **Campbell's** Healthy Request	140
w bacon 'n ham / 7-½ fl oz / **Campbell's** Microwave	230
w ham / 11 fl oz / **Campbell's** Old Fashioned Chunky	290
w ham / 9-⅝ fl oz / **Campbell's** Old Fashioned Chunky	250
Bean, frozen / black w ham / 6 fl oz / **Kettle Ready**	154
Bean, frozen / w ham / 6 fl oz / **Kettle Ready**	113
Beef, canned	
Campbell's / 8 fl oz	80
Campbell's Chunky / 10-¾ fl oz	200
Campbell's Chunky / 9-½ fl oz	170
Progresso / 9-½ fl oz	160
Progresso / 10-½ fl oz	180
Progresso Hearty / 9-½ fl oz	160
Barley / 9-½ fl oz / **Progresso**	140
Barley / 10-½ fl oz / **Progresso**	150
Cabbage / 1 cup / **Manischewitz**	62
Flavor noodle / 1.35 fl oz / **Campbell's** Micro Cup	130
Hearty / 7.50 oz / **Healthy Choice**	120

Minestrone / 9-½ fl oz / **Progresso**	170
Minestrone / 10-½ fl oz / **Progresso**	180
Noodle / 8 fl oz / **Campbell's**	70
Noodle / 8 fl oz / **Campbell's** Homestyle	80
Noodle / 9-½ fl oz / **Progresso**	170
Noodle and ground beef / 8 fl oz / **Campbell's**	90
Stroganoff / 10-¾ fl oz / **Campbell's** Chunky	320
Vegetable / 7.50 oz / **Healthy Choice** Chunky	110
Vegetable / 7.50 oz / **Healthy Choice** Chunky Micro Cup	110
Vegetable / 9-½ fl oz / **Progresso**	150
Vegetable / 10-½ fl oz / **Progresso**	170
w vegetables and pasta / 10-¾ fl oz / **Campbell's** Home Cookin'	140
w vegetables and pasta / 9-½ fl oz / **Campbell's** Home Cookin'	120
Beef flavor, mix	
and noodles / 7 fl oz / **Lipton** Cup-A-Soup	107
Mushroom / 8 fl oz / **Lipton**	38
Oriental noodle / 8 fl oz / **Lipton** Instant	176
Beef, frozen / w vegetable / 6 fl oz / **Kettle Ready**	86
Beefy mushroom, canned / 8 fl oz / **Campbell's**	60
Beefy onion, mix / 8 fl oz / **Lipton**	27
Borscht, canned or jars / 8 fl oz / **Manischewitz** Low Calorie	20
Borscht w beets, canned or jars / 8 fl oz / **Manischewitz**	80
Bouillon	
Beef, cube / 1 cube / **Wyler's**	6
Beef, instant / 1 tsp / **Lite-Line** Low Sodium	12
Beef, instant / 1 tsp / **Wyler's**	6
Chicken, cube / 1 cube / **Wyler's**	8
Chicken, instant / 1 tsp / **Lite-Line** Low Sodium	12
Chicken, instant / 1 tsp / **Wyler's**	8
Onion, instant / 1 tsp / **Wyler's**	10
Vegetable, instant / 1 tsp / **Wyler's**	6
Broccoli and cheese, mix / 6 fl oz / **Lipton** Cup-A-Soup	70
Broccoli, cream of, canned / 8 fl oz / **Campbell's**	80
Broccoli, creamy, mix / 6 fl oz / **Lipton** Cup-A-Soup	62
Broccoli, golden, mix / 6 fl oz / **Lipton** Cup-A-Soup Lite	42
Broccoli, cream of, frozen / 6 fl oz / **Kettle Ready**	94

CALORIES

Broth
Beef, canned
    Campbell's / 8 fl oz   16
    College Inn / 7 oz   16
    Health Valley No Salt / 6.9 oz   10
    Swanson / 7-¼ oz   18
Beef, mix / 1 packet / **Weight Watchers**   8
Chicken, canned
    Campbell's / 8 fl oz   30
    Campbell's Low Sodium / 10-½ fl oz   30
    College Inn / 7 fl oz   35
    College Inn Lower Salt / 7 fl oz   20
    Hain / 9 fl oz   30
    Hain No Salt / 9 fl oz   45
    Health Valley / 6.9 oz   20
    Health Valley No Salt / 6.9 oz   35
    Swanson / 7-½ oz   30
    Swanson Clear Natural Goodness / 7-¼ oz   20
Chicken, mix / 1 packet / **Weight Watchers**   8
Chicken and noodles, canned / 8 fl oz / **Campbell's**   45
Vegetable, canned / 9-½ fl oz / **Hain**   45
Vegetable, canned / 9-½ fl oz / **Hain** Low Salt   40
Cauliflower, cream of, frozen / 6 fl oz / **Kettle Ready**   93
Celery, cream of, canned / 8 fl oz / **Campbell's**   100
Cheddar-broccoli, frozen / 6 fl oz / **Kettle Ready**   136.7
Cheddar cheese, canned / 8 fl oz / **Campbell's**   110
Cheddar, creamy, frozen / 6 fl oz / **Kettle Ready**   158
Cheese, mix / ¾ cup / **Hain**   250
Cheese and broccoli, mix / ¾ cup / **Hain**   310
Chickarina, canned / 9-½ fl oz / **Progresso**   130
Chicken, canned
    Campbell's Old Fashioned Chunky / 10-¾ fl oz   180
    Campbell's Old Fashioned Chunky / 9-½ fl oz   150
    Progresso Homestyle / 9-½ fl oz   110
    Alphabet / 8 fl oz / **Campbell's**   80
    and stars / 8 fl oz / **Campbell's**   80
    Barley
        Campbell's / 8 fl oz   70
        Manischewitz / 1 cup   83
        Progresso / 9-¼ oz   100
Corn chowder / 10¾- fl oz / **Campbell's** Chunky   340
Corn chowder / 9-½ oz / **Campbell's** Chunky   300

CALORIES

Cream of / 8 fl oz / **Campbell's**	110
Cream of / 9-½ fl oz / **Progresso**	190
Gumbo / 8 fl oz / **Campbell's**	60
Gumbo w sausage / 10-¾ fl oz / **Campbell's** Home Cookin'	140
Gumbo w sausage / 9-½ fl oz / **Campbell's** Home Cookin'	120
Hearty	
Healthy Choice / 7.50 oz	150
Progresso / 9-½ fl oz	130
Progresso / 10-½ fl oz	130
Minestrone	
Campbell's Home Cookin' / 10-¾ fl oz	180
Campbell's Home Cookin' / 9-½ fl oz	160
Progresso / 9-½ fl oz	130
Progresso / 10-½ fl oz	140
Mushroom	
Campbell's Creamy / 8 fl oz	120
Campbell's Creamy Chunky / 10-½ fl oz	270
Campbell's Creamy Chunky / 9-⅜ fl oz	240
'n dumplings / 8 fl oz / **Campbell's**	80
Noodle	
Campbell's / 8 fl oz	60
Campbell's Chunky / 10-¾ fl oz	200
Campbell's Chunky / 9-½ fl oz	180
Campbell's Healthy Request / 8 fl oz	60
Campbell's Hearty Healthy Request / 8 fl oz	80
Campbell's Home Cookin' / 10-¾ fl oz	140
Campbell's Home Cookin' / 9-½ fl oz	110
Campbell's Homestyle / 8 fl oz	70
Campbell's Low Sodium / 10-¾ fl oz	170
Campbell's Microwave / 7-½ fl oz	100
Hain / 9-½ fl oz	120
Hain No Salt / 9-½ fl oz	120
Progresso / 9-½ fl oz	120
Progresso / 10-½ fl oz	120
Weight Watchers / 10.5 oz	80
Noodle, old fashioned / 7.5 oz / **Healthy Choice**	90
Noodle vegetable / 7.5 oz / **Healthy Choice**	160
Noodle vegetable / 7.5 oz / **Healthy Choice** Micro Cups	160

CALORIES

Noodle-O's / 8 fl oz / **Campbell's**	70
Nuggets w vegetables and noodles / 9-½ fl oz / **Campbell's** Chunky	170
Nuggets w vegetables and noodles / 10-¾ fl oz / **Campbell's** Chunky	190
Rice	
Campbell's Home Cookin' / 10-¾ fl oz	150
Campbell's Home Cookin' / 9-½ fl oz	130
Progresso / 9-½ fl oz	130
Progresso / 10-½ fl oz	120
w rice	
Campbell's / 8 fl oz	60
Campbell's Chunky / 9-½ fl oz	140
Campbell's Healthy Request / 8 fl oz	60
Campbell's Microwave / 7-½ fl oz	100
Healthy Choice / 7.50 oz	140
Vegetable	
Campbell's / 8 fl oz	70
Campbell's Chunky / 9-½ fl oz	170
Manischewitz / 1 cup	55
Progresso / 9-½ fl oz	140
Progresso / 10-½ fl oz	150
Chicken, mix	
Cream of / 6 fl oz / **Lipton** Cup-A-Soup	84
Creamy / 7 fl oz / **Lipton** Cup-A-Soup Lots-a-Noodles	179
Creamy w white meat / 6 fl oz / **Campbell's**	90
Florentine / 6 fl oz / **Lipton** Cup-A-Soup Lite	42
Hearty / 6 fl oz / **Lipton** Cup-A-Soup Supreme	106
Hearty country / 6 fl oz / **Lipton** Cup-A-Soup	69
Lemon / 6 fl oz / **Lipton** Cup-A-Soup Lite	48
Noodle	
Campbell's / 8 fl oz	100
Lipton Cup-A-Soup / 6 fl oz	48
Lipton Cup-A-Soup Hearty / 6 fl oz	69
Lipton Hearty / 8 fl oz	81
Noodle w meat / 6 fl oz / **Lipton** Cup-A-Soup	46
Noodle w white meat / 6 fl oz / **Campbell's**	90
w noodles / 6 fl oz / **Campbell's**	90
Rice / 6 fl oz / **Lipton** Cup-A-Soup	45
Vegetables / 6 fl oz / **Lipton** Cup-A-Soup	47

CALORIES

Chicken flavor, mix / 6 fl oz / **Lipton** Cup-A-Soup	110.2
Chicken flavor, mix / 6 fl oz / **Lipton** Cup-A-Soup Supreme Country Style	106.9
Chicken flavor, broth, mix / 6 fl oz / **Lipton** Cup-A-Soup	20
Chicken flavor, creamy vegetable, mix / 6 fl oz / **Lipton** Cup-A-Soup	93
Chicken flavor, noodle, microwavable cup / 1.35 fl oz / **Campbell's**	140
Chicken flavor, Oriental noodle, mix / 8 fl oz / **Lipton** Instant	180
Chicken, cream of, frozen / 6 fl oz / **Kettle Ready**	98
Chicken gumbo, frozen / 6 fl oz / **Kettle Ready**	94
Chicken noodle, frozen / 6 fl oz / **Kettle Ready**	94
Chili beef, canned	
Campbell's / 8 fl oz	140
Campbell's Chunky / 11 fl oz	290
Campbell's Chunky / 9-¾ fl oz	260
Campbell's Microwave / 7-½ fl oz	190
Chili, frozen / 6 fl oz / **Kettle Ready**	160
Chili, jalapeno, frozen / 6 fl oz / **Kettle Ready**	173
Clam chowder, canned,	
Manhattan style	
Campbell's Chunky / 10-¾ fl oz	160
Campbell's / 8 fl oz	70
Campbell's Chunky / 9-½ fl oz	150
Health Valley No Salt / 7-½ oz	100
Progresso / 9-½ fl oz	120
Snow's Condensed / 3-¾ oz	70
New England	
Campbell's / 8 fl oz	80
Campbell's Chunky / 10-¾ fl oz	290
Campbell's Chunky / 9-½ fl oz	260
Hain / 9-½ fl oz	150
Progresso / 9-¼ fl oz	190
Progresso / 10-½ fl oz	220
Snow's / 7-½ oz	140
Clam chowder, frozen	
Boston / 6 fl oz / **Kettle Ready**	130
Manhattan style / 6 fl oz / **Kettle Ready**	69
New England / 6 fl oz / **Kettle Ready**	116

CALORIES

Consomme, canned / 8 fl oz / **Campbell's**	25
Corn chowder, canned / 9-¼ fl oz / **Progresso**	200
Corn and broccoli chowder, frozen / 6 fl oz / **Kettle Ready**	102
Corn and vegetable, canned / 7-½ oz / **Health Valley**	70
Corn chowder, canned / 7-½ oz / **Snow's**	150
Creole, canned / 10-¾ fl oz / **Campbell's** Chunky	240
Creole, canned / 9-½ fl oz / **Campbell's** Chunky	220
Curly noodle w chicken, canned / 8 fl oz / **Campbell's**	80
Escarole in chicken broth, canned / 9-¼ fl oz / **Progresso**	30
Fish chowder, canned / 7-½ oz / **Snow's**	130
French onion, canned / 8 fl oz / **Campbell's**	60
Green pea, canned / 8 fl oz / **Campbell's**	160
Ham and bean, canned / 9-½ fl oz / **Progresso**	140
Ham 'n butter beans, canned / 10-¾ fl oz / **Campbell's** Chunky	280
Lentil, canned	
Campbell's Hearty Home Cookin' / 10-¾ fl oz	170
Campbell's Hearty Home Cookin' / 9-½ fl oz	140
Health Valley No Salt / 7-½ oz	170
Progresso / 9-½ fl oz	140
Progresso / 10-½ fl oz	140
Lentil, mix / ¾ cup / **Hain**	130
Lentil minestrone, mix / 1.87 oz dry / **Fearn**	160
Lentil vegetarian, canned / 9-½ fl oz / **Hain**	160
Lentil vegetarian, canned / 9-½ fl oz / **Hain** No Salt	160
w sausage, canned / 9-½ fl oz / **Progresso**	170
Lentil and carrots, canned / 7-½ oz / **Health Valley**	70
Macaroni and bean, canned / 9-½ fl oz / **Progresso**	140
Macaroni and bean, canned / 10-½ fl oz / **Progresso**	150
Minestrone, canned	
Campbell's / 8 fl oz	80
Campbell's Chunky / 9-½ fl oz	160
Campbell's Hearty Healthy Request / 8 fl oz	90
Campbell's Home Cookin' / 10-¾ fl oz	140
Campbell's Home Cookin' / 9-½ fl oz	120
Hain / 9-½ fl oz	160
Hain No Salt / 9-½ fl oz	160
Health Valley / 7-½ oz	80
Health Valley No Salt / 7-½ oz	130
Healthy Choice / 7.50 oz	160

CALORIES

Progresso / 9-½ fl oz	130
Progresso / 10-½ fl oz	120
Progresso Hearty / 9-¼ fl oz	110
Progresso Zesty / 9-½ fl oz	150
Minestrone, mix / ¾ cup / **Hain**	110
Minestrone, mix / 6 fl oz / **Manischewitz**	50
Minestrone, frozen / 6 fl oz / **Kettle Ready** Hearty	104
Mushroom, mix / ¾ cup / **Hain**	210
Mushroom, mix / ¾ cup / **Hain** No Salt	250
Mushroom, canned	
Barley	
Hain / 9-½ fl oz	80
Health Valley No Salt / 7-½ oz	100
Manischewitz / 1 cup	72
Cream of	
Campbell's / 8 fl oz	100
Campbell's Healthy Request / 8 fl oz	60
Campbell's Low Sodium / 10-½ fl oz	210
Progresso / 9-¼ fl oz	160
Weight Watchers / 10.5 oz	90
Creamy / 9-½ fl oz / **Hain**	120
Golden / 8 fl oz / **Campbell's**	70
Mushroom, cream of, frozen / 6 fl oz / **Kettle Ready**	85
Mushroom, cream of, mix / 6 fl oz / **Lipton** Cup-A-Soup	71
Nacho cheese, canned / 8 fl oz / **Campbell's**	110
Noodle, mix	
Campbell's / 8 fl oz	110
Campbell's Hearty / 8 fl oz	90
Lipton / 8 fl oz	82
Lipton Cup-A-Soup Ring / 6 fl oz	56
Lipton Giggle / 8 fl oz	72
Lipton Ring-O-Noodle / 8 fl oz	66
Noodle	
Oriental, mix / 8 fl oz / **Lipton** Instant	198
w chicken broth, canned / 1.35 fl oz / **Campbell's** Micro Cups	130
w vegetables, canned / 1.70 fl oz / **Campbell's** Micro Cups	180
w vegetables, mix / 8 fl oz / **Lipton** Hearty	75
w real chicken broth, mix / 8 fl oz / **Lipton**	62

CALORIES

Onion, mix	
Campbell's / 8 fl oz	30
Hain / ¾ cup	50
Hain No Salt / ¾ cup	50
Lipton / 8 fl oz	20
Lipton Cup-A-Soup / 6 fl oz	27
Onion	
Cream of, canned / 8 fl oz / **Campbell's**	100
Golden, w real chicken broth, mix / 8 fl oz / **Lipton**	62
Mushroom, mix / 8 fl oz / **Lipton**	41
Onion, French, frozen / 6 fl oz / **Kettle Ready**	42
Oriental, mix / 6 fl oz / **Lipton** Cup-A-Soup Lite	45
Oyster stew, canned / 8 fl oz / **Campbell's**	70
Pea, green, mix / 6 fl oz / **Lipton** Cup-A-Soup	113
Split	
Canned / 10-¾ fl oz / **Campbell's** Low Sodium	230
Canned / 7-½ oz / **Health Valley** No Salt	90
Canned / 9-½ fl oz / **Progresso**	160
Canned / 10-½ fl oz / **Progresso**	201
Mix / ¾ cup / **Hain**	310
Split w carrots, canned / 7-½ oz / **Health Valley**	50
Split w ham, canned	
Campbell's Chunky / 9-½ fl oz	210
Campbell's Chunky / 10-¾ fl oz	230
Campbell's Home Cookin' / 10-¾ fl oz	230
Campbell's Home Cookin' / 9-½ fl oz	200
Healthy Choice / 7.50 oz	170
Progresso / 9-½ fl oz	150
Progresso / 10-½ fl oz	160
Split w ham and bacon, canned / 8 fl oz / **Campbell's**	160
Split w ham, frozen / 6 fl oz / **Kettle Ready**	155
Pepper pot, canned / 8 fl oz / **Campbell's**	90
Pepper steak, canned / 10-¾ fl oz / **Campbell's** Chunky	180
Pepper steak, canned / 9-½ fl oz / **Campbell's** Chunky	160
Potato, cream of, canned / 8 fl oz / **Campbell's**	80
Potato leek, mix / ¾ cup / **Hain**	260
Potato leek, canned / 7-½ oz / **Health Valley** No Salt	130
Potato, cream of, frozen / 6 fl oz / **Kettle Ready**	120
Schav, canned / 1 cup / **Manischewitz**	11
Scotch broth, canned / 8 fl oz / **Campbell's**	80
Seafood chowder, canned / 7-½ oz / **Snow's**	130
Shrimp, cream of, canned / 8 fl oz / **Campbell's**	90

CALORIES

Sirloin burger, canned / 10-¾ fl oz / **Campbell's** Chunky	220
Sirloin burger, canned / 9-½ fl oz / **Campbell's** Chunky	200
Steak and potato, canned / 10-¾ fl oz / **Campbell's** Chunky	200
Steak and potato, canned / 9-½ fl oz / **Campbell's** Chunky	170
Teddy bear, canned / 8 fl oz / **Campbell's**	70
Tomato, canned	
Campbell's / 8 fl oz	90
Campbell's Healthy Request / 8 fl oz	90
Campbell's Zesty / 8 fl oz	100
Health Valley No Salt / 7-½ oz	130
Manischewitz / 1 cup	60
Progresso / 9-½ fl oz	120
Progresso / 10-½ fl oz	130
Tomato, mix / ¾ cup / **Hain**	220
Tomato, mix / 6 fl oz / **Lipton** Cup-A-Soup	103
Tomato	
and herb, mix / 6 fl oz / **Lipton** Cup-A-Soup Creamy Lite	66
Beef w rotini, canned / 9-½ fl oz / **Progresso**	170
Garden, canned	
Campbell's Home Cookin' / 10-¾ fl oz	150
Campbell's Home Cookin' / 9-½ fl oz	130
Healthy Choice / 7.50 oz	130
Rice, canned / 8 fl oz / **Campbell's** Old Fashioned	110
Tortellini, canned / 9-¼ fl oz / **Progresso**	130
Vegetable, canned / 7-½ oz / **Health Valley**	50
w tomato pieces, canned / 10-½ fl oz / **Campbell's** Low Sodium	190
Tomato bisque, canned / 8 fl oz / **Campbell's**	120
Tomato Florentine, frozen / 6 fl oz / **Kettle Ready**	106
Tortellini, canned / 9-½ fl oz / **Progresso**	90
Tortellini, creamy, canned / 9-¼ fl oz / **Progresso**	240
Tortellini in tomato, frozen / 6 fl oz / **Kettle Ready**	122
Turkey noodle, canned / 8 fl oz / **Campbell's**	70
Turkey vegetable, canned	
Campbell's / 8 fl oz	70
Campbell's Chunky / 9-⅜ fl oz	150
Weight Watchers / 10.5 oz	70
Turkey rice, canned / 9-½ fl oz / **Hain**	100

	CALORIES
Turkey rice, canned / 9-½ fl oz / **Hain** No Salt	120
Vegetable, canned	
Campbell's / 8 fl oz	90
Campbell's Chunky / 10-¾ fl oz	160
Campbell's Chunky / 9-½ fl oz	150
Campbell's Country Home Cookin' / 10-¾ fl oz	120
Campbell's Country Home Cookin' / 9-½ fl oz	100
Campbell's Healthy Request / 8 fl oz	90
Campbell's Hearty Healthy Request / 8 fl oz	110
Campbell's Homestyle / 8 fl oz	60
Campbell's Old Fashioned / 8 fl oz	60
Health Valley No Salt / 7-½ oz	110
Manischewitz / 1 cup	63
Progresso / 9-½ fl oz	90
Progresso 10-½ fl oz	80
Vegetable, mix	
Hain / ¾ cup	80
Hain No Salt / ¾ cup	80
Lipton / 8 fl oz	39
Manischewitz / 6 fl oz	50
Vegetable	
Barley, canned / 7-½ oz / **Health Valley**	60
Beef, canned	
Campbell's / 8 fl oz	70
Campbell's Chunky Low Sodium / 10-¾ fl oz	180
Campbell's Healthy Request / 8 fl oz	70
Campbell's Hearty Healthy Request / 8 fl oz	120
Campbell's Home Cookin' / 10-¾ fl oz	140
Campbell's Home Cookin' / 9-½ fl oz	120
Campbell's Microwave / 7-½ fl oz	100
Campbell's Old Fashioned Chunky / 10-¾ fl oz	190
Campbell's Old Fashioned Chunky / 9-½ fl oz	160
Healthy Choice / 7.50 oz	130
Chicken, canned	
Hain / 9-½ fl oz	120
Hain No Salt / 9-½ fl oz	130
Health Valley No Salt / 7-½ oz	125
Country, canned / 7.50 oz / **Healthy Choice**	120
Country, mix / 8 fl oz / **Lipton**	80
Country harvest, mix / 6 fl oz / **Lipton** Cup-A-Soup	95

CALORIES

Country style, mix / 6 fl oz / **Lipton** Cup-A-Soup Harvest	91
Five bean, canned / 7-½ oz / **Health Valley** No Salt	110
Garden, Oriental noodle, mix / 8 fl oz / **Lipton** Instant	200
Garden, canned / 7-½ oz / **Health Valley**	50
Italian, canned / 9-½ fl oz / **Hain**	160
Italian, canned / 9-½ fl oz / **Hain** Low Sodium	150
Lots-a-noodles, mix / 7 fl oz / **Lipton** Cup-A-Soup	123
Mediterranean, canned / 9-½ fl oz / **Campbell's** Chunky	170
Split pea, canned / 9-½ fl oz / **Hain**	170
Split pea, canned / 9-½ fl oz / **Hain** No Salt	170
Spring, mix / 6 fl oz / **Lipton** Cup-A-Soup	33
Vegetarian, canned	
Campbell's / 8 fl oz	80
Hain / 9-½ fl oz	150
Hain No Salt / 9-½ fl oz	150
Vegetarian, chunky, canned / 10.5 oz / **Weight Watchers**	100
w beef stock, canned / 10.5 oz / **Weight Watchers**	90
w five bean, canned / 7-½ oz / **Health Valley**	100
Vegetable, garden, frozen / 6 fl oz / **Kettle Ready**	85
Won ton, canned / 8 fl oz / **Campbell's**	40

Spaghetti and Spaghetti Dishes

CALORIES

Spaghetti in tomato sauce, canned	
Chef Boyardee ABC's and 123's / 7.5 oz	160
Chef Boyardee ABC's and 123's / 7 oz	160
Chef Boyardee Dinosaurs / 7.5 oz	160
Chef Boyardee Dinosaurs / 8.6 oz	200
Chef Boyardee Dinosaurs / 7 oz	160

CALORIES

Chef Boyardee Pac Man / 7.5 oz	150
Chef Boyardee Sharks / 7.5 oz	170
Chef Boyardee Smurfs / 7.5 oz	150
Chef Boyardee Tic Tac Toes / 7.5 oz	160
Chef Boyardee Tic Tac Toes / 7 oz	160
Chef Boyardee Turtles / 7.5 oz	150
Healthy Choice Rings / 7.5 oz	140
Healthy Choice Rings Micro Cups / 7.5 oz	140
w cheese / 7-⅜ oz / **Franco-American**	180
w cheese sauce	
Franco-American CircusO's / 7-⅜ oz	170
Franco-American SpaghettiO's / 7-½ oz	170
Franco-American SportyO's / 7-½ oz	170
Franco-American TeddyO's / 7-½ oz	170
w frankfurters / 1 cup / **Van Camp's**	243
w meat sauce / 7.50 oz / **Healthy Choice**	150
w meat sauce / 7.50 oz / **Healthy Choice** Micro Cups	150
w meatballs / 7-⅜ oz / **Franco-American**	220
Franco-American CircusO's / 7-⅜ oz	210
Franco-American SpaghettiO's / 7-⅜ oz	220
Franco-American SportyO's / 7-⅜ oz	210
Franco-American TeddyO's / 7-⅜ oz	210
w sliced franks / 7-⅜ oz / **Franco-American** SpaghettiO's	220
Spaghetti w sauce, frozen	
w beef and mushroom sauce / 12 oz / **Healthy Choice**	370
w beef sauce and mushrooms / 9 oz / **Le Menu** Light	280
w meat sauce	
Banquet Entree Express / 8.5 oz	220
Healthy Choice Entree / 10 oz	280
Stouffer's 12-⅞ oz	370
Stouffer's Lean Cuisine Entree / 11-½ oz	290
Weight Watchers / 10.5 oz	280
w meatballs	
Stouffer's / 12-⅝ oz	380
Stouffer's / 8.75 oz	300
Stouffer's Lean Cuisine Entree / 9-½ oz	280
Spaghetti and sauce, mix	
Hamburger Helper / ⅕ serv prepared	340

CALORIES

	CALORIES
Kraft Mild American / 1 cup	300
Kraft Tangy Italian / 1 cup	310
McCormick/Schilling / ¼ pkg prepared	32
w meat sauce / 1 cup / **Kraft**	360

Spices

CALORIES

1 teaspoon unless noted

	CALORIES
Allspice	5
Anise seed	7
Basil, fresh / 2 tbsp	1
Basil, ground	4
Bay leaf	2
Caraway seed	7
Cardamom, ground	6
Celery seed	10
Chervil, dried	2
Chili powder	8
Chives, fresh / 1 tsp chopped	0
Cinnamon, ground	5
Cloves, ground	7
Coriander leaf, dried	2
Coriander leaf, fresh / ¼ cup	1
Coriander seed	5
Cumin seed	5
Curry powder	5
Dill seed	7
Dill weed	3
Dill weed, fresh / 5 sprigs	0
Fennel seed	7
Fenugreek seed	12
Garlic powder	10
Ginger, fresh / ¼ cup sliced	17
Ginger, ground	6
Mace, ground	8

CALORIES

Marjoram, dried	2
Mustard seed	15
Nutmeg, ground	12
Onion powder	5
Oregano, ground	5
Paprika	5
Parsley, dried	1
Parsley, fresh	4
Pepper, black	5
Pepper, red or cayenne	6
Pepper, white	7
Poppy seed	15
Rosemary, dried	4
Saffron	2
Sage, ground	2
Savory, ground	4
Sesame seeds	16
Tarragon, ground	5
Thyme, ground	4
Turmeric, ground	8

Spreads

CALORIES

Chicken, canned / 2-⅛ oz / **Underwood** Chunky	150
Chicken, chunky, canned / 2-⅛ oz / **Underwood** Light	100
Chicken, smoky flavored, canned / 2-⅛ oz / **Underwood**	150
Chicken salad, canned / 1.9 oz / **Libby's**	90
Ham, deviled, canned / 2-⅛ oz / **Underwood**	220
Ham, deviled, canned / 2-⅛ oz / **Underwood** Light	120
Ham, deviled, smoked, canned / 2-⅛ oz / **Underwood**	190
Ham salad, canned / 1.9 oz / **Libby's**	70
Liverwurst, canned / 2-⅛ oz / **Underwood**	180
Pate, liver, canned / 2-⅛ oz / **Underwood** Sell's	190
Peanut butter: **2 tbsp unless noted**	
Bama Creamy	200

CALORIES

Bama Crunchy	200
Bama w Jelly	150
Estee	100
Hollywood Creamy	35
Hollywood Unsalted	35
Jif Creamy	180
Jif Crunchy	180
Nu Made Chunky	190
Nu Made Creamy	190
Peter Pan Creamy	190
Peter Pan Crunchy	190
Peter Pan Salt Free	190
Peter Pan Salt Free Crunch	190
Safeway Real Roast Chunky	190
Safeway Real Roast Creamy	190
Reese's Creamy	180
Reese's Crunchy	190
Skippy Creamy	190
Skippy Honey Roasted Chunky	190
Skippy Honey Roasted Creamy	190
Skippy Super Chunk	190
Smucker's Goober Grape	180
Smucker's Honey Sweetened	200
Smucker's Natural	200
Smucker's Natural No Salt	200
Roast beef, canned / 2-⅛ oz / **Underwood**	140
Roast beef, canned / 2-⅛ oz / **Underwood** Light	90
Roast beef, smoked, canned / 2-⅛ oz / **Underwood**	140
Sandwich spread / 1 tbsp / **Nu Made**	60
Sandwich spread / 1 oz / **Oscar Mayer**	67
Tuna salad, canned / 1.9 oz / **Libby's**	80
Turkey, chunky, canned / 2-⅛ oz / **Underwood** Light	75
Turkey salad, canned / 1.9 oz / **Libby's**	100

Sugar and Sweeteners

	CALORIES
Honey, strained or extracted / 1 tbsp	65
Honey, strained or extracted / 1 cup	1030
Fructose / 1 tsp	12
Sugar	
Brown, not packed / 1 cup	540
Brown, packed / 1 cup	820
Maple / 1 oz	100
Powdered, sifted / 1 cup	385
Powdered, unsifted / 1 cup	460
Powdered, unsifted / 1 tbsp	30
White, granulated / 1 cup	770
White, granulated / 1 tbsp	45
White, granulated / 1 tsp	15
Sugar substitute, granulated	
Equal / 1 packet	4
Equal / 1 tablet	0
Estee / 1 tsp	12
Pillsbury Sweet Sprinkle / 1 tsp	2
Sprinkly Sweet / 1 tbsp	2
Sugar Twin / 1 tsp	<2
Sweet 'N Low / 1 packet	4
Sweet 'N Low Brown Sugar / 1/10 tsp	2
Sweet 10 / 1/8 tbsp	0
Weight Watchers / 1 gram	4
Sugar substitute, liquid / **Pillsbury** Sweet Ten Liquid / 1/8 tsp	0

Syrups

CALORIES

1 tablespoon

Apricot / **Knott's Berry Farm**	50
Corn, dark / 1 tbsp / **Karo**	60
Corn, light / 1 tbsp / **Karo**	60
Fruit / **Smucker's**	50
Fruit, all flavors / **Knott's Berry Farm**	60
Light fruit / **Knott's Berry Farm**	25
Molasses, dark / **Brer Rabbit**	50
Molasses, light / **Brer Rabbit**	50
Molasses, robust flavor / **Grandma's**	68
Molasses, unsulphured / **Grandma's**	68
Pancake and waffle	
Aunt Jemima ButterLite	25
Aunt Jemima Lite	27
Aunt Jemima Original	55
Brer Rabbit Light and Dark	120
Knott's Berry Farm	55
Log Cabin Lite	25
Log Cabin	50
Log Cabin Country Kitchen	50
Pillsbury Hungry Jack Lite	50
Pillsbury Hungry Jack Regular	50
Weight Watchers Reduced Calorie	25

Tea

TEA BAGS

5 fl oz prepared unless noted

Nestea / 6 fl oz prepared	0
Salada	0
Apple orchard / **Bigelow**	5
Cinnamon stick / **Bigelow**	1
Constant Comment / **Bigelow**	1
Earl Grey / **Bigelow**	1
English Teatime / **Bigelow**	1
Fruit and almond / **Bigelow**	1
I Love Lemon / **Bigelow**	1
Lemon Lift / **Bigelow**	1
Mint Medley / **Bigelow**	1
Orange Pekoe / **Bigelow**	1
Orange & spice / **Bigelow**	1
Peppermint stick / **Bigelow**	1
Plantation mint / **Bigelow**	1
Sweet Dreams / **Bigelow**	1
Take-a-Break / **Bigelow**	3

ICED TEA

Canned: 8 fl oz unless noted

Lipton Diet / 6 fl oz	2
Shasta Non Carb / 12 fl oz	136

	CALORIES
Lemon-flavored w Vit. C / 6 fl oz, as packaged / **Lipton**	58
w lemon / ready to drink / **Nestea** Sugarfree	2
w lemon and sugar / ready to drink / **Nestea**	70
Dairy: 8 fl oz	
Lemon flavored w Vit. C / as packaged / **Lipton** Sugar Free Dairy	<1
Lemon flavored w Vit. C / as packaged / **Lipton** Presweetened Dairy	81
Lemon flavored w Vit. C / as packaged / **Lipton** Sugar Free	<1
Fountain syrup, lemon-flavored / 6 fl oz, as packaged / **Lipton** Sweetened	55
Instant, prepared: 8 fl oz	
Nestea	2
Nestea Decaffeinated	0
Lipton Decaffeinated	0
Lemon-flavored / **Lipton**	3
Raspberry-flavored / **Lipton**	3
Mix	
Lipton Decaf, Sugar Free / 8 fl oz	1
Lipton Decaf w Nutrasweet / 8 fl oz	3
Lipton Sugar Free / 8 fl oz	1
Lipton w Nutrasweet / 8 fl oz	3
Lipton Post Tea / 1 fl oz	<1
Nestea, Sugarfree / 8 fl oz prepared	4
All flavors / 8 fl oz prepared / **Nestea** Ice Teasers	6
Lemon-flavored / 6 fl oz / **Lipton** Post Tea	55
Lemon-flavored / 6 fl oz / **Lipton**	55
Lemon-flavored / 6 fl oz prepared / **Lipton** Decaf	55
Lemon-flavor / 8 fl oz prepared / **Nestea**	6
Lemon and sugar / 8 fl oz prepared / **Nestea**	70
Natural lemon flavor / 8.45 fl oz / **Lipton**	96
Natural lemon flavor / 8 fl oz prepared / **Nestea** Plunge Ice Tea, Sweetened	90
Natural lemon flavor / 8 fl oz prepared / **Nestea** Diet Plunge Ice Tea	8
Peach-flavored / 8 fl oz / **Lipton** Sugar Free	5
Raspberry-flavored / 8 fl oz / **Lipton** Sugar Free	5

Thickeners

CALORIES

	CALORIES
Cornstarch, 1 tbsp	
Argo	35
Cream	29

Toppings

CALORIES

2 tbsp unless noted

	CALORIES
Butterscotch	
Kraft / 1 tbsp	60
Smucker's	140
Smucker's Special Recipe	160
Caramel / 1 tbsp / **Kraft**	60
Caramel / **Smucker's**	140
Chocolate	
Estee / 1 tbsp	20
Hershey's / 1.4 oz	110
Kraft / 1 tbsp	50
Dark chocolate / **Smucker's** Special Recipe	130
Fudge / 1 oz / **Hershey's**	100
Fudge / **Smucker's**	130
Chocolate-flavored / **Smucker's**	130
Hot caramel / **Smucker's**	150
Hot fudge	
Kraft / 1 tbsp	70
Smucker's	110
Smucker's Light	70
Smucker's Special Recipe	150

CALORIES

Hot toffee fudge / **Smucker's**	110
Marshmallow / **Smucker's**	120
Marshmallow creme / 1 oz / **Kraft**	90
Peanut butter-caramel / **Smucker's**	150
Pecans in syrup / **Smucker's**	130
Pineapple / 1 tbsp / **Kraft**	50
Pineapple / **Smucker's**	130
Real cream / ¼ cup / **Kraft**	30
Smucker's Magic Shell / chocolate	190
Smucker's Magic Shell / chocolate fudge	190
Smucker's Magic Shell / chocolate nut	200
Strawberry / 1 tbsp / **Kraft**	50
Strawberry / **Smucker's**	120
Swiss milk chocolate fudge / **Smucker's**	140
Walnuts in syrup / **Smucker's**	130
Whipped	
Mix / 1 tbsp / **D-Zerta**, Reduced Calorie	8
Mix / 1 tbsp / **Dream Whip**	10
Kraft / ¼ cup	35
Dairy recipe / frozen / 1 tbsp / **Cool Whip** Extra Creamy	14
Nondairy / frozen / 1 tbsp	
Cool Whip	12
Cool Whip Lite	8
LaCreme	16
Pet	14

Vegetables

FRESH

	CALORIES
Alfalfa sprouts / 1 cup	10
Amaranth, raw / 1 cup	7
Amaranth, cooked / ½ cup	14
Artichokes, globe or French, cooked / 1 medium	55
Arugula, raw / 1 leaf	0
Asparagus	
Raw / 4 spears	14
Raw / ½ cup	16
Cooked, cuts and tips, drained / ½ cup	22
Spears, cooked, drained / 4 spears (½-in diam at base)	14
Balsam pear, leafy tips, cooked / ½ cup	10
Balsam pear, pods, cooked / ½ cup	12
Bamboo shoots, raw / ½ cup (½-in slices)	21
Bamboo shoots, cooked / 1 cup (½-in slices)	15
Beans	
Black, dry, cooked, drained / 1 cup	225
Great Northern, cooked, drained / 1 cup	210
Kidney, sprouted seeds, raw / ½ cup	27
Kidney, sprouted seeds, cooked, drained / 1 lb	152
Lima, immature, raw / 1 cup	176
Lima, immature, cooked, drained / 1 cup	208
Lima, dried, cooked, drained / 1 cup	260
Mung, sprouted seeds, raw / 1 cup	30

CALORIES

Mung, sprouted seeds, cooked, drained / 1 cup	25
Pea (navy), raw / ½ cup	35
Pea (navy), dry, cooked, drained / 1 cup	225
Pinto, dry, raw / 1 lb	280
Pinto, dry, cooked, drained / 1 cup	265
Snap (includes Italian, green and yellow), raw / 1 cup	35
Snap (includes Italian, green and yellow), cooked, drained / 1 cup	44
Beets, red	
Raw, sliced / ½ cup	30
Cooked, drained, diced or sliced / 1 cup	55
Cooked, drained, whole (2-in diam) / 2 beets	30
Beets, green	
Raw, 1-in pieces / ½ cup	4
Raw / 1 leaf	6
cooked, drained, leaves and stems / 1 cup	40
Borage, raw, 1-in pieces / ½ cup	9
Borage, cooked, drained / 1 lb	113
Broadbeans, raw / 1 cup	79
Broadbeans, cooked, drained / 1 lb	255
Broccoli	
Chopped, raw / ½ cup	12
Spear, raw / 1 spear	10
Cooked, drained / 1 medium spear	50
Cooked, drained, spears chopped (½-in pieces) / 1 cup	45
Brussels sprouts	
Raw / 1 medium	8
Raw / ½ cup	19
Cooked, drained, about 1-½-in diam / 7–8 sprouts or 1 cup	60
Butterbur, raw / 1 cup	13
Butterbur, cooked / 1 lb	39
Cabbage	
Raw / 1 head (5-¾-in diam)	215
Raw, shredded / ½ cup	8
Cooked, drained, shredded / ½ cup	16
Chinese (Pakchoi), raw, shredded / ½ cup	5
Chinese (Pakchoi), cooked, drained, shredded / 1 cup	20

CALORIES

Chinese (Petsai), raw, shredded / ½ cup	6
Chinese (Petsai), cooked, drained, shredded / 1 cup	16
Red, raw, shredded / ½ cup	10
Red, cooked, drained, shredded / ½ cup	5
Savoy, raw, shredded / ½ cup	10
Savoy, cooked, drained, shredded / ½ cup	18
Cardoon, raw, shredded / ½ cup	18
Cardoon, cooked / 1 lb	100
Carrots	
Raw / 1 carrot (2-½ oz)	31
Raw, shredded / ½ cup	24
Raw, baby / 1 medium carrot (2-¾ in)	4
Raw, baby / 1 large carrot (3-¼ in)	6
Cooked, drained, sliced / ½ cup	35
Cooked, drained, whole / 1 carrot (1-½ oz)	21
Cauliflower	
Raw / ½ cup (1-in pieces)	12
Raw / 3 flowerets	13
Cooked, drained / ½ cup (1-in pieces)	15
Cooked, drained / 3 flowerets	13
Celeriac, raw / ½ cup	31
Celeriac, cooked, drained / 1 lb	115
Celery	
Raw, large outer stalk, 8-in long, 1-½-in wide) / 1 stalk	5
Raw, diced / ½ cup	9
Cooked, diced / ½ cup	11
Chard, Swiss, raw, chopped / ½ cup	3
Chard, Swiss, cooked, drained, chopped / ½ cup	18
Chayote, raw / 1 cup (1-in pieces)	32
Chayote, cooked, drained / 1 cup (1-in pieces)	38
Chickpeas, cooked, drained / 1 cup	270
Chicory greens, raw, chopped / ½ cup	21
Chicory roots, raw / ½ cup (1-in pieces)	33
Chicory, Witloof, raw / ½ cup	7
Chives, raw, chopped / 1 tsp	0
Collards	
Raw, chopped / ½ cup	18
Cooked, drained, chopped / ½ cup	13
Corn	
Sweet, raw, white and yellow, kernels from 1 ear / about 3 oz	77

CALORIES

Sweet, raw, white and yellow, cut / ½ cup	66
Sweet, white and yellow, cooked, drained, kernels from 1 ear / 2-7/10 oz	83
Sweet, white and yellow, cooked, drained, cut / ½ cup	89
Cowpeas	
Green, raw / ½ cup	91
Green, cooked, drained / ½ cup	89
Immature seeds (blackeyed), cooked, drained / 1 cup	180
Leafy tips, raw, chopped / 1 cup	10
Leafy tips, cooked, drained, chopped / 1 cup	12
Young pods w seeds, raw / ½ cup	21
Young pods w seeds, cooked, drained / ½ cup	16
Cress, garden	
Raw / 1 sprig	0
Raw / ½ cup	8
Cooked, drained / ½ cup	16
Cucumber, raw, sliced / ½ cup	7
Cucumber, raw, unpeeled, whole / 1 (about 10-½ oz)	39
Dandelion greens, raw, chopped / ½ cup	13
Dandelion greens, cooked, drained, chopped / ½ cup	17
Dock or sorrel, raw, chopped / ½ cup	15
Eggplant, raw / ½ cup (1-in pieces)	11
Eggplant, cooked, drained / ½ cup (1-in cubes)	13
Endive, raw, chopped / ½ cup	4
Eppaw, raw / ½ cup	75
Fennel, bulb, raw, sliced / 1 cup	27
Garlic, raw / 1 clove	4
Ginger root, raw, sliced / ¼ cup	17
Gourd	
Dishcloth, raw / 1 cup (1-in slices)	19
Dishcloth, cooked, drained / 1 cup (1-in slices)	99
White flowered, raw / ½ cup (1-in cubes)	8
White flowered, cooked, drained / ½ cup (1-in cubes)	11
Horseradish	
Tree leafy tips, raw, chopped / ½ cup	6
Tree leafy tips, cooked, drained, chopped / ½ cup	13
Tree pods, raw, sliced / 1 cup	37
Tree pods, cooked, drained, sliced / 1 cup	42

Hyacinth-beans, raw / ½ cup	19
Hyacinth-beans, cooked, drained / ½ cup	22
Jerusalem artichoke, raw, sliced / ½ cup	57
Jew's ear, raw / 1 piece (about ¼ oz)	2
Jute, potherb, raw / ½ cup	5
Jute, potherb, cooked, drained / ½ cup	16
Kale, raw, chopped / ½ cup	17
Kale, cooked, drained, chopped / ½ cup	21
Kale, Scotch, raw, chopped / ½ cup	14
Kale, Scotch, cooked, drained, chopped / ½ cup	18
Kohlrabi, raw, sliced / ½ cup	19
Kohlrabi, cooked, drained, sliced / ½ cup	24
Leeks, raw, chopped / ¼ cup	16
Leeks, cooked, drained, chopped / ¼ cup	8
Lentils, sprouted, raw / ½ cup	40
Lettuce	
Butterhead, raw / 2 leaves (about ½ oz)	2
Butterhead, raw / 1 head	21
Cos or romaine, raw / 1 leaf (about ⅓ oz)	2
Cos or romaine, raw, shredded / ½ cup	4
Crisphead (including Iceberg) / 1 leaf (about ⅔ oz)	3
Crisphead (including Iceberg) / 1 head	70
Looseleaf, raw / 1 leaf (about ⅓ oz)	2
Looseleaf, raw, shredded / ½ cup	5
Mushrooms, raw / ½ cup pieces	9
Mushrooms, cooked, drained / ½ cup pieces	21
Mushrooms, Enoki, raw / 1 medium mushroom (3-⅜ in)	1
Mushrooms, Enoki, raw / 1 large mushroom (4-⅛ in)	2
Mustard greens, raw, chopped / ½ cup	7
Mustard greens, cooked, drained, chopped / ½ cup	11
Mustard spinach, raw, chopped / ½ cup	17
Mustard spinach, cooked, drained, chopped / ½ cup	14
New Zealand spinach, raw, chopped / ½ cup	4
New Zealand spinach, cooked, drained, chopped / ½ cup	11
Okra, raw, sliced / ½ cup	19
Okra, cooked, drained, sliced / ½ cup	25
Onions	
Raw, chopped / 1 tbsp	3
Raw, chopped / ½ cup	27
Cooked, drained, chopped / 1 tbsp	4

CALORIES

Cooked, drained, chopped / ½ cup	29
Spring, raw, chopped / ½ cup	13
Parsley, raw / 10 sprigs	4
Parsley, raw, chopped / ½ cup	11
Parsnips, raw, sliced / ½ cup	50
Parsnips, cooked, drained, sliced / ½ cup	63
Peas	
Edible podded, raw / ½ cup	30
Edible podded, cooked, drained / ½ cup	34
Green, raw / ½ cup	63
Green, cooked, drained / ½ cup	67
Mature seeds, sprouted, raw / ½ cup	77
Mature seeds, sprouted, cooked, drained / 1 lb	535
Peppers, chili, raw / 1 pepper	18
Peppers, chili, raw, chopped / ½ cup	30
Peppers (green and red)	
Sweet, raw / 1 pepper (about 3-in diam)	18
Sweet, raw, chopped / ½ cup	12
Sweet, cooked, drained / 1 pepper	13
Sweet, cooked, drained, chopped / ½ cup	12
Peppers (yellow), sweet, raw / 1 large pepper (5-in x 3-in diam)	50
Pokeberry shoots, raw / ½ cup	18
Pokeberry shoots, cooked, drained / ½ cup	16
Potatoes	
Baked in skin / 1 potato (4-¾-in long, 2-⅓-in diam)	220
Boiled in skin / ½ cup flesh	68
Mashed, w milk and butter / ½ cup	111
Microwave in skin / ½ cup flesh	78
Peeled, raw, diced / ½ cup	59
Pumpkin, raw, cubed / ½ cup	15
Pumpkin, cooked, mashed / ½ cup	24
Purslane, raw / 1 plant	1
Purslane, cooked, drained / ½ cup	10
Radicchio, raw / 1 medium leaf	2
Radishes, raw, sliced / ½ cup	10
Radishes, Oriental, raw, sliced / ½ cup	8
Radishes, Oriental, cooked, sliced / ½ cup	13
Radishes, white icicle, raw, sliced / ½ cup	7
Radish seeds, sprouted, raw / ½ cup	8
Rutabagas, raw, cubed / ½ cup	25

CALORIES

Rutabagas, cooked, drained, cubed / ½ cup	29
Salsify, raw, sliced / ½ cup	55
Salsify, cooked, drained, sliced / ½ cup	46
Seaweed	
Agar, raw / 1 lb	116
Irish moss, raw / 1 lb	222
Kelp, raw / 1 lb	195
Laver, raw / 1 lb	158
Spirulina, raw / 1 lb	120
Wakame, raw / 1 lb	206
Shallots, raw, chopped / 1 tbsp	7
Soybeans	
Green, raw / ½ cup	188
Green, cooked, drained / ½ cup	127
Mature seeds, sprouted, raw / 10 sprouts	12
Mature seeds, sprouted, cooked / ½ cup	38
Spinach, raw, chopped / ½ cup	6
Spinach, cooked, drained / ½ cup	21
Squash	
Summer, all varieties, raw, sliced / ½ cup	13
Summer, all varieties, cooked, sliced / ½ cup	18
Summer, crookneck, (includes straightneck), raw, sliced / ½ cup	12
Summer, crookneck, (includes straightneck), cooked, drained, sliced / ½ cup	18
Summer, scallop, raw, sliced / ½ cup	12
Summer, scallop, cooked, drained, sliced / ½ cup	14
Summer, zucchini, raw, sliced / ½ cup	9
Summer, zucchini, cooked, drained, sliced / ½ cup	14
Summer, zucchini, baby, raw / 1 medium (2-⅝-in x ⅝-in diam)	2
Winter, all varieties, raw, cubed / ½ cup	21
Winter, all varieties, cooked, baked, cubed / ½ cup	39
Winter, acorn, raw, cubed / 1 cup	56
Winter, acorn, cooked, baked, cubed / ½ cup	57
Winter, acorn, cooked, boiled, mashed / ½ cup	41
Winter, butternut, raw, cubed / ½ cup	32
Winter, butternut, cooked, baked, cubed / ½ cup	41
Winter, hubbard, raw, cubed / ½ cup	23
Winter, hubbard, cooked, baked, cubed / ½ cup	51
Winter, hubbard, cooked, boiled, mashed / ½ cup	35

CALORIES

Winter, spaghetti, raw, cubed / ½ cup	17
Winter, spaghetti, baked or boiled / ½ cup	23
Succotash, raw / 1 lb	451
Succotash, cooked, drained / ½ cup	111
Swamp cabbage, raw / 1 shoot	2
Swamp cabbage, cooked, drained, chopped / ½ cup	10
Sweetpotato leaves, raw / 1 leaf	6
Sweetpotato leaves, cooked, steamed / ½ cup	11
Sweet potatoes	
Raw / 1 potato (4-½ oz)	136
Baked in skin / 1 potato (4 oz)	118
Baked in skin, mashed / ½ cup	103
Boiled w o skin, mashed / ½ cup	172
Taro, raw, sliced / ½ cup	56
Taro, cooked, sliced / ½ cup	94
Taro leaves, raw / 1 leaf	4
Taro leaves, cooked, steamed / ½ cup	18
Taro shoots, raw, sliced / ½ cup	5
Taro shoots, cooked, sliced / ½ cup	10
Taro, Tahitian, raw, sliced / ½ cup	25
Taro, Tahitian, cooked, sliced / ½ cup	30
Tomatillos, raw / 1 medium (1-⅝-in diam)	11
Tomatoes	
Green, raw / 1 tomato (about 4-⅓ oz)	30
Red, ripe, raw / 1 tomato (about 4-⅓ oz)	24
Red, ripe, boiled / ½ cup	30
Red, ripe, stewed / 1 cup	59
Turnips, raw, cubed / ½ cup	18
Turnips, cooked, drained, cubed / ½ cup	14
Turnip greens, raw, chopped / ½ cup	7
Turnip greens, cooked, drained, chopped / ½ cup	15
Water chestnuts, Chinese, raw / 4 pieces	38
Watercress, raw / 1 sprig	0
Watercress, raw, chopped / ½ cup	2
Yam, raw, cubed / ½ cup	89
Yam, baked or boiled, cubed / ½ cup	79
Yambean (tuber portion), raw, sliced / 1 slice (⅛-in thick, 5-in diam)	2
Yambean, (tuber portion), cooked, drained / 1 lb	174

CANNED AND FROZEN

CALORIES

½ cup unless noted; 3.3 oz is usually about ½ cup

Artichoke hearts, frozen / 3 oz / **Birds Eye** Deluxe	30
Artichoke hearts, frozen / 3 oz / **Seabrook**	30
Asparagus, canned	
Cut / **Green Giant**	18
Cut / **Green Giant** 50% Less Salt	18
Spears / **Green Giant**	18
Spears and tips / **Del Monte**	20
Tipped / **Del Monte**	20
White / **Green Giant**	16
Asparagus, frozen	
Cut / 3.3 oz / **Birds Eye**	25
Cut / **Green Giant** Harvest Fresh	25
Cut / 3.3 oz / **Seabrook**	25
Spears / 3.3 oz / **Birds Eye**	25
Spears / 3.3 oz / **Seabrook**	25
Bean salad, canned / **Green Giant** Three Bean	70
Beans, baked, canned	
B&M / 8 oz	240
Campbell's Homestyle / 8 oz	220
Campbell's Old Fashioned / 8 oz	230
Green Giant	130
Van Camp's / 1 cup	260
Van Camp's Deluxe / 1 cup	320
Barbecue / 8 oz / **B&M**	280
Barbecue / 7-⅞ oz / **Campbell's**	210
Barbecue / 4 oz / **Hunt's** Big John's Beans	170
Hot and spicy / 8 oz / **B&M**	240
Maple / 8 oz / **B&M**	240
Maple / 8 oz / **Friends**	240
Pork and molasses / **Seneca**	140
Pork and tomato sauce / **Seneca**	140
Tomato / 8 oz / **B&M**	230
Vegetarian / 8 oz / **B&M** 50% Less Sodium	230
Vegetarian / 7-¾ oz / **Campbell's**	170
Vegetarian / **Seneca**	130

	CALORIES
Vegetarian / 1 cup / **Van Camp's**	206
w brown sugar / 1 cup / **Van Camp's**	290
w frankfurters / 1 cup / **Van Camp's** Chilee Weenee	309
w frankfurters / 7 oz / **Luck's**	300
w frankfurters / **Van Camp's** Beanee Weenee	326
w pork / 8 oz / **B&M**	240
w pork / 8 oz / **Campbell's**	200
w pork / 4 oz / **Hunt's**	135
w pork / 1 cup / **Van Camp's**	216
w pork in tomato sauce / **Green Giant**	90
w pork and tomato sauce / 7-½ oz / **Luck's**	240
Beans, black, canned / **Green Giant** in Brine	90
Beans, black, canned / 4 oz / **Progresso**	90
Beans, butter, canned	
Green Giant in Brine	70
Van Camp's / 1 cup	162
Speckled w pork / 7-½ oz / **Luck's**	230
Beans, butter, frozen / speckled, 3.3 oz / **Seabrook**	120
Beans, cannellini, canned / white kidney / 4 oz / **Progresso**	80
Beans, chick, canned / 4 oz / **Progresso**	110
Beans, fava, canned / **Progresso**	90
Beans, garbanzo, canned **Green Giant** in Brine	90
Beans, garbanzo, canned / **Green Giant** in Brine, 50% Less Salt	90
Beans, great northern, canned / **Green Giant** in Brine	80
Beans, great northern, canned / w pork / 7.5 oz / **Luck's**	230
Beans, green, canned	
Almondine / **Green Giant**	45
Cut / **Del Monte**	20
Cut / **Del Monte** No Salt	20
Cut / **Green Giant**	16
Cut / **Green Giant** 50% Less Salt	16
Cut and french / **Seneca** Natural Pack	20
Cut and whole / **Seneca**	20
French / **Seneca**	20
French style / **Del Monte**	20
French style / **Del Monte** No Salt	20
French style / **Green Giant**	16
French style, seasoned / **Del Monte**	20
Italian cut / **Del Monte**	25

CALORIES

Kitchen cut / **Green Giant**	16
Whole / **Del Monte**	20
Beans, green, frozen	
Birds Eye Deluxe Petite / 2.6 oz	20
Green Giant Plain Polybag	14
Health Valley	25
and spaetzle / 3.3 oz / **Birds Eye** International	100
Cut / 3 oz / **Birds Eye**	25
Cut / 3 oz / **Birds Eye** Portion Pack	25
Cut / **Green Giant** Harvest Fresh	16
Cut / 3 oz / **Seabrook**	25
Cut, in butter sauce / **Green Giant**	30
French cut / 3 oz / **Seabrook**	25
French style / 3 oz / **Birds Eye**	25
French style w almonds / 3 oz / **Birds Eye**	50
in butter sauce / 5.5 oz / **Green Giant**	60
Italian / 3 oz / **Birds Eye**	30
Italian / 3 oz / **Seabrook**	30
Mushroom casserole / 4.75 oz / **Stouffer's**	160
Whole / 3 oz / **Birds Eye** Deluxe	25
Whole / 4 oz / **Birds Eye** Farm Fresh	30
Whole / 3 oz / **Seabrook**	25
Beans, green, microwave / **Del Monte** Vegetable Classics	50
Beans, green, cut, microwave / **Green Giant**	12
Beans, kidney, canned	
Red / **Green Giant** in Brine	90
Red / **Green Giant** in Brine, 50% Less Salt	90
Red / 4 oz / **Hunt's**	100
Red / 4 oz / **Progresso**	100
Red, dark / 7.5 oz **Ranch Style**	170
Red, dark / 1 cup / **Van Camp's**	182
Red, light / 1 cup / **Van Camp's**	184
Red, New Orleans style / 1 cup / **Van Camp's**	178
Red, small / 4 oz / **Hunt's**	90
Red, special cook / 7-½ oz / **Luck's**	190
Red w pork / 8 oz / **Friends**	270
Red w pork / 7-½ oz / **Luck's**	240
Beans, lima, canned	
Del Monte	70
Seneca	80

CALORIES

Giant w pork / 7-½ oz / **Luck's**	240
w pork / 7-½ oz / **Luck's**	240
Beans, lima, frozen	
Health Valley	25
Baby / 3.3 oz / **Birds Eye**	130
Baby / **Green Giant** Harvest Fresh	80
Baby / 3.3 oz / **Seabrook**	130
Baby butter / 3.3 oz / **Seabrook**	140
Fordhook / 3.3 oz / **Birds Eye**	100
Fordhook / 3.3 oz / **Seabrook**	100
in butter sauce / **Green Giant**	100
Tiny / 3.3 oz / **Seabrook**	110
Beans, navy, Old fashioned, canned / 7-½ oz / **Ranch Style**	160
Beans, navy, w pork, canned / 7-½ oz / **Luck's**	230
Beans, October, seasoned w pork, canned / 7-½ oz / **Luck's**	230
Beans, pea, baked, canned / 8 oz / **B&M**	270
Beans, pea, w pork, canned / 8 oz / **Friends**	260
Beans, pinto, canned	
Green Giant in Brine	90
Progresso	110
Ranch Style / 7-½ oz	160
and great northern / 7-½ oz / **Luck's**	230
Onions w pork / 7-½ oz / **Luck's**	250
Seasoned w pork / 7 oz / **Luck's**	200
w jalapeno / 7-½ oz / **Ranch Style**	180
Beans, pinto, frozen / 3.2 oz / **Seabrook**	160
Beans, red, canned / 1 cup / **Van Camp's**	194
Beans, red, canned / ½ cup / **Green Giant** in Brine	90
Beans, wax, canned	
Cut / **Del Monte**	20
Cut / **Seneca**	20
French style / **Del Monte**	20
Beans, wax, frozen / 3 oz / **Seabrook**	25
Beans, yellow-eye, canned / 8 oz / **B&M**	260
Beans, yellow-eye, canned, w pork / 7-½ oz / **Luck's**	240
Beets, canned	
All cuts / **Seneca**	35
Harvard / **Seneca**	80
Pickled, crinkle sliced / **Del Monte**	80

Pickled, sliced and whole / **Seneca**	80
Pickled, sliced w onion / **Seneca**	80
Sliced / **Del Monte**	35
Sliced / **Del Monte** No Salt	35
Sliced and whole / **Seneca**	35
Tiny, whole / **Del Monte**	35
Whole / **Del Monte**	35
Beets, green w potatoes and mushrooms in sauce / microwave / **Green Giant**	60
Broccoli, frozen	
Green Giant Valley Combinations	80
Health Valley	25
Baby carrots and water chestnuts / 4 oz / **Birds Eye** Farm Fresh	45
Baby spears / 3.3 oz / **Birds Eye** Deluxe	30
Chopped / 3.3 oz / **Birds Eye**	25
Chopped / 3.3 oz / **Seabrook**	25
Cut / 3.2 oz / **Birds Eye**	25
Cut / 3 oz / **Birds Eye** Portion Pack	20
Cut / **Green Giant** Harvest Fresh	16
Cut / **Green Giant** Plain Polybag	18
Cut / 3.3 oz / **Seabrook**	25
Cut, in butter sauce / 4-½ oz / **Green Giant**	45
Cut, in cheese sauce / 5 oz / **Green Giant**	80
Florets / 3.3 oz / **Birds Eye** Deluxe	25
Spears / 3.3 oz / **Birds Eye**	25
Spears, baby / 3.3 oz / **Birds Eye**	30
Spears / **Green Giant** Harvest Fresh	20
Spears / **Green Giant** Select	18
Spears / 3.3 oz / **Seabrook**	25
Spears, baby / 3.3 oz / **Seabrook**	30
Spears in butter sauce / **Green Giant**	40
Spears, whole / 4 oz / **Birds Eye** Farm Fresh	30
w beans, pearl onions and peppers / 4 oz / **Birds Eye** Farm Fresh	35
w carrots and rotini in cheese sauce / 5-½ oz / **Green Giant**	100
w cauliflower and carrots / 4 oz / **Birds Eye** Farm Fresh	35
w cauliflower and carrots / 4 oz / **Green Giant**	30
w cauliflower and carrots in butter / **Green Giant**	30

w cauliflower and carrots in butter sauce / 3.3 oz / **Birds Eye**	45
w cauliflower and carrots in cheese sauce / 5 oz / **Birds Eye** For One	110
w cauliflower and carrots in cheese sauce / 5 oz / **Green Giant**	80
w cauliflower and red peppers / 4 oz / **Birds Eye** Farm Fresh	30
w cauliflower and carrots w cheese sauce / 4-½ oz / **Birds Eye**	110
w cauliflower medley / **Green Giant** Valley Combinations	640
w cheese sauce / 5 oz / **Birds Eye**	130
w cheese sauce / **Green Giant**	60
w corn and red peppers / 4 oz / **Birds Eye** Farm Fresh	60
w peppers, bamboo shoots and straw mushrooms / 4 oz / **Birds Eye** Farm Fresh	30
w red peppers / **Green Giant** Select	25
w rice au gratin / 5-¾ oz / **Birds Eye** For One	180
Brussels sprouts, frozen	
Birds Eye / 3.3 oz	35
Seabrook / 3.3 oz	35
Baby w cream sauce / 4-½ oz / **Birds Eye**	130
in butter sauce / **Green Giant**	40
w cauliflower and carrots / 4 oz / **Birds Eye** Farm Fresh	40
Carrots, canned	
Diced / **Del Monte**	30
Sliced / **Del Monte**	30
Sliced and diced / **Seneca**	20
Whole / **Del Monte**	30
Carrots, frozen	
Seabrook / 3.3 oz	40
Baby w peas and pearl onions / 3.3 oz / **Birds Eye** Deluxe	50
Baby, whole / 3.3 oz / **Birds Eye** Deluxe	40
Baby, whole / **Green Giant** Harvest Fresh	18
Parisiene / 2.6 oz / **Birds Eye** Deluxe	30
Sliced / 3.2 oz / **Birds Eye**	35

CALORIES

Whole, baby / **Green Giant** Select	20
Cauliflower, can or jar, hot and spicy / 1 oz / **Vlasic**	4
Cauliflower, frozen	
Birds Eye / 3.3 oz	25
Seabrook / 3.3 oz	25
Florets / **Green Giant** Plain Polybag	12
in cheese sauce / 5-½ oz / **Green Giant**	80
w carrots and snow pea pods / 4 oz / **Birds Eye** Farm Fresh	40
w cheese sauce / 5 oz / **Birds Eye**	130
w cheese sauce / **Green Giant**	60
w zucchini, carrots and red peppers / 4 oz / **Birds Eye** Farm Fresh	30
Collard greens, canned, chopped w pork / 7-½ oz / **Luck's**	90
Collard greens, frozen, chopped / 3.3 oz / **Seabrook**	25
Corn, golden, canned	
Cream style / **Del Monte**	80
Cream style / **Del Monte** No Salt	80
Cream style / **Green Giant**	100
Cream style / **Seneca**	80
Delicorn / **Green Giant**	80
Mexicorn / **Green Giant**	70
Whole kernel	
Del Monte	70
Del Monte No Salt	80
Green Giant	70
Green Giant 50% Less Salt	70
Green Giant Niblets	80
Green Giant No Salt, No Sugar	80
Green Giant Sweet Select	60
Seneca	80
Seneca Natural Pack	80
Whole kernel, vacuum packed / **Del Monte**	90
Whole kernel, vacuum packed / **Del Monte** No Salt	90
Corn, golden, frozen	
Birds Eye Sweet / 3.3 oz	80
Health Valley	80
Baby cob / 2.6 oz / **Birds Eye** Deluxe	25
Cob / 4.4 oz / **Seabrook**	120
Cream style / **Green Giant**	110

CALORIES

in butter sauce / 4.5 oz / **Green Giant**	120
in butter sauce / **Green Giant** Niblets	100
On cob	
Birds Eye / 1 ear	120
Birds Eye Big Ears / 1 ear	160
Birds Eye Little Ears / 2 ears	130
Green Giant / 2 half ears	120
Green Giant Half Ears / 2 ears	90
Green Giant Nibblers / 2 ears	120
Green Giant Niblet Ears / 1 ear	120
Green Giant Sweet Select / 1 ear	90
Ore-Ida / 1 ear	190
Ore-Ida Mini Cob / 1 ear	90
Whole kernel	
Birds Eye Deluxe Petite / 2.6 oz	70
Birds Eye Portion Pack / 3 oz	70
Green Giant Harvest Fresh	80
Green Giant Niblets	90
Green Giant Sweet Select	60
Seabrook 3.3 oz	80
Whole kernel, sweet / 3.3 oz / **Birds Eye** Deluxe	80
in butter sauce / 3.3 oz / **Birds Eye**	90
Soufflé / 4 oz / **Stouffer's**	160
Corn, beans, carrots and pasta in tomato sauce / microwave / **Green Giant**	80
Corn, golden	
Whole kernel / microwave / **Green Giant**	80
and carrots / microwavable / **Del Monte** Vegetable Classics	70
Sante Fe style / microwavable / **Del Monte** Vegetable Classics	90
Corn, white, canned	
Cream style / **Del Monte**	90
Whole kernel / **Del Monte**	70
Whole kernel / **Green Giant**	80
Corn, white, frozen	
Green Giant Select	90
in butter sauce / **Green Giant**	100
Whole kernel / **Green Giant** Harvest Fresh	90
Whole kernel / 3.3 oz / **Seabrook**	80
Garden duet / microwavable / **Del Monte** Vegetable Classics	90

Garlic puree / 1 tsp / **Progresso**	4
Kale, chopped, frozen / 3.3 oz / **Seabrook**	25
Mixed, canned	
Del Monte	40
Green Giant Garden Medley	35
Seneca	40
Mixed, frozen	
Birds Eye / 3.3 oz	60
Birds Eye Portion Pack / 3 oz	50
Green Giant Harvest Fresh	40
Green Giant Plain Polybag	40
Health Valley	70
Ore-Ida Stew Vegetables / 3 oz	50
Seabrook / 3.3 oz	65
Breaded / 3 oz / **Ore-Ida**	160
California style / **Green Giant**	25
Chinese style / 3.3 oz / **Birds Eye** Stir Fry	35
Heartland style / **Green Giant**	25
in butter sauce / **Green Giant**	60
Italian style / 3.3 oz / **Birds Eye** International	100
Japanese style / 3.3 oz / **Birds Eye** International	90
Japanese style / 3.3 oz / **Birds Eye** Stir Fry	30
Le Sueur style / **Green Giant** Valley Combinations	70
Manhattan style / **Green Giant**	25
New England style / 3.3 oz / **Birds Eye** International	130
New England style / **Green Giant**	70
Oriental style / 3.3 oz / **Birds Eye** International	70
Pasta Primavera style / 3.3 oz / **Birds Eye** International	120
San Francisco style / 3.3 oz / **Birds Eye** International	100
San Francisco style / **Green Giant**	25
Santa Fe style / **Green Giant**	70
Seattle style / **Green Giant**	25
w cheese sauce / **Green Giant**	60
Western style / **Green Giant**	60
Mixed, microwave / **Green Giant**	35
Mixed, Dijon, microwave / **Del Monte** Vegetable Classics	70

	CALORIES
Mushrooms, canned: ¼ cup	
B in B	12
Green Giant	12
Green Giant Whole Straw	12
Seneca	35
w garlic / **B in B**	12
Mushrooms, frozen	
Breaded / 2.67 oz / **Ore-Ida**	120
Creamy / 1 pkg / **Green Giant** Garden Gourmet	220
Whole / 2.6 oz / **Birds Eye** Deluxe	20
Mustard greens, chopped, frozen / 3.3 oz / **Seabrook**	20
Okra	
Breaded, frozen / 3 oz / **Ore-Ida**	170
Cut, frozen / 3.3 oz / **Seabrook**	25
Whole, frozen / 3.3 oz / **Seabrook**	30
Onions, frozen	
Chopped / 2 oz / **Ore-Ida**	20
Chopped / 1 oz / **Seabrook**	8
Onion rings, fried / 2 oz / **Ore-Ida** Onion Ringers	150
Small w cream sauce / 5 oz / **Birds Eye**	140
Small, whole / 4 oz / **Birds Eye**	40
Small, whole / 3.3 oz / **Seabrook**	35
Pea pods, Chinese, frozen / 2 oz / **Seabrook**	20
Pea pods, snow, frozen / 3 oz / **Birds Eye** Deluxe	35
Peas, blackeyed, canned	
Green Giant in Brine	90
Ranch Style / 7.7 oz	180
Ranch Style / 7.5 oz	170
and corn / 7.5 oz / **Luck's**	210
Seasoned w pork / 7 oz / **Luck's**	230
Peas, blackeye, frozen / 3.3 oz / **Seabrook**	130
Peas, crowder, w pork, canned / 7.5 oz / **Luck's**	210
Peas, crowder, frozen / 3.2 oz / **Seabrook**	130
Peas, green, canned	
Green Giant 50% Less Salt	50
Green Giant Early	50
Green Giant Sweet	50
Green Giant Tender	50
Seneca	60
Seneca Natural Pack	60
and carrots / **Seneca**	50

CALORIES

Seasoned / **Del Monte**	60
Sweet / **Del Monte**	60
Sweet / **Del Monte** No Salt	60
Sweet / **Del Monte** Small	50
w carrots / **Del Monte**	50
w tiny pearl onions / **Green Giant**	50
Peas, green, frozen	
Birds Eye / 3.3 oz	80
Birds Eye Deluxe Tiny / 3.3 oz	60
Birds Eye Portion Pack / 3 oz	70
Green Giant Harvest Fresh	30
Green Giant Harvest Fresh, Sweet	50
Green Giant Select	60
Health Valley	80
and carrots / 3.3 oz / **Seabrook**	60
and onions / 3.3 oz / **Seabrook**	70
Baby / **Green Giant** Harvest Fresh	60
in butter sauce / **Green Giant**	80
in butter sauce / 4.5 oz / **Green Giant**	90
Regular / 3.3 oz / **Seabrook**	80
Sweet / **Green Giant** Plain Polybag	50
Tiny / 3.3 oz / **Seabrook**	60
w cream sauce / 5 oz / **Birds Eye**	180
w mushrooms / **Green Giant** Select	60
w pasta parmesan / 5.5 oz / **Green Giant**	160
w pearl onions / 3.3 oz / **Birds Eye**	70
w pearl onions and cheese sauce / 5 oz / **Birds Eye**	140
w potatoes and cream sauce / 5 oz / **Birds Eye**	190
Peas and mushrooms / microwavable / **Del Monte** Classics	70
Peas, snap, canned / 7.5 oz / **Luck's**	220
Peas, sugar, snap, frozen / 2.6 oz / **Birds Eye** Deluxe	45
Peas, sugar, snap w carrots and water chestnuts, frozen / 3.2 oz / **Birds Eye** Farm Fresh	50
Peppers, green, frozen / 1 oz / **Seabrook**	6
Peppers, red, frozen / 1 oz / **Seabrook**	8
Potatoes, canned	
Seneca	45
Sliced / **Del Monte**	45
Whole / **Del Monte**	45
Whole / 4 oz / **Hunt's**	70

Potatoes, frozen

Au gratin / 5.5 oz / **Birds Eye** For One	240
Au gratin / 3.8 oz / **Stouffer's**	110
Diced and hash-shred / 4 oz / **Seabrook**	80

French fried

Ore-Ida Zesties / 3 oz	160
Ore-Ida Cottage Fries / 3 oz	130
Ore-Ida Country Style / 3 oz	110
Ore-Ida Crinkle Cuts, Microwave / 3.5 oz	190
Ore-Ida Crispy Crunchers / 3 oz	180
Ore-Ida Deep Fries, Crinkle Cuts / 3 oz	160
Ore-Ida Deep Fries French Fries / 3 oz	170
Ore-Ida Golden Crinkles / 3 oz	120
Ore-Ida Golden Fries / 3 oz	120
Ore-Ida Golden Twirls / 3 oz	160
Ore-Ida Lites, Crinkle Cuts / 3 oz	90
Ore-Ida Pixie Crinkles / 3 oz	140
Ore-Ida Shoestrings / 3 oz	150
Seabrook Cottage Cut / 2.8 oz	110
Seabrook Regular / 3 oz	120
Seabrook Shoestring / 3 oz	140
Seabrook Crinkle Cut / 3 oz	120

Fried

Ore-Ida Crispers / 3 oz	220
Ore-Ida Crispy Crowns / 3 oz	190
Ore-Ida Tater Tots / 3 oz	160
Ore-Ida Tater Tots, Microwave / 4 oz	210
Fried w bacon flavor / 3 oz / **Ore-Ida** Tater Tots	150
Fried w onion / 3 oz / **Ore-Ida** Tater Tots	150

Hash browns

Ore-Ida Cheddar Browns / 3 oz	90
Ore-Ida Golden Patties / 2.5 oz	130
Ore-Ida Microwave / 2 oz	110
Ore-Ida Potatoes O'Brien / 3 oz	60
Ore-Ida Shredded / 3 oz	70
Ore-Ida Southern Style / 3 oz	70
Ore-Ida Toaster Hash Browns / 1.75 oz	100

Scalloped / 3.8 oz / **Stouffer's**	90
Stuffed w broccoli and cheese / 5.63 oz / **Ore-Ida**	160
Stuffed w vegetable primavera / 6.13 oz / **Ore-Ida**	160
Twice baked butter flavor / 5 oz / **Ore-Ida**	200

CALORIES

Twice baked cheddar cheese / 5 oz / **Ore-Ida**	210
Twice baked sour cream and chives / 5 oz / **Ore-Ida**	190
w broccoli in cheese sauce / 5.5 oz / **Green Giant**	130
Wedges / 3 oz / **Ore-Ida** Home Style	110
Whole, boiled / 3.3 oz / **Seabrook**	60
Potatoes au gratin, microwavable / ¾ cup / **Del Monte** Vegetable Classics	190
Potatoes, escalloped / microwavable / ¾ cup / **Del Monte** Vegetable Classics	190
Potatoes, nacho / microwavable / ¾ cup / **Del Monte** Vegetable Classics	170
Potatoes, mix	
American cheese / ⅙ serv prepared / **Betty Crocker** Homestyle	140
Au gratin / ⅙ serv prepared / **Betty Crocker**	140
Au gratin / mix prepared / **Kraft** Potatoes and Cheese	130
Au gratin, broccoli / ⅙ serv prepared / **Betty Crocker** Homestyle	130
Au gratin, broccoli / mix prepared / **Kraft** Potatoes and Cheese	150
Au gratin / prepared / **Pillsbury**	140
Bacon and cheddar / ⅙ serv prepared / **Betty Crocker** Twice Baked	210
Cheddar 'n Bacon / ⅙ serv prepared / **Betty Crocker**	140
Cheddar and bacon / ½ cup prepared / **Pillsbury**	140
Cheddar cheese / ⅙ serv prepared / **Betty Crocker** Homestyle	140
Cheddar w onion / ⅙ serv prepared / **Betty Crocker** Twice Baked	190
Hash browns / ⅙ serv prepared / **Betty Crocker**	160
Herbed butter / ⅙ serv prepared / **Betty Crocker** Twice Baked	220
Julienne / ⅙ serv prepared / **Betty Crocker**	130
Mashed	
Country Store / ⅓ cup flakes	70
Pillsbury Hungry Jack / prepared	130
Pillsbury Idaho Granules / prepared	120
Pillsbury Idaho Spuds / prepared	130
Betty Crocker / prepared	130

CALORIES

	CALORIES
Pancakes / 3 cakes, 3-in diam / **Pillsbury**	90
Scalloped / ⅙ serv prepared / **Betty Crocker**	140
Scalloped / prepared / **Kraft** Potatoes and Cheese	140
Scalloped cheese / prepared / **Pillsbury**	150
Scalloped w cheese / ⅙ serv prepared / **Betty Crocker**	140
Scalloped w cheese / ⅙ serv prepared / **Betty Crocker** Homestyle	140
Scalloped w ham / ⅕ serv prepared / **Betty Crocker**	160
Scalloped w ham / prepared / **Kraft** Potatoes and Cheese	150
Scalloped, white sauce / prepared / **Pillsbury**	150
Smokey cheddar / ⅙ serv prepared / **Betty Crocker**	140
Sour cream 'n chives / ⅙ serv prepared / **Betty Crocker**	140
Sour cream and chives / ⅙ serv prepared / **Betty Crocker** Twice Baked	200
Sour cream and chives / prepared / **Pillsbury**	150
Sour cream w chives / prepared / **Kraft** Potatoes and Cheese	150
Two cheese / prepared / **Kraft** Potatoes and Cheese	130
Potatoes au gratin, microwave / **Green Giant**	120
Pumpkin, canned / **Del Monte**	35
Pumpkin, canned / **Libby's**	42
Sauerkraut, canned	
Del Monte	25
Seneca	20
Vlasic Old Fashioned / 1 oz	4
Spinach, canned	
Seneca	25
Chopped / **Del Monte**	25
Whole leaf / **Del Monte**	25
Whole leaf / **Del Monte** No Salt	25
Spinach, frozen	
Green Giant Plain Polybag	25
Health Valley	25
Chopped / 3.3 oz / **Birds Eye**	20
Chopped / **Green Giant** Harvest Fresh	25
Chopped / 3.3 oz / **Seabrook**	20
Creamed / 3 oz / **Birds Eye**	60
Creamed / **Green Giant**	70

Creamed / 4.5 oz / **Stouffer's**	170
Leaf / 3.2 oz / **Birds Eye** Portion Pack	20
Leaf / 3.3 oz / **Seabrook**	20
Leaf in butter sauce / **Green Giant**	40
Leaf, whole / 3.3 oz / **Birds Eye**	20
Soufflé / 4 oz / **Stouffer's**	140

Squash, frozen

Winter, cooked / 4 oz / **Birds Eye**	45
Summer / 3.3 oz / **Seabrook**	18
Winter / 4 oz / **Seabrook** Winter	45
Zucchini / 3.3 oz / **Seabrook**	16

Succotash, canned, whole kernel / **Seneca**	80
Succotash, frozen / 3.3 oz / **Seabrook**	100

Tomato paste, canned

Contadina / 2 oz	50
Del Monte / ¾ cup	150
Del Monte / ¾ cup	150
Del Monte No Salt / 6 oz	150
Hunt's / 2 oz	45
Hunt's / 4 oz	45
Hunt's No Salt Added / 2 oz	45
Progresso / 6 oz	150
Italian / 2 oz / **Contadina**	65
Italian style / 2 oz / **Hunt's**	50
w garlic / 2 oz / **Hunt's**	50

Tomato puree, canned

Progresso	45
Heavy concentrate / **Progresso**	50

Tomatoes, canned

Crushed / 4 oz / **Hunt's** Angela Mia	35
Crushed / **Progresso**	40
Crushed, Italian flavored / 4 oz / **Hunt's**	40
Pearl, Italian style / **Contadina**	25
Pear-shaped, Italian style / 4 oz / **Hunt's**	20
Peeled / 4 oz / **Hunt's**	20

Stewed

Contadina	35
Del Monte	35
Del Monte Cajun Style	30
Del Monte Chunky Pasta	45
Del Monte Italian Style	30

Del Monte Mexican Style	35
Del Monte No Salt	35
Del Monte Original Style	35
Del Monte Original Style, No Salt	35
Hunt's / 4 oz	35
Hunt's No Salt / 4 oz	35
Stewed, Italian style / **Contadina**	35
Stewed, Italian style / 4 oz / **Hunt's**	40
Wedges / **Del Monte**	30
Whole	
Del Monte	25
Hunt's / 4 oz	20
Hunt's No Salt / 4 oz	20
Whole, Italian style / 4 oz / **Hunt's**	25
Whole, Italian style / **Progresso**	18
Whole, peeled / **Contadina**	25
Whole, peeled / **Del Monte**	25
Turnip greens	
w diced turnip, canned / 7.5 oz / **Luck's**	80
Chopped, frozen / 3.3 oz / **Seabrook**	20
w diced turnips, frozen / 3.3 oz / **Seabrook**	20

Vegetables, frozen: 4.6 oz

Chow Mein in Oriental sauce / **Birds Eye** Custom Cuisine	80
w Dijon sauce, for chicken or fish / **Birds Eye** Custom Cuisine	70
w herb sauce, for chicken or shrimp / **Birds Eye** Custom Cuisine	90
w mushroom sauce, for beef / **Birds Eye** Custom Cuisine	60
w Oriental sauce, for beef / **Birds Eye** Custom Cuisine	90
w pasta in cheese sauce / **Birds Eye** Custom Cuisine	150
w pasta in Stroganoff sauce / **Birds Eye** Custom Cuisine	120
w rice in wine sauce, for chicken / **Birds Eye** Custom Cuisine	100
w tomato basil sauce, for chicken / **Birds Eye** Custom Cuisine	110

CALORIES

Zucchini, canned / **Progresso**	50
Zucchini, canned in tomato sauce / **Del Monte**	30
Zucchini, frozen, breaded / 3 oz / **Ore-Ida**	150
Zucchini, frozen w carrots, pearl onions and mushrooms / 4 oz / **Birds Eye** Farm Fresh	30

Vegetable Juices

CALORIES

6 fl oz unless noted

Beefamato / **Mott's**	80
Carrot / **Hain**	80
Carrot / **Hollywood**	80
Tomato	
Campbell's	40
Del Monte	35
Libby's	35
Welch's	35
Tomato and chile cocktail / **Snap-E-Tom**	40
Vegetable	
Mott's	40
Smucker's Hearty / 8 fl oz	58
Smucker's Hot and Spicy / 8 fl oz	58
V-8	35
V-8 No Salt	35
V-8 Spicy Hot	35

Wines and Distilled Spirits

4 fl oz

	CALORIES
Aurore / **Great Western** (1987)	92
Baco Noir / **Great Western** (1987)	82
Baco Noir Nouveau / **Great Western** (1988)	80
Barbera / **Sebastiani**	87
Beaujolais / **Hiram Walker**	96
Blush / **Great Western** Premium	90
Bordeaux, red claret / **Hiram Walker**	96
Burgundy	
Gallo	88
Gallo Hearty	87
Gallo Resv.	85
Great Western	84
Taylor	87
Red / **Hiram Walker**	96
Sparkling	
Gold Seal	105
Great Western	102
Henri Marchant	104
Hiram Walker	116
Taylor	98
White / **Hiram Walker** Chablis	90
Cabernet / **Gallo**	88
Cabernet Sauvignon / **Gallo**	89
Catawba	
Pink / **Gold Seal**	133

CALORIES

Pink / **Great Western**	129
Pink / **Taylor**	112
Red / **Gold Seal**	132
White / **Gold Seal**	126
Chablis	
Gallo Blanc	82
Gold Seal	84
Great Western	81
Taylor	82
Blush / **Gallo**	86
Pink / **Gallo**	82
Champagne	
Gold Seal Blanc de Blancs	88
Gold Seal Brut	94
Gold Seal Extra Dry	103
Gold Seal Natural	86
Great Western Extra Dry	96
Henri Marchant Brut	93
Henri Marchant Extra Dry	104
Henri Marchant Natural	86
Hiram Walker Brut	100
Hiram Walker Extra Dry	116
Taylor Brut	93
Taylor Extra Dry	96
Brut / **Great Western**	91
Pink / **Gold Seal**	102
Pink / **Henri Marchant**	102
Pink / **Taylor**	98
Rose / **Great Western**	100
Chardonnay	
Gallo (1990)	91
Great Western (1987)	81
Sebastiani	94
Chenin Blanc / **Gallo** (1990)	81
Chianti / **Hiram Walker**	100
Cold Duck	
Great Western	111
Henri Marchant	104
Taylor	106
Colombard, French / **Gallo** (1990)	83
Concord, red / **Gold Seal**	128

CALORIES

Delaware, pink / **Gold Seal**	130
Dubonnet / **Hiram Walker**	160
Dutchess / **Great Western** (1987)	85
Gewurtztraminer / **Gallo** (1988)	83
Gewurtztraminer / **Great Western** (1988)	85
Grenache, white / **Gallo** (1990)	80
Labrusca, red concord / **Gold Seal**	127
Lake Country	
Chablis / **Taylor**	85
Chablis, blush / **Taylor**	97
Gold / **Taylor**	97
Niagara / **Taylor**	101
Pink / **Taylor**	101
Pink, soft / **Taylor**	92
Red / **Taylor**	97
Red, soft / **Taylor**	97
Very Berry / **Taylor**	89
Very Punch / **Taylor**	89
White / **Taylor**	72
White, soft / **Taylor**	89
Liebfraumitch / **Hiram Walker**	84
Madeira / **Hiram Walker**	160
Merlot / **Sebastiani**	86
Muscatel / **Hiram Walker**	196
Port	
Great Western	170
Hiram Walker	200
Taylor	173
Taylor Light	161
Ruby / **Hiram Walker**	184
Tawny / **Hiram Walker**	184
Tawny / **Taylor**	174
Tawny / **Taylor** Light	160
Rhine	
Gallo	89
Great Western	90
Taylor	89
Hiram Walker	96
Riesling	
Gallo (1988)	80
Great Western (1987)	90

CALORIES

Great Western (BS 1988)	127
Great Western (LH 1988)	102
Hiram Walker	90
Rose	
Great Western	95
Hiram Walker	95
Taylor	87
Red / **Gallo**	91
Rose of Isabella / **Great Western** (1988)	97
Sangria / **Taylor**	128
Sauterne	
Gold Seal Dry	91
Hiram Walker	116
Hiram Walker Dry	108
Taylor	93
White / **Gold Seal**	96
Sauvignon / **Sebastiani** Cabernet	83
Sauvignon Blanc / **Gallo** (1990)	79
Seyval Blanc / **Great Western** (1987)	84
Seyval Blanc / **Great Western** (LS 1987)	82
Sherry	
Great Western Solera	144
Great Western Solera, Dry	134
Hiram Walker	185
Hiram Walker Dry	162
Taylor Dry	135
Taylor Light Dry	124
Cream	
Great Western Solera	166
Hiram Walker	200
Taylor	179
Taylor Empire	191
Taylor Light	166
Golden / **Taylor**	159
Golden / **Taylor** Light	146
Sylvaner / **Hiram Walker**	90
Vermouth	
Dry	
Great Western	119

CALORIES

Hiram Walker	136
Taylor	116
Sweet	
Hiram Walker	180
Taylor	162
Great Western	140
Vidal Ice / **Great Western** (1987)	162
Vidal Ice / **Great Western** (1988)	200
Vignoles	
Great Western (LH 1988)	113
Great Western (1987)	85
Great Western (BS 1988)	132
Zinfandel	
Gallo (1986)	92
Sebastiani	86
White / **Gallo** (1991)	71

Yeast

	CALORIES
Baker's, dry, active / 1 pkg	20
Brewer's, dry / 1 tbsp	25
Dry, active / 1 packet / **Fleischmann's**	20
Dry, active, rapid rise / 1 packet / **Fleischmann's**	20
Fresh / .6 oz cake / **Fleischmann's**	16
Household / 2 oz cake / **Fleischmann's**	60

Yogurt

	CALORIES
Banana berry / 4-⅖ oz / **Light n' Lively** Lowfat	130
Black cherry	
Breyers Lowfat / 8 oz	260
Knudsen Nonfat / 6 oz	70
Light n' Lively Lowfat / 8 oz	230
Light n' Lively Nonfat / 8 oz	100
Blueberry	
Breyers Lowfat / 8 oz	250
Knudsen Nonfat / 6 oz	70
Light n' Lively Free Nonfat / 4-⅖ oz	50
Light n' Lively Lowfat / 8 oz	240
Light n' Lively Lowfat / 4-⅖ oz	130

CALORIES

Light n' Lively Nonfat / 8 oz	90
Mountain High / 1 cup	220
Boysenberry / 8 oz / **Knudsen** Lowfat	240
Cherry	
Knudsen Lowfat / 8 oz	240
Light n' Lively Lowfat / 4-⅔ oz	140
Yoplait Custard Style / 6 oz	180
Cherry vanilla / 1 cup / **Lite-Line**	240
Double chocolate / 4 oz / **Yoplait** Pudding	180
Fruit flavors	
Yoplait Custard Style / 6 oz	190
Yoplait Custard Style / 4 oz	130
Yoplait Fat Free / 6 oz	150
Yoplait Light / 6 oz	80
Yoplait Light / 4 oz	60
Yoplait Original / 6 oz	190
Yoplait Original / 4 oz	120
Grape / 4-⅔ oz / **Light n' Lively** Lowfat	130
Lemon	
Dannon Low Fat / 8 oz	200
Knudsen Lowfat / 8 oz	240
Knudsen Nonfat / 6 oz	70
Light n' Lively Nonfat / 8 oz	100
Lime / 8 oz / **Knudsen** Lowfat	240
Milk chocolate / 4 oz / **Yoplait** Pudding	180
Mixed berry / 8 oz / **Breyers** Lowfat	250
Mixed berry / 6 oz / **Yoplait** Custard Style	180
Peach	
Breyers Lowfat / 8 oz	250
Knudsen Lowfat / 8 oz	240
Knudsen Nonfat / 6 oz	70
Light n' Lively Lowfat / 8 oz	240
Light n' Lively Lowfat / 4-⅔ oz	130
Light n' Lively Nonfat / 8 oz	100
Lite-Line / 1 cup	230
Pineapple	
Breyers Lowfat / 8 oz	250
Knudsen Nonfat / 6 oz	70
Light n' Lively Lowfat / 8 oz	230
Light n' Lively Lowfat / 4.4 oz	130

CALORIES

Plain

Breyers Lowfat / 8 oz	140
Dannon Low Fat / 8 oz	140
Dannon Non Fat / 8 oz	110
Knudsen / 8 oz	200
Knudsen Lowfat / 8 oz	160
Lite-Line Lowfat, Swiss Style / 1 cup	140
Meadow Gold Lowfat / 1 cup	160
Mountain High / 1 cup	200
Weight Watchers Nonfat / 1 cup	90
Yoplait Nonfat / 8 oz	120
Yoplait Original / 6 oz	130
Raspberry / 8 oz / **Knudsen** Lowfat	240
Raspberry / 1 cup / **Meadow Gold** Lowfat, Sundae Style	250

Red raspberry

Breyers Lowfat / 8 oz	250
Knudsen Nonfat / 6 oz	70
Light n' Lively Free Nonfat / 4-⅔ oz	50
Light n' Lively Lowfat / 8 oz	230
Light n' Lively Lowfat / 4-⅔ oz	130
Light n' Lively Nonfat / 8 oz	90

Strawberry

Breyers Lowfat / 8 oz	250
Knudsen Lowfat / 8 oz	250
Knudsen Nonfat / 6 oz	70
Light n' Lively Free Nonfat / 4-⅔ oz	50
Light n' Lively Lowfat / 8 oz	240
Light n' Lively Lowfat / 4-⅔ oz	130
Light n' Lively Nonfat / 8 oz	90
Lite-Line / 1 cup	240

Strawberry banana

Breyers Lowfat / 8 oz	250
Knudsen Lowfat / 8 oz	240
Knudsen Nonfat / 6 oz	70
Light n' Lively Free Nonfat / 4-⅔ oz	50
Light n' Lively Lowfat / 8 oz	260
Light n' Lively Lowfat / 4-⅔ oz	140
Light n' Lively Nonfat / 8 oz	100
Strawberry fruit basket / 6 oz / **Knudsen** Nonfat	70

Strawberry fruit cup

Light n' Lively Free Nonfat / 4-⅔ oz	50

CALORIES

Light n' Lively Lowfat / 8 oz	240
Light n' Lively Lowfat / 4-⅗ oz	130
Light n' Lively Nonfat / 8 oz	90
Ultimate 90 / 1 cup / **Weight Watchers**	90
Vanilla	
Dannon Lowfat / 8 oz	200
Knudsen Lowfat / 8 oz	240
Knudsen Nonfat / 6 oz	70
Yoplait Custard Style / 6 oz	180
Yoplait Custard Style / 4 oz	130
Yoplait Nonfat / 8 oz	180
Yoplait Original / 6 oz	180
Yoplait Pudding / 4 oz	150
Vanilla bean / 8 oz / **Breyers** Lowfat	230
Wild berry / 4-⅗ oz / **Light n' Lively** Lowfat	140

FROZEN BARS

Chocolate / 1 bar / **Dole** Yogurt Bars	70
Strawberry / 1 bar / **Dole** Yogurt Bars	70
Strawberry banana / 1 bar / **Dole** Yogurt Bars	60

FROZEN YOGURT

Regular

Black cherry / ½ cup / **Breyers**	140
Black cherry / ½ cup / **Sealtest** Free Nonfat	110
Chocolate	
Baskin-Robbins Lowfat / ½ cup	140
Baskin-Robbins Nonfat / ½ cup	110
Breyers / ½ cup	150
Häagen-Dazs / 3 fl oz	130
Sealtest Free Nonfat / ½ cup	110
Double chunk chocolate / ½ cup / **Frusen Glädjé**	160
Peach	
Breyers / ½ cup	140
Häagen-Dazs / 3 fl oz	120
Sealtest Free Nonfat / ½ cup	100
Praline almond / ½ cup / **Frusen Glädjé**	170
Raspberry / ½ cup / **Baskin-Robbins** Lowfat	120

Red raspberry / ½ cup / **Breyers**	140
Red raspberry / ½ cup / **Sealtest** Free Nonfat	100
Strawberry	
Baskin-Robbins Nonfat / ½ cup	110
Breyers / ½ cup	140
Frusen Glädjé / ½ cup	120
Häagen-Dazs / 3 fl oz	120
Sealtest Free Nonfat / ½ cup	100
Strawberry banana / ½ cup / **Breyers**	130
Vanilla	
Baskin-Robbins Lowfat / ½ cup	120
Baskin-Robbins Nonfat / ½ cup	100
Breyers / ½ cup	140
Frusen Glädjé / ½ cup	130
Häagen-Dazs / 3 fl oz	130
Sealtest Free Nonfat / ½ cup	100
Vanilla almond crunch / 3 fl oz / **Häagen-Dazs**	150

Soft: 1 fl oz

Chocolate / **Häagen-Dazs**	30
Chocolate / **Häagen-Dazs** Non Fat	30
Coffee / **Häagen-Dazs**	28
Raspberry / **Häagen-Dazs**	30
Strawberry / **Häagen-Dazs** Non Fat	25
Vanilla / **Häagen-Dazs**	28

Restaurant Calorie Guide

To be sure, it is difficult to know the calories in restaurant food because recipes and specialties can differ greatly. However, here is a general dining-out calorie guide, based on figures for typical restaurant foods including American and ethnic foods, as compiled by the U.S. Department of Agriculture's continuing food consumption surveys, conducted mostly during 1985 and 1986. Agriculture officials use these calorie counts in estimating the nutritional value of the American diet.

It is important to point out that these government figures for restaurant foods are *approximate*—typical of what experts expect to find in restaurant dishes. Obviously, the calorie counts for restaurant foods cannot be precise because recipes and portions vary. Agriculture nutritionists calculate the calories in typical serving sizes, using classic recipes from standard cookbooks. The ingredients are quite similar from restaurant to restaurant in a dish like chicken curry or a reuben sandwich or paella, for example. Often, restaurant recipes are primarily distinguished not by a difference in basic high-calorie ingredients, but by spices, flavoring and other ingredients of little caloric importance.

Although these calorie counts are not absolute, they are some of the most authoritative available and fill a critical gap for calorie watchers who frequently eat out. At very least, the figures help guide you to dishes that are traditionally lower in calories and enable you to compare the over-all caloric expectations in various types of restaurants. Governmental authorities have enough confidence in the general accuracy of the figures to use them in assessing the nation's caloric energy intakes. Additionally, the author made further calculations for Japanese sushi and tempura, using basic information from the USDA and measurements obtained in a typical Japanese restaurant.

All of the portions are *average*, the size government analysts expect typical restaurants to serve. More precise measurements, such as one cup, 3 ounces, etc., are given when available to help you better judge the serving size.

The calorie counts in fast foods, obtained from the companies, are based on standardized restaurant chain recipes and serving sizes and vary only slightly, if at all, throughout the country.

Restaurants

AMERICAN

Includes regional cooking and delicatessen Jewish foods

Apple cobbler / ½ cup	235
Baked Alaska / 1 piece	350
Banana split	80
Boston baked beans / ½ cup	155
Blintz, cheese / 1 blintz	139
Blintz, fruit / 1 blintz	125
Caesar salad / 1 cup	160
Carrot cake / 1/12 of 10-in cake	550
Cheesecake / 1/12 of 9-in cake	406
Chicken a la king / ¾ cup	345
Chicken croquettes / 3 oz	222
Chicken fricasse / ¾ cup	290
Chicken w dumplings / 1 cup	373
Chicken and noodles / ¾ cup	275
Chicken salad / ¾ cup	314
Clams, raw / 1 clam	12
Clams raw / half dozen on half shell	72
Clams, breaded, fried / 3 oz or about ½ cup	158
Codfish balls / 1 piece	227
Codfish, creamed / ¾ cup	250
Coleslaw / ½ cup	115
Corned beef hash / 1 cup	344

CALORIES

Crabs, steamed / 1 medium, Chesapeake Bay	17
Crab cake / 1 cake or 4 oz	203
Crab Imperial / ¾ cup	281
Crab salad / ¾ cup	205
Crayfish tails / 3 oz	88
Crayfish tails / 1 tail	5
Deviled crab / ¾ cup	250
Flounder, stuffed w crab / 7-½ oz	310
Green pepper, stuffed / ½ pepper	200
Ham salad / ¾ cup	298
Hush puppies / 1 piece	73
Julienne salad wo dressing / 1 cup	73
Julienne salad wo dressing / 1 salad	300
Julienne salad w dressing / 1 cup	510
Kidney bean salad / ½ cup	175
Knish, cheese / 1 knish	208
Knish, potato / 1 knish	204
Liver, chopped w egg and onion / ¾ cup	225
Lobster, steamed or broiled in shell / 1 lb	105
Lobster tail	
1 small	45
1 medium	95
1 large	170
Lobster, stuffed and baked / 14 oz w o shell	750
Lobster Newburg / ¾ cup	454
Lobster Norfolk / ¾ cup	333
Lobster salad / ¾ cup	102
Matzo balls / one matzo	50
Matzo ball soup / 1 cup	120
Meat loaf / 1 medium slice (3-½ oz)	240
Mussels, cooked	
1 small	10
½ cup	120
Oysters, fried, breaded / 1 medium	25
Potato, baked / 1 medium	130
Salmon croquettes / 1 croquette	272
Salmon salad / ¾ cup	320
Shoe-fly pie / ⅛ of 9-inch pie	392
Shrimp, stuffed / 1 shrimp	30
Shrimp, creole / 1 cup	300
Shrimp gumbo w rice / 1 cup	300

Shrimp jambalaya w rice / 1 cup	300
Shrimp salad / ¾ cup	210
Smoked salmon / 1 piece (about ⅔ oz)	35
Sundae, fruit	330
Tuna salad / ¾ cup	290
Turkey salad / ¾ cup	314
Vegetables, batter-fried	
Broccoli / 1 cup	160
Cauliflower / ½ cup	83
Eggplant / 1 stick	45
Okra / ½ cup	88
Onion rings	
1 large ring	40
1 medium ring	25
Zucchini / 1 slice	25

Breakfast or Brunch Foods

Eggs	
Fried / 1 egg	100
Hard or soft boiled / 1 egg	80
Poached / 1 egg	80
Scrambled / 1 egg	110
Benedict / 1 egg	335
Omelets, two eggs	
Plain	215
Cheese	295
Ham	350
Ham and cheese	450
Spanish	328
Western	358
Corn meal mush, fried / 1 slice	85
Croissant, fresh / 1 croissant	205
Danish pastry / 1 piece	270
Grits / ⅔ cup	83
Pancakes / 1 cake, 6-in diam	162
Quiche Lorraine / ⅛ of 9-in diam	593
Spinach quiche / ⅛ of 9-in diam	335
Waffles / 2 pieces, 4-in squares	204

Salad Bar

Bacon bits / 1 tbsp	27
Beets, pickled, canned / ⅛ cup	18
Broccoli / ⅛ cup	3
Carrots / ⅛ cup	6
Cheese	
Cheddar / 2 tbsp	21
Cottage / ½ cup	116
Parmesan / 2 tbsp	45
Chickpeas / 2 tbsp	21
Cucumber / 2 tbsp	2
Egg, chopped / 2 tbsp	27
Lettuce / ¼ cup	18
Mushrooms, sliced / 2 tbsp	3
Onions / 2 tbsp	3
Pepper, green / 2 tbsp	3
Potato salad / ½ cup	180
Sprouts, alfalfa / 2 tbsp	2
Tomato / 2 slices	3

Salad Dressings: 1 tbsp

Blue	75
French	79
Italian	78
Italian, low calorie	7
Oil/vinegar	72
Thousand Island	56

Sandwiches

Bacon and cheese	439
Bacon and egg	391
Bacon, lettuce and tomato	346
Bologna	260
Cheese	275
Cheeseburger, plain on bun	323
Chicken salad	279
Chili dog	413
Club (bacon, tomato, chicken)	502

CALORIES

Corn dog	278
Corned beef	250
Crabcake	318
Egg	230
Egg salad	290
Fish on bun	375
Ham	260
Ham and cheese	381
Ham and cheese, grilled	417
Ham and egg	269
Ham salad	258
Hero, ham and cheese	445
Hoagie, cheese	440
Hot dog, plain	263
Hot dog w condiments	296
Pastrami	338
Peanut butter	280
Peanut butter and jelly	315
Pig in blanket	278
Reuben	535
Roast beef	341
Salami	238
Sausage	345
Sloppy Joe on bun	387
Steak	438
Steak and cheese	543
Submarine, regular	560
Submarine, steak, w tomato	438
Turkey salad	218
Tuna salad	374

CHINESE

Bean sprouts, fried / ¼ cup	40
Beef chow mein w noodles / 1 cup	405
Beef chop suey w noodles / 1 cup	405
Beef chow mein wo noodles / ¾ cup	204
Beef and broccoli / ¾ cup	185
Beef and green beans / ½ cup	130
Beef and vegetables, stir fried / ¾ cup	115
Bird's nest soup / 1 cup	30

	CALORIES
Chicken chow mein w noodles / 1 cup	287
Chicken chow mein wo noodles / ¾ cup	145
Chinese barbecue pork or roast pork / ¾ cup	340
Chinese pancake / 1 cake	60
Chow mein noodles / ½ cup	110
Dim sum / 1 dumpling	55
Egg drop soup / 1 cup	65
Egg foo yung, pork / 1 patty	100
Egg foo yung, shrimp / 1 patty	175
Egg roll w meat / 1 (2-¼ oz)	120
Egg roll w shrimp: 1 (2-¼ oz)	106
Egg roll, vegetarian: 1 (2-¼ oz)	103
Fried rice w bean sprouts / ½ cup	160
Fried rice w shrimp / ¾ cup	215
Hot and sour soup / 1 cup	100
Lo mein w meat / 1 cup	285
Lychee, fresh / 1 fruit	8
Pancake / 1 pancake	60
Pepper beef / 1 cup	240
Pork chop suey w noodles / 1 cup	430
Pork chop suey wo noodles / ¾ cup	223
Rice cake / 1 oz	80
Shrimp chop suey w noodles / 1 cup	235
Shrimp chow mein w noodles / 1 cup	265
Shrimp chow mein wo noodles / ¾ cup	141
Shrimp w lobster sauce / ¾ cup	216
Stir fried vegetables / ½ cup	85
Sweet and sour shrimp w sauce / ¾ cup	460
Sweet and sour pork w pineapple / ¾ cup	475
Sweet and sour soup / 1 cup	30
Won ton chips / 1 piece	10
Won ton, fried / 1 piece	20
Won ton, meat-filled, fried / 1 piece	60
Won ton soup / 1 cup	210

ENGLISH

Beef Wellington / 1 slice (4 oz)	325
Brunswick stew / ¾ cup	300
Scone / 1 regular	150
Shepherd's pie / 1 cup	304

CALORIES

Welsh rarebit / ½ cup	205
Yorkshire pudding / 3-in square	170

FRENCH AND CONTINENTAL

Beef Bourguignon / ¾ cup	194
Beef burgundy / ¾ cup	230
Beef stroganoff / ¾ cup	308
Beef stroganoff w noodles / 1 cup	342
Bouillabaisse / 1 cup	230
Brioche / 1 medium	270
Cheese fondue / ¼ cup	125
Cheese souffle / 1 cup	205
Chicken cordon bleu / 8 oz	437
Chocolate eclair / 1 eclair	220
Chocolate mousse / ½ cup	175
Crepe, fruit-filled / 1 crepe	95
Crepe, filled w poultry or meat w sauce / 1 crepe	250
Escargots / 1 snail	8
Fish timbale or mousse / ¾ cup	272
French horn / 1 piece	135
Frog legs / 1 fried leg	60
Hollandaise sauce / 2 tbsp	135
Meringue / 1 piece (4x2x2 in)	85
Swedish meatballs / ¾ cup	275

GERMAN

Apple strudel / 1 piece (about 3 oz)	280
Frankfurters and sauerkraut / 1 frank w kraut	158
German potato salad / ½ cup	110
Sauerbraten / 1 piece 3x2x¾-in or 3-½ oz	190
Weiner schnitzel / 1 piece (about 3-½ oz)	280

GREEK

Baklava / 1 piece	332
Gyros sandwich	215
Pita bread	
1 small	165

1 large	265
Spanakopita / 1 serving	255

INDIAN

Chapati / 1 piece	73
Chutney / 1 tbsp	28
Curry, beef / ¾ cup	345
Curry, shrimp / ¾ cup	232
Curry, chicken / ¾ cup	302
Curried chick peas and potatoes / ½ cup	111
Paratha (fried bread) / 1 piece (about 1 oz)	96
Puri bread / 1 piece	115

ITALIAN

Antipasto	
1 small	125
1 large	250
1 cup	150
Bread sticks / 1 medium	40
Calzone, meat and cheese / ½ calzone (about 7-½ oz)	736
Cannoli / 1 piece	234
Chicken cacciatore / ¾ cup	345
Chicken tetrazzini / 1 cup	210
Clams casino	
1 large	100
1 small	50
Eggplant parmesan / ½ cup	190
Garlic bread / 1 medium slice	100
Gnocchi, cheese / 1 cup	125
Fettucine Alfredo / 1 cup	270
Manicotti, cheese w meat sauce / 1 manicotti	235
manicotti, cheese w tomato sauce / 1 manicotti	223
Lasagna / 1 cup	350
Lasagna, meatless / 1 piece (2-½ in x 4-in)	317
Pasta salad, vegetable / ¾ cup	253
Pizza	
Cheese, thin crust / ⅛ of 12-in pizza	163
Cheese, thick crust / ⅛ of 12-in pizza	203
Meat, cheese, thin crust / ⅛ of 12-in pizza	210

Meat, cheese, thick crust / ⅛ of 12-in pizza	250
Vegetarian, thin crust / ⅛ of 12-in pizza	150
Vegetarian, thick crust / ⅛ of 12-in pizza	192
Polenta / ⅔ cup	165
Ratatouille / ½ cup	73
Ravioli, cheese-filled w tomato sauce / 1 cup	338
Ravioli, cheese-filled w tomato beef sauce / 1 cup	360
Ravioli, meat-filled w tomato sauce / 1 cup	386
Rigatoni w sausage / ¾ cup	260
Rissoto / ½ cup	180
Spaghetti w meat sauce / 1 cup	255
Spaghetti w tomato sauce / 1 cup	155
Spaghetti w meatballs and tomato sauce / 1 cup	330
Spaghetti w meatballs, tomato sauce and cheese / 1 cup	225
Spaghetti w red clam sauce / 1 cup	225
Spaghetti carbonara / 1 cup	372
Tortellini (meat-filled) w tomato sauce / 1 cup	262
Veal parmigiana / 1 piece (about 6 oz)	350
Veal scallopini / 1 slice (about 3-½ oz)	255
Ziti / 1 cup	350

JAPANESE

Japanese pickles (tsukemono) / ¼ cup	7
Japanese pickled cabbage / ¼ cup	7
Japanese radish (daikon) / ½ cup	14
Kim chee / 1 cup	30
Miso soup / 1 cup	78
Sashimi, tuna / 1 cubic inch	25
Sashimi / 1 2-in piece (⅓ oz)	12
Sukiyaki / ¾ cup	130
Sushi, roll: 1 piece (⅙ roll usually)	
w cucumber (kappa maki)	30
w tuna (tekka maki)	32
California roll	35
Sushi: 1 piece	
Eel (anago)	80
Flounder	55
Salmon	50
Shrimp (ebi)	45
Tuna (maguro)	50

Yellowtail	54
Seaweed and soy sauce / ½ cup	20
Tempura, fish cake / 10 oz	466
Tempura	
Shrimp / 1 jumbo shrimp	70
Softshell crab / 1 crab (2-¼ oz)	215
Vegetable / 1 cup or about (2-¼ oz)	100
1 small piece	20
1 large piece	40
Teriyaki, chicken / 6-½ oz	257
Teriyaki, steak / 6-½ oz	317
Tofu, stir fried / ½ cup	66
Tofu, deep fried / 1 oz	75
Tofu w beef and vegetables / ¾ cup	200

LATIN AMERICAN

Arroz con pollo / 1 cup wo bones	185
Black bean soup / 1 cup	116
Cheese, white (queso del pais blanco) / 1 cubic in	25
Cuban sandwich	672
Diplomat pudding / ½ cup	395
Flan / 1 custard cup	195
Gazpacho / 1 cup	56
Guava nectar / ½ cup	65
Guava paste / 1 medium piece (1 oz)	90
Octopus salad / ¾ cup	277
Paella / 1 cup	350
Plantain, fried (tostones) / ½ cup	210
Plantain, ripe, fried / 2-in piece	50
Pumpkin pudding, Puerto Rican / 1 piece, (2-½ in x 2 in x 1- in)	185
Red beans, stewed / ½ cup	185
Rice and beans / ⅔ cup	150
Seviche / ¾ cup	122
Veal marengo / 1 cup	200
Yucca, white, boiled / ½ cup	110
Zarzuela / ¾ cup	310

MEXICAN

1 whole item unless otherwise noted

	CALORIES
Burrito,	
Beef and beans	290
Beef, beans and cheese	388
Bean and cheese	286
Chalupe, chicken and cheese	311
Chiles rellenos	218
Chili con carne	
Beans / 1 cup	311
Beans and rice / 1 cup	308
Chili con queso	
¼ cup	135
1 tbsp	35
Chimichanga, beef and cheese / about 4 oz	282
Chimichanga, chicken and sour cream / about 4 oz	214
Enchilada	
Cheese	164
Beef and beans	192
Beef and cheese	235
Chicken	168
Chicken and cheese	214
Guacamole / ½ cup	240
Nachos, cheese and bean / 1 piece	50
Quesadilla	190
Refried beans / ½ cup	210
Taco	
Bean and cheese	144
Beef and cheese	180
Chicken and cheese	148
Taco salad / 1 cup	202
Tamale	183
Taquito	185
Tortilla, corn, plain	32
Tortilla, flour, plain	118
Tostada	
Bean and cheese	144
Beef and cheese	180
Chicken and cheese	148

CALORIES

MIDDLE EASTERN

Cabbage rolls / 1 roll	100
Grape leaves, stuffed w rice / 1 roll	145
Hummus / 1 oz (about 1-¾ tbsp)	45
Kibbe / 1 cup	375
Lamb shishkabob	
1 medium	115
1 large	225
Turkish coffee / 4 fl oz	45

MIDDLE EUROPEAN

Noodles, Romanoff / 1 cup	270
Pierogi / 1 pastry	105
Potato pancakes / 1 medium	105
Rice pilaf / ¾ cup	200
Shav soup / 1 cup	60
Veal Goulash / 1 cup	200
Veal Paprikash / ½ cup	230

WINES AND BAR DRINKS

1 typical drink

Bacardi	118
Black Russian	255
Bloody Mary	125
Bourbon and soda	105
Brandy, straight / 1 fl oz	65
Brandy Alexander	180
Daiquiri	113
Gibson	158
Gimlet	132
Gin / 1 jigger	110
Gin and tonic	170
Gin rickey	115
Grasshopper	165
Hot buttered rum	180
Mai Tai	310

Manhattan	130
Margarita	170
Martini	160
Mint julep	155
Old fashioned	155
Pina colada	230
Rum / 1 jigger	100
Sangria	155
Scotch and soda	105
Screwdriver	182
Singapore sling	228
Sloe gin fizz	120
Stinger	282
Tequila sunrise	190
Tom Collins	120
Vodka / 1 jigger	100
Whiskey / 1 jigger	105
Whiskey sour	122
White Russian	268

Wine

Dry, dinner wines / 1 wine glass (3-½ fl oz)	70
Dessert wines (Marsala, port, tokay, madeira, sherry, sweet vermouth) / 1 wine glass (3-½ fl oz)	150
Wine spritzer	60

Fast Foods

Fast Foods

1 serving unless noted

ARBY'S

	CALORIES
Arby's Sauce / ½ oz	15
Au Jus / 4 oz	7
Bacon Platter	860
Biscuit, Bacon	318
Biscuit, Ham	323
Biscuit, Plain	280
Biscuit, Sausage	460
Blueberry Muffin	200
Cheesecake	306
Chicken Breast Sandwich	489
Chicken Cordon Bleu Sandwich	658
Chicken Fajita Pita Sandwich	272
Chocolate Chip Cookie	130
Cinnamon Nut Danish	340
Croissant, Bacon and Egg	389
Croissant, Ham and Cheese	345
Croissant, Mushroom and Cheese	493
Croissant, Plain	260
Croissant, Sausage and Egg	519
Egg Platter	460
Fish Fillet Sandwich	537
Grilled Chicken Barbecue Sandwich	378
Grilled Chicken Deluxe Sandwich	426

CALORIES

Ham Deluxe Light Sandwich	255
Ham Platter	518
Ham 'n Cheese Sandwich	330
Horsey Sauce / ½ oz	55
Maple Syrup / 1-½ oz	120
Polar Swirl, Butterfinger	457
Polar Swirl, Heath	543
Polar Swirl, Oreo	482
Polar Swirl, Peanut Butter Cup	517
Polar Swirl, Snickers	511
Potatoes	
Baked with Butter and Sour Cream	463
Broccoli 'n Cheddar Baked	417
Cakes	204
Cheddar Fries	399
Curly Fries	337
Deluxe Baked	621
French Fries	246
Mushroom 'n Cheese Baked	515
Plain Baked	240
Roast Beef 'n Cheddar Sandwich	451
Roast Beef Bac'N Cheddar Deluxe Sandwich	532
Roast Beef Deluxe Light Sandwich	294
Roast Beef French Dip 'N Swiss Sandwich	425
Roast Beef French Dip Sandwich	345
Roast Beef Giant Sandwich	530
Roast Beef Junior Sandwich	218
Roast Beef Philly 'N Swiss Sandwich	498
Roast Beef Regular Sandwich	353
Roast Beef Super Sandwich	529
Roast Chicken Club Sandwich	513
Roast Chicken Deluxe Light Sandwich	263
Roast Chicken Deluxe Sandwich	373
Roast Turkey Deluxe Light Sandwich	260
Salad Chef	210
Salad Chef Light	205
Salad Chicken Cashew	590
Salad Dressings	
Blue Cheese / 2 oz	295
Buttermilk Ranch / 2 oz	349
Creamy French Weight Watchers / 1 oz	48

CALORIES

Creamy Italian Weight Watchers / 1 oz	29
Croutons / ½ oz	59
Honey French / 2 oz	322
Italian Light / 2 oz	23
Thousand Island / 2 oz	298
Salad Garden	149
Salad Garden Light	109
Salad Roast Chicken Light	184
Salad Side Light	25
Sausage Platter	640
Shakes	
Chocolate	451
Jamocha	368
Vanilla	330
Soups	
Beef with Vegetables and Barley	96
Boston Clam Chowder	207
Cream of Broccoli	180
French Onion	67
Lumberjack Mixed Vegetable	89
Old Fashioned Chicken Noodle	99
Pilgrim's Corn Chowder	193
Split Pea with Ham	200
Tomato Florentine	84
Wisconsin Cheese	287
Sub Deluxe Sandwich	482
Toastix	420
Turkey Deluxe Sandwich	399
Turnover, Apple	303
Turnover, Blueberry	320
Turnover, Cherry	280

ARTHUR TREACHER'S FISH & CHIPS

Chicken, Fried	369
Chicken Sandwich	413
Chips French Fries	276
Chowder	112
Cole Slaw	123
Fish, Broiled / 6 oz	245
Fish, Fried / 2 pieces	355

Fish Sandwich	440
Krunch Pup	203
Lemon Luv	276
Shrimp, Fried	381

BURGER KING

Breakfast Buddy w Sausage, Egg and Cheese	255
Burger Buddies	349
Cheeseburger	318
Cheeseburger, Bacon, Double	507
Cheeseburger, Bacon, Double Deluxe	584
Cheeseburger, Deluxe	390
Cheeseburger, Double	483
Chicken Sandwich	685
Chicken Sandwich, BK Broiler	267
Chicken Tenders / 6 pieces	236
Croissan'wich w Bacon, Egg and Cheese	353
Croissan'wich w Ham, Egg and Cheese	351
Croissan'wich w Sausage, Egg and Cheese	534
Filet of Fish Sandwich, Ocean Catch	479
French Fries, Medium, Salted	372
French Toast Sticks	538
Hamburger	272
Hamburger Deluxe	344
Hash Browns	213
Ice Cream Bar, Snickers	220
Muffins, Blueberry Mini	292
Onion Rings	339
Pies	
Apple	311
Cherry	360
Lemon	290
Salad, Chef wo Dressing	178
Salad, Chicken Chunky wo Dressing	142
Salad Dressings: 2 oz	
Bleu Cheese	300
French Newman's Own	290
Italian Light, Reduced Calorie, Newman's Own	170
Olive Oil and Vinegar, Newman's Own	310
Ranch, Newman's Own	350

CALORIES

Thousand Island, Newman's Own	290
Salad, Garden wo Dressing	95
Salad, Side wo Dressing	25
Sauces: 1 oz	
A M Express Dip	84
Barbecue Dipping	36
Honey Dipping	91
Ranch Dipping	171
Sweet and Sour Dipping	45
Shakes	
Chocolate	326
Chocolate w Syrup Added	409
Strawberry w Syrup Added	394
Vanilla	334
Whopper	
Double Sandwich	844
Double Sandwich w Cheese	935
Sandwich	614
Sandwich w Cheese	706

CARL'S JR.

American Cheese / 1 oz	60
Bacon / 2 strips	45
Blueberry Muffin	340
Bran Muffin	310
Breakfast Burrito	430
Cheeseburger, Bacon, Western	730
Cheeseburger, Bacon, Western, Double	1030
Cheeseburger, Southwestern	590
Cheesecake	310
Chicken Club Sandwich, Charbroiler	570
Chicken Sandwich, Charbroiler BBQ	310
Chicken Sandwich, Sante Fe	540
Chicken Strips / 6 pieces	260
Chili Dog, All-Star	720
Chocolate Chip Cookies	330
Cinnamon Rolls	460
CrissCut Fries	330
Danish	520
English Muffin w Margarine	190

CALORIES

Fish Sandwich, Carl's Catch	560
French Fries, Regular	420
French Toast Dips	490
Fudge Brownie	430
Fudge Moussecake	400
Hamburger	320
Hamburger, Carl's Original	460
Hamburger, Famous Star	610
Hamburger, Super Star	820
Hash Brown Nuggets	270
Hot Cakes w Margarine	510
Hot Dog, All-Star	540
Onion Rings	520
Potatoes	
Bacon and Cheese	730
Broccoli and Cheese	590
Cheese	690
Lite	290
Sour Cream and Chives	470
Roast Beef Club Sandwich	620
Roast Beef Sandwich Deluxe	540
Salad, Chicken To Go	200
Salad Dressings: 1 oz	
Blue Cheese	150
French, Reduced Calorie	40
House	110
Italian	120
Thousand Island	110
Salad, Garden To Go, Small	50
Salsa / 1 oz	8
Sausage	190
Scrambled Eggs	120
Shakes, Regular	350
Sunrise Sandwich	300
Swiss Cheese / 1 oz	60
Zucchini	390

CHURCH'S FRIED CHICKEN

Chicken	
Dark meat, one average portion	305

CALORIES

White meat, one average portion	327
Breast	283
Leg	172
Thigh	319
Wing	279
Snack, one large piece chicken	316
Dinner roll	83
Coleslaw / 3 oz	83
Corn on the cob, buttered / 9 oz	165
French fries / 3 oz	256
Jalapeno pepper	4
Pie, Apple / 3 oz	300
Pie, Pecan / 3 oz	367

DAIRY QUEEN/BRAZIER

Banana Split	510
Blizzard, Heath / Regular	820
Blizzard, Heath / Small	560
Blizzard, Strawberry / Regular	740
Blizzard, Strawberry / Small	500
Breeze, Heath / Regular	680
Breeze, Heath / Small	450
Breeze, Strawberry / Regular	590
Breeze, Strawberry / Small	400
Buster Bar	450
Cones	
Chocolate / Large	350
Chocolate / Regular	230
Dipped Chocolate / Regular	330
Vanilla / Large	340
Vanilla / Regular	230
Vanilla / Small	140
Yogurt / Large	260
Yogurt / Regular	180
Cup, Yogurt / Large	230
Cup, Yogurt / Regular	170
Dilly Bar	210
DQ Frozen Cake Slice	380
DQ Homestyle Ultimate Burger	700
DQ Sandwich	140
French Fries / Large	390

CALORIES

French Fries / Regular	300
French Fries / Small	210
Hamburger	310
Hamburger, Double	460
Hamburger, Double with Cheese	570
Hamburger with Cheese	365
Hot Dog	280
Hot Dog, ¼-lb Super Dog	590
Hot Dog with Cheese	330
Hot Dog with Chili	320
Hot Fudge Brownie Delight	710
Malt, Vanilla / Regular	610
Mr. Misty / Regular	250
Nutty Double Fudge	580
Onion Rings / Regular	240
Peanut Buster Parfait	710
QC Chocolate Big Scoop	310
QC Vanilla Big Scoop	300
Salad Dressings: 2 oz	
French, Reduced Calorie	90
Thousand Island	225
Salad, Garden wo Dressing	200
Salad, Side wo Dressing	25
Sandwiches	
Beef BBQ	225
Chicken Fillet, Breaded	430
Chicken Fillet, Breaded with Cheese	480
Chicken Fillet, Grilled	300
Fish Fillet	370
Fish Fillet with Cheese	420
Shakes	
Chocolate / Regular	540
Vanilla / Large	600
Vanilla / Regular	520
Sundaes	
Chocolate / Regular	300
Strawberry, Waffle Cone	350
200 Yogurt, Strawberry / Regular	

DUNKIN' DONUTS

Apple-Filled w Cinnamon Sugar Yeast Donut	250
Bavarian-Filled w Chocolate Frosting Yeast Donut	240
Blueberry-Filled Yeast Donut	210
Chocolate Chunk Cookie	200
Chocolate Chunk Cookie w Nuts	210
Chocolate Frosted Yeast Ring	200
Croissant, Almond	420
Croissant, Chocolate	440
Croissant, Plain	310
Glazed Buttermilk Ring	290
Glazed Chocolate Ring	324
Glazed Coffee Roll	280
Glazed French Cruller	140
Glazed Whole Wheat Ring	330
Glazed Yeast Ring	200
Jelly-Filled Yeast Donut	220
Lemon-Filled Yeast Donut	260
Muffins	
Apple 'n Spice	300
Banana Nut	310
Blueberry	280
Bran w Raisins	310
Corn	340
Cranberry Nut	290
Oat Bran	330
Oatmeal Pecan Raisin Cookie	200
Plain Cake Ring	270

HARDEE'S

Bacon and Egg Biscuit	410
Bacon Biscuit	360
Bacon Egg and Cheese Biscuit	460
Big Cookie	250
Big Country Breakfast, Bacon	660
Big Country Breakfast, Country Ham	670
Big Country Breakfast, Ham	620
Big Country Breakfast, Sausage	850

CALORIES

Big Deluxe Burger	500
Big Twin	450
Biscuit 'n Gravy	440
Blueberry Muffin	400
Canadian Rise 'n Shine Biscuit	470
Cheeseburger	320
Cheeseburger, Bacon	610
Cheeseburger/Quarter Pounder	500
Chicken Biscuit	430
Chicken	
Breast	460
Leg	220
Thigh	520
Wing	280
Chicken Stix / 6 pieces	210
Chicken Stix / 9 pieces	310
Cinnamon 'n Raisin	320
Cone	20
Cool Twist Cone, Chocolate	200
Cool Twist Cone, Vanilla	190
Cool Twist Cone, Vanilla and Chocolate	190
Cool Twist Sundae, Caramel	330
Cool Twist Sundae, Hot Fudge	320
Cool Twist Sundae, Strawberry	260
Cool Twist Yogurt, Chocolate	170
Cool Twist Yogurt, Vanilla	160
French Fries	
Big Fry / 5.5 oz	500
Crispy Curls	300
Large / 4 oz	360
Regular / 2.5 oz	230
Gravy / 5 oz	60
Ham and Egg Biscuit	370
Ham Biscuit	320
Ham, Country and Egg Biscuit	400
Ham, Country Biscuit	350
Ham, Egg and Cheese Biscuit	420
Hamburger	270
Hash Rounds	230
Hot Dog, All Beef	300
Margarine, Butter Blend / ⅕ oz	35

CALORIES

Mashed Potatoes / 4 oz	70
Mashed Potatoes / 12 oz	220
Mushroom 'n Swiss Burger	490
Oat Bran Raisin Muffin	440
Pancakes: 3 cakes	280
w One Sausage Pattie	430
w Two Bacon Strips	350
Rise 'n Shine Biscuit	320
Salads	
Chef	240
Chicken 'n Pasta	230
Cole Slaw / 4 oz	320
Cole Slaw / 12 oz	990
Garden	210
Side	20
Sandwiches	
Big Roast Beef	300
Chicken Fillet	370
Chicken, Grilled	310
Fisherman's Fillet	500
Hot Ham 'n Cheese	330
Roast Beef / Regular	260
Turkey Club	390
Sausage and Egg Biscuit	490
Sausage Biscuit	440
Shakes	
Chocolate	460
Strawberry	440
Vanilla	400
Steak and Egg Biscuit	550
Steak Biscuit	500
Syrup / 1-½ oz	120
Turnover, Apple	270

JACK IN THE BOX

Breakfast Jack	307
Cheeseburger	315
Cheeseburger, Bacon Bacon	705
Cheeseburger / Double	467
Cheeseburger, Ultimate	942

Cheesecake	309
Chicken Strips / 4 pieces	285
Chicken Strips / 6 pieces	451
Double Fudge Cake	288
Egg Rolls / 3 pieces	437
Egg Rolls / 5 pieces	753
French Fries	
Jumbo	396
Regular	351
Small	219
Grape Jelly	38
Hamburger	267
Hamburger, Grilled, Sourdough	712
Hash Browns	156
Jumbo Jack	584
Jumbo Jack with Cheese	677
Onion Rings	380
Pancake Platter	612
Pancake Syrup	121
Salad, Chef	325
Salad Dressings	
Bleu Cheese	262
Buttermilk House Dressing	362
French, Reduced Calorie	176
Thousand Island	312
Salad, Side	51
Salad, Taco	503
Sandwiches	
Chicken and Mushroom	440
Chicken Fajita Pita	292
Chicken Supreme	641
Fish Supreme	510
Grilled Chicken Fillet	408
Ham and Turkey Melt	592
Old Fashioned Patty Melt	713
Pastrami Melt	600
Sirloin Cheesesteak	621
Sourdough Breakfast	450
Steak Fajita Melt	433
Sauces: 1 oz	
BBQ	44

CALORIES

Guacamole	55
Salsa	8
Sweet and Sour	40
Sausage Crescent	584
Scrambled Egg Platter	559
Scrambled Egg Pocket	431
Seasoned Curly Fries	358
Sesame Breadsticks	70
Shakes	
Chocolate	330
Strawberry	320
Vanilla	320
Supreme Crescent	547
Taco	187
Taco, Super	281
Taquitos / 5 pieces	362
Taquitos / 7 pieces	511
Tortilla Chips	139
Turnover, Apple	348

KENTUCKY FRIED CHICKEN

Buttermilk Biscuit	235
Chicken Littles Sandwich	169
Chicken Nuggets / 6 pieces	284
Coleslaw	114
Colonel's Chicken Sandwich	482
Corn On The Cob	90
Extra Crispy Chicken	
Breast Center	344
Breast Side	379
Drumstick	205
Thigh	414
Wing	231
French Fries	244
French Fries, Crispy Fries	294
Hot and Spicy Chicken	
Breast Center	382
Breast Side	398
Drumstick	207
Thigh	412

Wing	244
Hot Wings / 6 pieces	471
Lite 'N Crispy Chicken	
Breast Center	220
Breast Side	204
Drumstick	121
Thigh	246
Mashed Potatoes and Gravy	71
Original Recipe Chicken	
Breast Center	260
Breast Side	245
Drumstick	152
Thigh	287
Wing	172
Sauces	
Barbeque / 1 oz	35
Honey / ½ oz	49
Mustard / 1 oz	36
Sweet and Sour / 1 oz	58

LONG JOHN SILVER'S

Brownie, Walnut	440
Chicken	
Baked, Light Herb / 3 pieces	130
Baked w rice, green beans, slaw and roll	570
Plank / one piece	130
Planks / 2 pieces	270
Planks / 2 pieces and fries	440
Planks / 3 pieces w fries, slaw and 2 hush puppies	860
Sandwich, Baked wo sauce	310
Sandwich, Batter-dipped / 2 pieces wo sauce	440
Clams / 6 oz w fries, slaw and 2 hush puppies	910
Coleslaw, drained on fork	140
Cookie, Chocolate Chip	230
Cookie, Oatmeal Raisin	160
Corn Cobbette / one piece w prep	140
Fish	
Baked Light w lemon crumbs / 2 pieces w rice and small salad wo dressing	270
Baked w lemon crumbs / 3 pieces	150

Baked w lemon crumbs / 3 pieces w rice, green beans, slaw and roll	580
Batter-dipped / one piece	210
and chicken / one each and fries	510
and chicken / one fish, 2 chicken w fries and slaw	930
and fries / 2 pieces	580
Homestyle / one piece	110
Long John's Homestyle / 3 pieces w fries and slaw	780
& More / 2 pieces w fries and slaw	860
Sandwich, Batter-dipped / one piece wo sauce	380
Shrimp and chicken w fries and slaw	1130
Shrimp and clams w fries and slaw	1200
and shrimp w fries and slaw	1070
Fries / one order	170
Hush Puppy / 1 piece	70
Pie, Apple	320
Pie, Cherry	360
Pie, Lemon	340
Roll	110
Salad, Ocean Chef wo dressing	150
Salad, Seafood wo dressing	380
Salad, Small wo dressing	11
Salad Dressing, Creamy Italian / 1 oz	30
Salad Dressing, Ranch / 1 oz	180
Salad Dressing, Sea Salad / 1 oz	140
Sauces	
Honey Mustard / .42 oz	20
Malt Vinegar / .28 oz	1
Seafood / .42 oz	14
Sweet 'n Sour / .42 oz	20
Tartar / .42 oz	50
Seafood chowder w cod / 7 oz	140
Seafood gumbo w cod / 7 oz	120
Shrimp / 10 pieces w fries, slaw and 2 hush puppies	710
Shrimp / Batter-dipped / one piece	25
Shrimp Scampi, Baked w rice, green beans, slaw and roll	560
Vegetable, Green beans	20
Vegetable, Rice	160
Children's Menu	
Chicken Planks / 2 pieces and fries	510

Fish, chicken, fries and hush puppy	580
Fish / one piece, fries and hush puppy	450

McDONALD'S

Bacon, Egg and Cheese Biscuit	440
Big Mac	500
Biscuit with Biscuit Spread	260
Breakfast Burrito	280
Cheeseburger	305
Chicken Fajitas	185
Chicken McNuggets	270
Cone, Vanilla Frozen Yogurt	105
Cookies, Chocolaty Chip	330
Cookies, McDonaldland	290
Danish	
Apple	390
Cinnamon Raisin	440
Iced Cheese	390
Raspberry	410
Egg McMuffin	280
English Muffin with Spread	170
Filet-O-Fish	370
French Fries	
Large	400
Medium	320
Small	220
Hamburger	255
Hash Brown Potatoes	130
Hotcakes with Margarine and Syrup	440
McChicken	415
McLean Deluxe	320
McLean Deluxe with Cheese	370
Muffin, Apple Bran / Fat Free	180
Pie, Apple	260
Quarter Pounder	410
Quarter Pounder with Cheese	510
Salad	
Bacon Bits	15
Chef	170
Chicken Chunky	150

CALORIES

Croutons	50
Garden	50
Side	30
Salad Dressing	
Bleu Cheese / ½ oz	50
Ranch / ½ oz	55
Red French, Reduced Calorie / ½ oz	40
Thousand Island / ½ oz	45
Vinaigrette Lite / ½ oz	12
Sauces	
Barbecue / 1.12 oz	50
Honey / .5 oz	45
Hot Mustard / 1.05 oz	70
Sweet 'N Sour / 1.12 oz	60
Sausage	160
Sausage Biscuit	420
Sausage Biscuit with Egg	505
Sausage McMuffin	345
Sausage McMuffin with Egg	430
Scrambled Eggs / 2	140
Shake	
Chocolate	320
Strawberry	320
Vanilla	290
Sundae	
Hot Caramel w Frozen Yogurt	270
Hot Fudge w Frozen Yogurt	240
Strawberry w Frozen Yogurt	210

PIZZA HUT

2 slices / medium pizza unless noted

Hand-Tossed	
Cheese	518
Pepperoni	500
Super Supreme	556
Supreme	540
Pan Pizza	
Cheese	492
Pepperoni	540

CALORIES

Super Supreme	563
Supreme	589
Personal Pan Pizza Pepperoni / whole	675
Personal Pan Pizza Supreme / whole	647
Thin 'n Crispy	
Cheese	398
Pepperoni	413
Super Supreme	463
Supreme	459

PONDEROSA

Apple Rings, Spiced / 4 oz	100
Apples	80
Apples, Canned / 4 oz	90
Applesauce / 4 oz	80
Banana	87
Banana Chips / 1/10 oz	25
Banana Pudding / 1 oz	52
Beans, Baked / 4 oz	170
Beans, Green / 3-1/2 oz	20
Beets, Diced / 5 oz	55
Breadsticks, Italian	100
Broccoli / 1 oz	9
Cabbage, Green / 1 oz	9
Cabbage, Red / 1 oz	1
Cantaloupe	13
Carrots / 3-1/2 oz	31
Carrots / 1 oz	12
Cauliflower / 1 oz	8
Cauliflower, Breaded / 4 oz	115
Celery / 1 oz	4
Cheese, Shredded, Imitation / 1 oz	90
Cherry Peppers / 2 pieces	7
Chicken Breast	98
Chicken Salad / 3-1/2 oz	213
Chicken Wings / 2 pieces	213
Chopped Steak / 4 oz	225
Chopped Steak / 5-3/10 oz	296
Chow Mein Noodles / 1/5 oz	25
Coconut Shredded / 1/5 oz	25

CALORIES

Corn / 3-½ oz	90
Cottage Cheese / 4 oz	120
Crackers	
Meal Mates, Sesame / 2	45
Melba Snacks / 2	18
Ritz / 2	40
Saltine / 2	25
Sesame Breadsticks / 2	35
Croutons / 1 oz	115
Cucumber / 1 oz	4
Eggs, Diced / 2 oz	94
Fish	
Baked, Bake 'R Broil	230
Baked Scrod	120
Broiled Halibut	170
Broiled Roughy	139
Broiled Salmon	192
Broiled Swordfish	271
Broiled Trout	228
Fried	190
Nuggets	31
Fruit Cocktail / 4 oz	97
Garbanzo Beans / 1 oz	102
Gelatin, Plain / 4 oz	71
Granola / ⅕ oz	24
Grapes / 10	34
Gravy, Brown / 2 oz	25
Gravy, Turkey / 2 oz	25
Ham Diced / 2 oz	120
Honeydew Melon	25
Hot Dog	144
Ice Milk, Chocolate / 3-½ oz	152
Ice Milk, Vanilla / 3-½ oz	150
Kansas City Strip	138
Lemon	3
Lettuce / 1 oz	5
Macaroni and Cheese / 1 oz	17
Macaroni Salad / 3-½ oz	335
Margarine, Whipped / 1 tbsp	34
Meatball	58
Mousse, Chocolate / 1 oz	78

CALORIES

Mousse, Strawberry / 1 oz	74
Mushrooms / 1 oz	8
New York Strip / 10 oz	314
New York Strip / 8 oz	384
Okra, Breaded / 4 oz	124
Olive, Black	4
Olive, Green	3
Onion Rings, Breaded / 4 oz	213
Onion, Green	7
Onions, Red and Yellow / 1 oz	11
Orange	45
Pasta Salad, Pre-Made / 3-½ oz	269
Peaches, Canned / 4 oz	70
Peanuts, Granulated / ⅕ oz	30
Pears, Canned / 4 oz	98
Peas / 3-½ oz	67
Peppers, Green / 1 oz	6
Pickles, Dill Spears / .14 oz	0
Pickles, Sweet Chips / .14 oz	4
Pineapple, Fresh	11
Pineapple Tidbits / 4 oz	95
Porterhouse	640
Potato Salad / 3-½ oz	126
Potato Wedges / 3-½ oz	130
Potatoes	
Baked	145
French Fried	120
Mashed	62
Radishes / 1 oz	4
Ribeye	282
Rice Pilaf / 4 oz	160
Roll, Dinner	184
Roll, Sourdough	110
Salad, Cole Slaw / 1 oz	150
Salad Dressing: 1 oz unless noted	
Blue Cheese	130
Creamy Italian	103
Cucumber, Reduced Calorie	69
Italian, Reduced Calorie	31
Parmesan Pepper	150
Ranch	147

CALORIES

Salad Oil / 1 tbsp	120
Sweet 'n Tangy	122
Thousand Island	113
Sauce	
BBQ / 1 tbsp	25
Cheese / 2 oz	52
Cocktail / 1 oz	34
Spaghetti / 4 oz	110
Sweet and Sour / 1 oz	37
Tartar / 1 oz	85
Shells, Pasta / 2 oz	78
Shortening, Liquid / 1 oz	249
Shrimp, Fried / 7 pieces	231
Shrimp Mini / 6 pieces	47
Sirloin / 1	241
Sirloin Tips / 1	473
Sour Cream / 1 tbsp	26
Spaghetti / 2 oz	78
Spinach / 1 oz	7
Spread, Cheese / 1 oz	98
Spread, Cheese, Herb and Garlic / 1 tbsp	100
Sprinkles, Chocolate / .18 oz	24
Sprinkles, Rainbow / .18 oz	24
Sprouts, Alfalfa / 1 oz	10
Sprouts, Bean / 1 oz	10
Steak Kabobs, meat only	153
Steak Sandwich	408
Strawberries / 2 oz	14
Strawberry Glaze / 1 oz	37
Stuffing / 4 oz	230
Sunflower Seeds / .2 oz	31
T-Bone	444
Teriyaki Steak	174
Tomatoes / 1 oz	6
Topping	
Caramel / 1 oz	100
Chocolate / 1 oz	89
Strawberry / 1 oz	71
Whipped / 1 oz	80
Tortilla Chips / 1 oz	150
Turkey-Ham Salad / 3-½ oz	186

Turkey, Julienne / 1 oz	29
Wafer, Vanilla / 2	35
Watermelon	111
Winter Mix / 4-½ oz	25
Yogurt, Fruit / 4 oz	115
Yogurt, Vanilla / 4 oz	110
Zucchini / 1 oz	5
Zucchini, Breaded / 4 oz	102

ROY ROGERS

Biscuit	231
Breakfast Crescent Sandwich	401
w Bacon	431
w Ham	557
w Sausage	449
Brownie	264
Cheeseburger	563
Cheeseburger, Bacon	581
Chicken	
Breast	324
Breast and Wing	466
Leg	117
Thigh	282
Thigh and Leg	399
Wing	142
Cole Slaw	110
Crescent Roll	287
Danish	
Apple	249
Cheese	254
Cherry	271
Egg and Biscuit Platter	394
Egg and Biscuit Platter w Bacon	435
Egg and Biscuit Platter w Ham	442
Egg and Biscuit Platter w Sausage	550
French Fries	268
French Fries / Large	357
Hamburger	456
Pancake Platter w Syrup and Butter	452
Pancake Platter w Syrup, Butter and Bacon	493

CALORIES

Pancake Platter w Syrup, Butter and Ham	506
Pancake Platter w Syrup, Butter and Sausage	608
Potato Hot Topped	
Plain	211
w Bacon 'n Cheese	397
w Broccoli 'n Cheese	376
w Oleo	274
w Sour Cream 'n Chives	408
w Taco Beef 'n Cheese	463
Roy Rogers Barbecue Burger	611
Salad Bar	
Bacon Bits / 1 tbsp	24
Broccoli / ½ cup	20
Cheddar Cheese / ¼ cup	112
Chinese Noodles / ¼ cup	55
Chopped Eggs / 2 tbsp	55
Croutons / 2 tbsp	132
Cucumbers / 5–6 slices	4
Green Peas / ¼ cup	7
Green Peppers / 2 tbsp	4
Lettuce / 1 cup	10
Macaroni Salad / 2 tbsp	60
Mushrooms / ¼ cup	5
Potato Salad / 2 tbsp	50
Shredded Carrots / ¼ cup	12
Sliced Beets / ¼ cup	16
Sunflower Seeds / 2 tbsp	101
Tomatoes / 3 slices	20
Salad Dressing: 2 tbsp	
Bacon 'n Tomato	136
Blue Cheese	150
Italian, Lo Cal	70
Ranch	155
Thousand Island	160
Sandwich	
Roast Beef	317
Roast Beef / Large	360
Roast Beef w Cheese	424
Roast Beef / Large w Cheese	467
Shake	
Chocolate	358

Strawberry	315
Vanilla	306
Strawberry Shortcake	447
Sundae	
Caramel	293
Hot Fudge	337
Strawberry	216

TACO BELL

Beef MexiMelt	266
Burrito	
Bean Fiesta	226
Bean w Red Sauce	447
Beef	493
Chicken	334
Combination	407
Supreme	503
Chicken MexiMelt	257
Chilito	383
Cinnamon Twists	171
Enchirito w Red Sauce	382
Jalapeno Peppers / 3-½ oz	20
Mexican Pizza	575
Nachos	346
Nachos Bell Grande	649
Nachos Supreme	367
Pintos 'n Cheese w Red Sauce	190
Salad Dressing, Ranch / 2-⅗ oz	236
Sauce	
Green / 1 oz	4
Guacamole / 7/10 oz	34
Nacho Cheese / 2 oz	103
Pico De Gallo / 7/10 oz	6
Red / 1 oz	10
Salsa / ⅖ oz	18
Sour Cream / 7/10 oz	46
Taco / ⅖ oz	2
Taco Hot / ⅖ oz	3
Taco	183
Taco Bell Grande	355

Taco	
Chicken, Soft	213
Fiesta	127
Fiesta, Soft	147
Salad	905
Salad wo Shell	484
Soft	225
Soft Supreme	272
Steak, Soft	218
Supreme	230
Tostada, Fiesta	167
Tostada w Red Sauce	243

WENDY'S

Cheddar Cheese / 1 oz	110
Cheeseburger, Bacon Jr	430
Cheeseburger, Jr	310
Cheeseburger, Kids Meal	300
Chicken	
Breast Fillet	220
Club Sandwich	506
Fillet, Grilled	100
Nuggets / 6 pieces	280
Sandwich	440
Sandwich, Grilled	340
Chili / 9 oz	220
Fish Fillet Sandwich	460
French Fries / 3-⅕ oz	240
Hamburger, Jr	260
Hamburger, Kids Meal	260
Hamburger Patty / ¼ lb	180
Hamburger, Plain Single	340
Kaiser Bun	200
Potatoes	
Hot Stuffed, Bacon and Cheese	520
Hot Stuffed, Broccoli and Cheese	400
Hot Stuffed, Cheese	420
Hot Stuffed, Chili and Cheese	500
Hot Stuffed, Plain	270
Hot Stuffed, Sour Cream and Chives	500

Salad Bar

Alfalfa Sprouts / 1 oz	8
Alfredo Sauce / 2 oz	35
Applesauce, Chunky / 1 oz	22
Bacon Bits / ½ oz	40
Bananas / 1 oz	28
Breadstick	30
Broccoli / 1-½ oz	12
Cantaloupe / 2 oz	20
Carrots / 1 oz	12
Cauliflower / 2 oz	14
Cheddar Chips / 1 oz	160
Cheese Ravioli w sauce / 2 oz	45
Cheese Sauce / 2 oz	39
Cheese, Shredded, Imitation / 1 oz	90
Cheese Tortellini w sauce / 2 oz	60
Chef Salad	130
Chicken Salad / 2 oz	120
Chives / 1 oz	71
Chow Mein Noodles / ½ oz	74
Cole Slaw / 2 oz	70
Cottage Cheese / 3-⅗ oz	108
Croutons / ½ oz	60
Cucumbers / ½ oz	2
Eggs, Hard Cooked / 7/10 oz	30
Fettucini / 2 oz	190
Garbanzo Beans / 1 oz	46
Garden Salad	70
Garlic Toast	70
Green Peas / 1 oz	21
Green Peppers / 3/10 oz	10
Honeydew Melon / 2 oz	20
Jalapeno Peppers / ½ oz	2
Lettuce, Iceberg / 2 oz	8
Lettuce, Romaine / 2 oz	9
Mushrooms / .59 oz	4
Olives, Black / 1 oz	35
Oranges / 2 oz	26
Parmesan Cheese / 1 oz	130
Parmesan Cheese, Imitation / 1 oz	80
Pasta Medley / 2 oz	60

CALORIES

Pasta Salad / 2 oz	35
Peaches / 2 oz	31
Pepperoni, Sliced / 1 oz	140
Picante Sauce / 2 oz	18
Pineapple Chunks / 3-½ oz	60
Potato Salad / 2 oz	125
Pudding, Butterscotch / 2 oz	90
Pudding, Chocolate / 2 oz	90
Red Onions / ³∕₁₀ oz	2
Red Peppers, Crushed / 1 oz	120
Refried Beans / 2 oz	70
Rice, Spanish / 2 oz	70
Rotini / 2 oz	90
Seafood Salad / 2 oz	110
Sour Cream Topping, Imitation / 1 oz	58
Spaghetti, Meat Sauce / 2 oz	60
Spaghetti Sauce / 2 oz	28
Strawberries / 2 oz	17
Sunflower Seeds and Raisins / 1 oz	140
Taco Chips / 1-⅖ oz	260
Taco Meat / 2 oz	110
Taco Salad	530
Taco Sauce / 1 oz	16
Taco Shell	45
Three Bean Salad / 2 oz	60
Tomatoes / 1 oz	6
Tortilla, Flour	110
Tuna Salad / 2 oz	100
Turkey-Ham / 1 oz	35
Watermelon / 2 oz	18
Salad Dressing	
Bacon and Tomato, Reduced Calorie / ½ oz	45
Blue Cheese / ½ oz	90
Celery Seed / ½ oz	70
French / ½ oz	60
French, Sweet Red / ½ oz	70
Hidden Valley Ranch / ½ oz	50
Italian Caesar / ½ oz	80
Italian, Golden / ½ oz	45
Italian, Reduced Calorie / ½ oz	25
Salad Oil / 1 oz	250

CALORIES

Thousand Island / ½ oz	70
Wine Vinegar / ½ oz	2
Sandwich Bun	160
Sauce for Nuggets	
Barbecue / 1 oz	50
Honey / ½ oz	45
Sweet and Sour / 1 oz	45
Sweet Mustard / 1 oz	50
Single Hamburger w Everything	420
Sour Cream / 1 oz	60
Steak Sandwich	440
Swiss Deluxe, Jr	360
Wendy's Big Classic	570

WHITE CASTLE

Bun Only	74
Cheese Only	31
Cheeseburger Sandwich	200
Chicken Sandwich	186
Fish wo Tartar Sandwich	155
French Fries	301
Hamburger Sandwich	161
Onion Chips	329
Onion Rings	245
Sausage and Egg Sandwich	322
Sausage Sandwich	196

Index

A

Acerola cherries, 107
  juice, fresh, 120
Alfalfa
  seeds, 129
  sprouts, 285
Almonds, 181, 182–83
  butter, 132
  extract, 102
  meal, 104
Amaranth, 129
  flour/pasta, 129
  raw, 285
American food (restaurants),
  325–29
Apples, 107
  baby desserts, 2
  baby fruit, 3
  baby juice, 5
  butter, 153
  can/frozen, 109–10
  –cinnamon bread mix, 21
  cobbler, restaurant, 325
  dried, 113
  jr. baby, 9
  jr. baby desserts, 8

juice drinks/–flavored beverages, 115
  muffin mixes, 177
  pie filling, can, 201
  pie/pastry snacks, 204
  pies, frozen, 199, 200
  snack cake, 34, 35
  snacks, 113
  sweet rolls, 236
  turnovers, 237
Applesauce
  baby, 3
  cake, 27
  cans/jars, 109–111
  jr. baby, 8, 9
Apricots, 107
  baby, 3–4
  can, 111
  dried, 113
  jr. baby, 9
  juice/nectar, 121–22
  pie filling, can, 201
  roll–up, 113
Arby's menu, 341–43
Arthur Treacher's menu, 343—44
Artichoke, 285
  hearts, frozen, 293

369

Index

Index

Index

Index

Index

Index

ABOUT THE AUTHOR

JEAN CARPER is a well-known authority on health and nutrition. She is a former award-winning medical correspondent for Cable News Network in Washington D.C. and currently writes a nationally syndicated newspaper column. She is the author of eighteen books, most recently the best-selling *The Food Pharmacy* and the *New York Times* bestseller, *Food—Your Miracle Medicine*.

BANTAM'S BEST IN HEALTH AND NUTRITION

____56476-5 HIGH SPEED HEALING: The Fastest, Safest and
Most Effective Shortcuts to Lasting Relief,
Prevention Magazine $6.99/$7.99 Canada

____56508-7 THE PILL BOOK, 6th Edition,
Harold M. Silverman, Pharm. D. $6.99/$8.99

____56579-6 THE NATURAL HEALTH GUIDE TO ANTIOXIDANTS,
Nancy Bruning and the Editors
of *Natural Health* Magazine $4.99/$6.50

____27775-8 CONTROLLING CHOLESTEROL,
Kenneth H. Cooper, M.D. $6.50/$8.50

____28937-3 OVERCOMING HYPERTENSION,
Kenneth H. Cooper, M.D. $6.99/$7.99

____27751-0 YEAST SYNDROME,
Trowbridge, M.D. and Walker $5.95/$6.95

____28498-3 THE BANTAM MEDICAL DICTIONARY $6.99/$8.99

____34524-9 THE FOOD PHARMACY, Jean Carper $13.95/$17.95

____29378-8 RECIPES FOR DIABETICS, Billie Little $5.99/$6.99

____27245-4 THE ANXIETY DISEASE,
David V. Sheehan, M.D. $5.99/$7.50

____34721-7 JANE BRODY'S NUTRITION BOOK,
Jane Brody $15.95/$18.95

____34350-5 JEAN CARPER'S TOTAL NUTRITION,
Jean Carper $13.95/$16.95

____34556-7 MINDING THE BODY, MENDING THE MIND,
Joan Borysenko, M.D. $12.95/$16.95

____27435-X THE VITAMIN BOOK, Silverman, M.D.,
Romano, M.D., and Elmer, M.D. $5.99/$6.99

____29192-0 THE PILL BOOK GUIDE TO EVERYTHING
YOU NEED TO KNOW ABOUT PROZAC,
Jonas, M.D., Shambury $4.99/$5.99

- -

Ask for these books at your local bookstore or use this page to order.

Please send me the books I have checked above. I am enclosing $____ (add $2.50 to
cover postage and handling). Send check or money order, no cash or C.O.D.'s, please.

Name _____

Address _____

City/State/Zip _____

Send order to: Bantam Books, Dept. HN 21, 2451 S. Wolf Rd., Des Plaines, IL 60018
Allow four to six weeks for delivery.
Prices and availability subject to change without notice.   HN 21 4/95

Bantam's Best in Diet, Health, and Nutrition